HIJACK THE AGING PROCESS

This all-encompassing book will show seniors how to grow younger not older.

Jokes are included throughout to encourage you to have many good belly laughs, for humor is healthy.

Lee Belshin

Lee Belshin, M.S.

Foreword

What do you get when you team up a standup comic with a health educator? "Me." And I will prove that it is your good fortune that this book has materialized, for I will now share with you the most amazing discovery of this century.

The Fountain of Youth has been discovered. All we have to do is partake of it. I personally have been sharing many of the studies described within which outline paths you can take for a happier, healthier future.

Millions die each year from diseases that could and should be prevented. I began to devote more time to encourage people to take advantage of the many studies that would assure them a long and healthy life. But, I soon realized I needed to reach a bigger audience and I was barely scratching the surface.

I decided to write books to rally more people to get in the act and tap into the Fountain of Youth that exists within them. These books are free from medical jargon and will guide you to healthier living. You will find the latest current thinking on how you may reduce the probability of a heart attack or cancer. But best of all, by combining Health and Humor you can:

Hijack the Aging Process.

So there you have it, evidence of the many years of study and research to find the Fountain of Youth. Yes, a portion of my life, with the backup of many dedicated medical professionals, has been spent to put you on track to live a healthy and happy life.

No longer should we think of seniors 80 or even 100 as being old. As gerontologists amass information on the aging process and understand more about their life span, they think that a senior has a good chance of reaching 125 years.

How exciting for seniors to be offered a place in this most desired lineup of people and quite a large group it is. Current estimates are that 450,000 are 100 years old and growing like greased lightning.

But where can I find the nearest location to join this group? I can see you packing and getting ready to join them. Well, here is the good news. You do not have to travel at all. It is right within us and always has been. Every time you exercise, eat healthy foods and have a good belly laugh, or adjust to a stressful situation you are replenishing the Fountain of Youth. This book will guide you to make the right choices based on up to date and reliable information.

As a typical type 'A' personality which will be discussed in future chapters, I decided to come out of retirement and fulfill a lifetime fantasy as a stand-up comedian.

Although I dedicated many hours of research to provide high level information on how to slow down the aging process, I did not air enough data on humor.

Now, this book provides you evidence that healthy laughter may very well be a vital factor for the graying senior. I will also share with you hundreds of jokes that I used in my role as a standup comic.

ACKNOWLEDGEMENT

This book has been made possible by the support and encouragement of many individuals in the medical profession and related fields. I would like to express gratitude to Dr. Edward B. Johns, professor emeritus of the UCLA School of Public Health who encouraged me to stay active in the field of Health Education.

Special thanks to Dean T. Mason, M.D., Editor of the American Heart Journal. Ralph de Vere White, M.D., Chairman of the department of Urology at the University of California at Davis. Meyer Friedman, M.D., the discoverer of type A behavior and its relationship to the heart. And William B. Kannel, M.D., Medical Director of the Framingham Study.

The information provided by John Yudkin, M.D., of London. Mrs. Phillip Gillon of the Hasdassah Hospital Israel, and the Health Officials in North Karelia were very helpful to me in doing research for my books and magnanimous in their support.

To Frank McCourt author and the only Irishman I knew who could sing "Bei Mir Bist Du Shane" in Yiddish. I was fortunate to meet him at several writers' conferences and exchanging many humorous stories and experiences with him. He was a great source of inspiration and encouraged me to do standup comedy.

Larry Whitaker chose to become involved as the producer of this book because he was impressed with the solid information within. He also realized from his own experience as a CEO for an international company that our citizens, old and young, have extremely poor health habits. Nationally, we are an unhealthy country and headed for disaster. He knew that he had the skills and technical knowledge to help disperse the inside facts for healthful living contained in this book.

Thanks to retired NASA Chemist Dr. Nancy Whitaker, PhD., for all of her detailed editing and scientific contributions.

Table of Contents

CHAPTER 1 HUMOR

LAUGHERS LAST LONGER

Studies reveal that mirthful laughter stimulates the immune system helping to resist diseases. It produces many of the same effects as aerobic exercise (that is the type of exercise that should push up your heart rate and keep it up for a sustained period of time) as it causes the tissue that makes up the inner lining of blood vessels to expand allowing for increased blood flow.

As a cardiologist at the Medical College of Wisconsin States, "Laughter could be an inexpensive and potentially beneficial therapy. It has been shown that it reduces stress hormones -- the bad guys that hinder the immune system and increases the number of blood platelets which can block arteries."

Sidney Smith, M.D., cardiologist at the University of North Carolina School of medicine states, "Time and time again physicians see that patients with a positive outlook seem to do better." Laughter relaxes the body and can scale down problems associated with coronary artery disease as high blood pressure and stroke. It also reduces the effects of ulcers and arthritis.

Other studies in Loma Vista by Lee Berk, PhD, an assistant professor of pathology and laboratory medicine and his associate Stanley Tan, M.D., at Loma Linda University School of Medicine, indicate that after exposure to humor there is a general increase in activity within the immune system. This includes an increase in the number and activity level of natural killer cells that attack viral infected cells, and some types of cancer and tumor cells.

They also found that it is a good buffer to negative stress hormones. Advising seniors to look for excuses to laugh may be sound medical advice to prevent health problems. The brain is connected to and sends messages constantly to the heart. Sending positive and humorous ones is like giving it a soothing massage. Also, it is impossible to think a negative thought if you are laughing. Laughter stimulates both sides of the brain to boost learning. A University of Maryland medical study suggests that a good sense of humor and the ability to laugh at stressful situations helps to mitigate the damaging physical effects of distressing emotions. It also stated, "We don't know yet why laughing protects the heart, but we do know that mental stress is associated with impairment of the endothelium, the protective barrier lining our blood vessels. This can cause a series of inflammatory reactions that lead to fat and cholesterol build up in the coronary arteries and ultimately to a heart attack."

According to Paul E. McGee, PhD, a development psychologist specializing in humor, laughter fights infection. It activates key immune system components including antibodies, natural killer cells and T-cells (a type of white blood cell that is of key importance to the immune system).

There is a strong bond between laughter and your relationships at the work place at home and with friends. Shared laughter is very effective in keeping a marriage upbeat. Undoubtedly it helped my wife and me. But I have to admit that our relationship was often put in the danger zone when I, as I am sure many comedians do; try out new jokes on their wife. Example:

> The other night as she stepped out of the shower I shouted, "You should use Slim-Fast instead of soap the next time you take a shower. It could take two inches of your tush." She did not think that was funny and couldn't wait to get even. The next morning as I was putting on my underwear, a cloud of smoke rose up in the air. I yelled out, "What did you do, put talcum powder in my shorts?" She yelled back, "No Miracle-Gro."

You cannot stay angry or mad if you are laughing. That makes me think, if you laugh, you will never get hardening of the attitudes "If you can find humor in anything, you can survive it."

Extensive research on laughter began in 1976 after the New England Journal of Medicine published an article on Norman Cousins who was a well-known author. He was diagnosed with acute inflammation of the spine which had affected most of the body and told was given a 1 to 500 chance of continuing to live very long and told to get his estate in order. The first thing he did was to fire his doctor, and get hold of movies of the Marx brothers and Candid Camera. He then checked in to a hotel to watch them as he reasoned that negative thoughts and attitudes caused his problem and that he needed positive thoughts to cure his disease. Yes, it worked. He lived 16 more cheerful years after his serious illness was diagnosed, and 26 years after his first heart attack.

William Fry Jr., M.D.,[1] who has done research on the physiology of laughter for over 30 years, lends support to Cousin's notion that laughter is like internal jogging and that it has a positive effect on blood pressure and respiration. It relaxes all the muscles in the body. Taking time to laugh at funny movies or other things that cook up a good belly laugh is a healthy way to combat stress as well as anger. He also claimed it took 10 minutes on a rowing machine for his heart rate to reach the level it would after just one minute of hearty laughter.

Marvin E. Herring, M.D., of the New Jersey School of Osteopathic Medicine, states: "the thorax, heart, lungs, diaphragm, abdomen and even the liver are given a massage during a hearty laugh."

Further research has shown that one minute of anger can decrease your immune system for up to 10 hours. One minute of laughter can boost your immune system for 24 hours. Now that news is something to laugh about. It triggers the release of endorphins which are the body's natural pain killers. It breaks down emotions that are stressed out. There is no way that you can feel dismal or anger when you are laughing. It is the greatest stress buster that prevents that feeling of being

---

[1] Dr. William Fry {cited in Jane Brody,} Personal Health, "New York Times, 7 April 1988.

overwhelmed. It helps you to relax and able to see things that are driving you up a wall in a less threatening way.

Humankind was given a sense of humor for a reason. We were born with the gift of laughter. Babies smile during the first weeks of life and laugh out loud within months of birth. By the time they reach nursery school he or she will laugh about 300 times a day. Children laugh more than adults. One researcher found that four year olds laugh about every four minutes. Adults laugh an average of 17 minutes a day.

Research reveals that laughter contributes "big time" to a happy marriage. Laura Bush said one of the reasons that she married her husband was, like her father, he has a good sense of humor, and can always make her laugh. Employers look upon it as a most positive quality to bring to the work place. It is a natural medicine. It is a contagious emotion that makes us feel chipper. Haven't you felt better after a hearty laugh?

Sure enough, the awareness of the benefits of laughter was known in age old times. As early as the 13th century surgeons used it to distract pain. Israel now trains medical clowns to improve their skills through humor and clowning to communicate with patients in a way that other members of the staff are unable to do.

Henry de Monroeville, a French surgeon during the thirteenth century wrote, "Let the surgeon take care to regulate the whole regimen of the patient's life for joy, and allow everyone else to tell him jokes."

Ancient Greeks sent sick people to the home of comedians.

Need more back up to convince you of the power of humor?

Voltaire said, "The art of medicine consists of keeping the patient amused while nature heals the disease."

Plato: "Even the God's love jokes."

Koran: "He deserves paradise who makes his companions laugh."

The Talmud, which is a collection of Jewish laws and traditions, itself, has descriptions of many humorous and ironic situations and comments. It recommends to teachers to begin their classroom studies each day by employing humor.

Mark Twain said in 1894, "Humor is the great thing. The saving thing. The minute it crops up all our irritations and resentments slip away and a sunny spirit takes place."

Henry W. Beecher, a 19th century American clergyman, said, "A person without humor is like a wagon without springs, jolted by every pebble on the road."

All public speakers will readily agree that beginning a talk with a humorous story will go a long way in winning the audience's attention and holding it for the rest of their presentation.

Comedian Yakov Smirnoff, said, "Everybody laughs the same in every language because laughter is a universal connection."

Abraham Lincoln had an immense stock of jokes, and he often used them to distract people he knew he couldn't immediately satisfy.

Former President Ronald Reagan, and now Barack Obama, interjected a lot of humor into their speeches, with great audience approval.

Dwight D. Eisenhower said, "A sense of humor is a part of the heart of leadership, of getting along with people, and getting things done."

Ella Wheeler, in an 1883 poem, expressed it so well, "Laugh and the world laughs with you. Weep and you weep alone."

Blessed are they who laugh at themselves for they shall never cease to be amused--Anonymous.

I always get a good laugh from the audience when I tell them that my first job as a standup comic was at Beermann's in Lincoln, California. I was so good that I did six shows and the place closed. Of course, I was not the reason. The audience loved it when I made fun of myself, and it was a good ice breaker to start the show.

Unfortunately, as we age we laugh less. Remember, "You don't stop laughing because you grow old. You grow old because you stop laughing."

Now that I think of it, before I do my gigs, I should discuss the many healthy pay-offs from laughing. It should encourage the audience to come up with hardy belly laughs whether I am funny or not.

Reminds me when I did my first performance. You can imagine how nervous I was, and just as I started a woman about my age stood up, held her purse up high and shouted out, "I will give free sex to anyone who can guess what I have in my purse." A man in the back yelled back, "AN ELEPHANT." She responded, "Close enough."

Read on and you will get the message that each time you exercise, eat a healthy meal, handle stress, and share a good joke, you are depositing a little of this elixir from the Fountain of Youth. This will repay you downstream with high interest.

Laughter can now be considered a sure thing to help us to attain membership in the centenarian club.

According to a study reported in the June 5, 2010 Science Daily, a sense of humor helps to keep people healthy, and increases their chances of living well beyond their retirement.

"Laughers do Last Longer." This book will encourage you to have many good belly laughs, which will help you to mock the life expectancy tables. It will include jokes that received a hearty applause from my standup comedy performances. But laughter alone will not continuously replenish your Fountain of Youth. So read on. This book will show you how to live a healthy, happy life, and grow older later -- much later.

HUMOR IS HEALTHY

As a young boy I would, without exception, go to the movies every Sunday. After all, where else could you find entertainment for two hours at a cost of 12 cents, and if you could afford to spend another penny, you could purchase enough candy to last you through the double feature, newsreel and comedy flick.

Afterwards, I would run home to join my father and his two brothers, to sit in front of a king size radio, and listen to the Jack Benny show. They would roar with laughter and put aside the gloominess they felt during the depression. As many others, they could only find part time jobs and felt insecure as to what the future would look like. The daily headlines in the newspapers were not reassuring. But for a moment during this doleful period, they could giggle, laugh and lighten up as they and millions of Americans listened to the comedy programs.

As the comedians made evident during rough times, laughter gives us the courage, strength, and hope, for the future. It helps us to relax and recharge. It is difficult to be angry or sad when you are having a good laugh. Have you noticed when others laugh that you want to join the crowd? It is definitely contagious. It has social benefits as well as mental and physical ones.

It, undoubtedly, had a dual benefit; for most comedians far exceeded their life expectancy. Yes, the benefits of humor work both ways. Now let us look at the top masters of comedy that contributed so much to the health of our nation.

Jack Benny

(2-14-1894 to 12-26-1974)

He charmed us as a comedian, actor on radio, television, and earlier on vaudeville. He was known for being ultra conservative with the dollar and will always be remembered in the scene when a mugger demanded his money or his life. He responded after a long pause -- "Wait, wait I am thinking!" He also entertained us with the violin which he learned to play at age six. He used it in vaudeville acts that paid $7.50 per show.

He served in the Navy during World War I, and entertained the troops with his violin. He really loved playing the violin and was quoted as saying: "If God came to me and said, 'If I could make you the greatest violin player, but you could never tell another joke.' I honestly would have to think about which choice I would make."

He had a great supporting cast including his wife Mary Livingston, Phil Harris, Rochester, and Dennis Day and of course, Jack Benny will always be remembered by his feud with Fred Allen, as well as his declaring that his age was "39".

Some of Jack's favorite jokes are:

"*My wife and I have been married 47 years and not once have we had an argument serious enough to consider divorce. Murder, yes, but divorce, never.*"

"*I went to see one of those X-rated movies the other night, and I couldn't believe my eyes, so I stayed to see it a second time.*"

"*I gambled at the crap table the other night and finally lost $8, but during that time the house gave me two cigars and four drinks. So it was a lot cheaper than renting a room.*"

"*Abraham Lincoln would walk five miles through the snow bare foot -- that's so he could save three cents. That is my kind of a guy.*"

"*George Burns and I have a lot in common. The other night I went to an X-rated movie, and we both fell asleep.*"

"*Give me golf clubs, fresh air, a beautiful partner and you can keep the clubs and the fresh air.*"

He came through with his beguiling humor at a time when the nation was in dire need for humor. He also was able to mock the actuarial tables.

Jack Benny lived to age 80

Eddie Cantor

(1-31-1892 to 10-10-1964)

Orphaned at age three, he was still able to become a successful writer, comedian, and singer who also helped us through rough times. He reduced the anger and anxiety that prevailed through the depression and World War II. He made us feel as if we were a member of his family by revealing intimate stories about his wife Ida and five daughters. His rolling eyes and song and dance routines most likely led to his nick name, Banjo Eyes.

At age 16 he won five dollars at an amateur singing contest and was hired as a singing waiter in Coney Island. That first paycheck mushroomed into a sizable estate which was lost during the crash of 1929.

No other entertainer proved as accomplished in as many fields as he did in the 1920's and 30's.

are: Some of Eddie's favorite jokes and quotes are:

"It takes twenty years to become an overnight success."

"A wedding is a funeral where you smell your own flowers."

"Marriage is an attempt to solve problems together which you didn't ever have when you were alone."

"Slow down and enjoy life. It's not only the scenery you miss by going so fast. You miss the sense of where you are going and why."

"When I see the ten most wanted lists: I always have this thought: if we'd made them feel wanted earlier they wouldn't be wanted now."

"If I was the best man at the wedding, why is she marrying him?"

Eddie lived to age 72

Red Skelton

(7-18-1913 to 9-17-1997)

His father was a clown and died before Red was born. Ed Wynn saw him selling newspapers and used him in an act. He left home at the age of ten then worked at a medicine show until going on to vaudeville at age 17. He was considered one of the greatest clowns and was later inducted into the International Clown Hall. While serving in the army during World War II, he had a nervous breakdown and was discharged in 1945.

He entertained many of his fellow servicemen and joked that he was the only celebrity that went into the service as a private and came out with the same rank.

He made his mark in radio, television, movies and live appearances. He did not like to cling to a script or a time limit, which created a lot of friction with his sponsors especially when he entertained at the big clubs. They wanted a snappy close, so the gamblers would get back to the tables. He was often rebuked for this and let it be known that for every ten minutes he went over it cost them a fortune. He once responded when criticized for not having a script so he could stay with a time limit, "God tells me what to do." His sponsor handed him a hundred blank sheets and said, "Tell God to fill in the pages."

He loved to entertain and the money was secondary to him. He would often stay late to tell jokes to other members of the cast. He said, "If you ever make a room full of people laugh, it's like a drug derived energy from laughter."

He never had to discuss jokes about the use of drugs or use the "F" words to get laughs from his audiences. He always ended his performances by saying, "God Bless."

Johnny Carson was one of his writers. This gave him more time to write books and paint clowns. Some of his favorite jokes were:

"Recipe for a perfect marriage is dining and dancing twice a week. The wife goes Tuesdays and I go Thursdays."

"My wife and I always sleep in separate beds; hers is in California and mine in Texas."

"We always hold hands, if I let go she goes shopping."

"My wife told me the car wasn't running well; there was water in the carburetor." I asked where the carburetor was. She told me, "in the lake."

"She got a mud pack, and it looked great for two days; then the mud fell off."

"Remember. Marriage is the number one cause of divorce."

Red Skelton lived to age 84

Bob Hope

(5-29-1903 to 7-27-2003)

He was quoted as saying, "I left England at the age of four when I found out that I could not be king." From the age of 12 he worked a variety of comedy acts at local board walks and entered a contest and won with an impersonation of Charlie Chaplin. His gigs on radio, movies, television, and on special events, had the world in stitches at a time when this form of refreshment was so much needed.

He transported his talent overseas and hosted 199 USO shows including many in danger zones. In 1943, he stopped at the bedside of a wounded soldier who was in a coma for two months. The soldier suddenly opened his eyes and said, "Hey, Bob Hope, when did you get here?" He left the area as he did not want the troops to see his tears. He returned later to present the soldier with the Purple Heart. He entertained troops during World War II, Korean War, Viet Nam, and the Gulf War. Congress gave him a special award -- Honorary Veteran. He said later of all his awards he appreciated this one the most.

He was known for his charitable giving and support of the Eisenhower Medical Center for which his Bob Hope Classic distributed, in 2009, $1,538,000.

Hope celebrated his 100 year old birthday party with several other notable centenarians: Irving Berlin, famous composer, who lived to age 101. Adolph Zukor, father of future films, who also lived to age l03. George Burns, well known actor, who lived to age l00. Hal

Roach, brilliant comedy producer, who lived to age 100. George Abbot, famous actor and writer, who lived to 108 and Spanish Senor Wonces, the skilled ventriloquist, who likewise lived to 108.

Wow. If I were an attorney I would rest my case. What other line of work could claim as many centenarians? The band of people who attended this party clearly point out that humor and other forms of entertainment works both ways. It is not only healthy for the comedian but also for the listener.

There were many other famous comedians who were not invited to Hope's party but, as his guests, they also mimic the actuarial tables.

He said at his party, "I know that I am getting old when the candles cost more than the cake."

Some of his favorite jokes are:

"*The airlines are really getting security conscious. You can still fly, but they won't tell you where you're going.*"

"*The other day, at the L.A. Airport, they searched Racquel Welch for three hours as she was getting off the plane. What bugged her most was that six of the guards were from a different airport.*"

"*I do benefits for all religions. I don't want to blow it all on a technicality.*"

"*I grew up with six brothers. That's how I learned to dance waiting for the bathroom.*"

"*I don't feel old. In fact, I don't feel anything until noon--then I take a nap.*"

Bob Hope lived to age 100

Rodney Dangerfield

(11-22-1919 -- 10-5-2004)

He was the son of a Vaudevillian who he would say, "Was never home. He was out making kids." He also said that his mother brought him up all wrong. This proved later to be erroneous as he became a successful comedian. He started as a teenager writing jokes for comedians and at age 19 became one himself. His career was far from being a "bed of roses" and he became a waiter, for which he was fired. He even tried being an acrobatic diver, but gave it up to become a salesman of aluminum siding so he could feed his family.

It took a long time, but he finally developed an image of being rejected and cast off by others. His jokes reveal this feeling:

"When I was born, the doctor went into the waiting room and said to my father, 'I'm sorry. We did everything we could but he pulled through.' "

"My wife made me join a bridge club. I jump off next Tuesday."

"I'm so ugly that when I worked in a pet shop people kept asking, 'how big will he get.' "

"One year they wanted to make me poster boy for birth control."

Rodney Dangerfield lived to age 85

1-19

(7-12-1908 to 3-27-2002).

He was an Emmy winning comedian, actor, and popular star on radio. His series on the Texaco Star Theatre did well and paved the way for his recognition as a TV star. His performance put it in the number one slot in Nielsen ratings, and received continuously an 80% rating. It was such a big hit that there was less traffic on the streets and fewer tickets sold at the theaters when his show was on. Many places closed down for an hour, so patrons could see their favorite program. It was mentioned in his biography that the water levels took a drastic drop after his show was broadcast so people could go to the bathroom.

He was credited with the popularity of TV and the massive sale of sets. As busy as he was, he always took time to entertain on military bases and for many charitable events. Among his favorite jokes were:

"*A young man fills out an application for a job and does well until he gets to the last question. Who should we notify in case of an accident? He mulls it over and then writes 'anybody in sight.'* "

"*The company accountant is shy and retiring. He's shy a quarter of a million dollars. That's why he's retiring.*"

"*He's so old that when he orders a three - minute egg, they ask for the money up front.*"

"My doctor told me that jogging could add years to my life. I think he was right. I feel ten years older already."

"Folks who don't know why America is the Land of Promise should be here during an election campaign."

"What is this, an audience or an oil painting?"

"Motivation is when your dreams put on work clothes."

"It is amazing how fast later comes when you buy now."

"A man of indeterminate age checked with a doctor to see if the doctor could tell him how old he was. After a quick examination the doctor said 'According to this examination I'm alone in this room.'"

"Your marriage is in trouble if your wife says, 'You're only interested in one thing, and you can't remember what it is.'"

He had millions of jokes. His book Milton Berle's, Private Joke File had over 10,000 of his best gags, anecdotes and one-liners.

Milton Berle lived to age 94

Henny Youngman

(3-16-1906) to (10-24-1998).

He was known as the master of one-liners. He played the violin was a band leader, stand-up comic, and performed in many theaters, nightclubs and was very popular at the Borscht Belt.

Some of his favorite jokes are:

> *"A doctor had a stethoscope up to a man's chest. The man asks, 'Doc, how do I stand', the doctor says, 'That's what puzzles me.'"*

> *"I had a lovely room in the hotel. It had a big bathroom and bedroom. It's a little inconvenient though. They're in separate buildings."*

> *"If you had your life to live over again, do it overseas."*

> *"You know what I did before I was married? Anything that I wanted to."*

> *"I take my wife everywhere I go, but she keeps coming back."*

Henny Youngman lived to age 92

Groucho Marx

(10-2-1890) to (8 -19-1977)

He often performed with brothers Harpo (who did not speak), Chico (as a comical Italian) and sometimes Zeppo. He always posed with a slanted walk, greased mustache, bushy brow, and cigar. He is best known for his one-liner performance on the very popular quiz show on radio and television. He performed on Vaudeville and in many movies,

He may be gone but certainly not forgotten. To this day, glasses with make-believe noses and mustaches are purchased at novelty and other stores. Two albums of the popular British rock band, Queen's, A **Day at the Races** (1976) and **A Night at the Opera** (1975) are named after the Marx Brothers' films.

Furthermore, one of the "0"s in the legendary "Hollywood" sign is dedicated to Groucho.

Some of his favorite jokes were:

"I would never belong to a club that would have me as a member."

"How do you feel about women's rights? I like either side of them."

"Women should be obscene and not heard."

"Politics doesn't make strange bedfellows; marriage does."

"I've had a perfectly wonderful evening. But this wasn't it."

"Don't look now, but there is one too many in this room; and I think it is you."

"I didn't like the play, but then I saw it under adverse conditions. The curtain was up."

"I never forget a face, but in your case, I'll be glad to make an exception."

"Those are my principles. If you don't like them, I have others."

Groucho Marx lived to age 86

George Burns

(1-20-l896) to (3-9-1996)

Even in his late 90's he maintained his exceptional ability to make us laugh. He had a distinguished career on Vaudeville, films, radio, and television. He never made it big time until he met and married Gracie Allen. They developed a humorous show for which he wrote most of the scripts.

As many of the other comedians we discussed, he came from a humble background and left school early to go into show business. George started by singing with other young members of his family at age seven. He had many to choose for his group of singers since he was born into a family of 12. They sang in saloons, on ferry boats, and brothels.

To this day, whenever the name George Burns comes up, right away one pictures him with a big cigar in his mouth. Then the most obvious question comes up, "How come he lived to 100 outliving several of his doctors, who admonished him for his poor health practices?" Medical researchers are at a loss to explain why. Not only George Burns, but other centenarians who were couch potatoes, ate a lot of red meat, smoked, and avoided exercise still seemed to live a long life.

Until this mystery can be unraveled, it makes good sense to listen to the majority of medical advice put forward in this book. It will give you a much greater chance to reach the 100-plus mark, and to agree that old age is a season of joy.

Some of his favorite jokes were:

"Happiness is having a large, loving, caring, close-knit family in another city."

"In those days, the best pain killer was ice; it wasn't addictive, and it was particularly effective if you poured some whiskey over it."

"I don't worry about getting old, I'm old already. Only young people worry about getting old."

"Sincerity is everything. If you can fake that, you've got it made."

George Burn lived to age 100

There were many other comedians who lived long lives. Myron Cohen lived to 84, Sid Caesar to 94. Many more will provide further proof that humor is healthy. In fact the average age death of the comedians discussed in this chapter was 87. That is amazing, since the life expectancy at that time was in the late 40's.

In American Vaudeville, and especially at the well-known Borscht Belt, many of the Jewish comedians such as Eddie Cantor, Jack Benny, Milton Berle, Henry Youngman, and the Marx brothers, among others, entertained the audience with the type of humor that was common place in the lives of Eastern Europeans. They portrayed themselves as slightly daffy and outlandish. They were the new generation of the Jewish comedians who performed in prior centuries.

As improbable as it may seem, many Jews used this type of humor to survive amid the Holocaust.

Making fun of the experiences and prejudices that the new emigrants were subjected to through their situational comedy was a forerunner to the acts of Jerry Seinfeld, and others.

There are many more seniors certainly noteworthy for proving the golden years can be not only the most entertaining but the most productive.

Growing younger each year, not older

The key to successful living is to pay as little attention to it as possible.

Judith Regan

Let us look at some others who have illustrated how chronological age has never been a reliable indicator of health or fitness.

1. Clint Eastwood, a legendary figure in both the United States and Europe, turned 85 years young on May 31, 2015, and still has that Adonis look. He has set his sights on age 105 and was recently quoted as saying, "He dreams of making films for two more decades."

2. Harry Belafonte, a prostate cancer survivor, was active in the music industry until he died at age 88.

3. Victor Borge was still playing the piano and entertaining us with his humorous antics until he died at age 91. He commented that his piano playing was improving as he grew older. He said even though "I walk slower I see more." He was often quoted as saying, "Laughter is the shortest distance between two people."

4. Lucille Ball, at 70, returned to television in a new comedy series that was very popular. Her reruns still draw a large audience on TV. She lived to 78.

5. At age 84, Ernest Borgnine drove to Alaska. He commented on the O'Reilly Factor TV program, "Aging is all in the mind. Just get up and go." He was active until his demise at age 95.

6. Arlene Francis, actress and television personality, was a panelist on the "What's My Line?" show. She lived to age 93.

7. Walter Cronkite had not lost any of his charm and ability to communicate with an audience even though he was in his late 70's. Sadly, he did not get his wish to become the oldest astronaut in space and surpass the record of John Glenn. He lived to age 92.

8. Senator Storm Thurman was still active at 99. He lived to be 100.

9. Kirk Douglas, at 99, still has that chipper look.

10. Olivia De Havilland is doing fine at age 99.

11. Tony Martin, until he died at 98, was still entertaining us with his comforting voice.

12. Art Linkletter, a popular American radio and television personality, lived to 97.

13. Bob Sheppard recently died at 99. He retired in 2007 after being the voice you heard announcing the Yankees baseball games for over a half of a century.

14. Phyllis Diller was known for her distinctive laugh, and kept us laughing well into her 80's. She did not become a standup comic until age 37, after raising five children .She claimed that doing comedy added many years to her life. She lived to age 95.

The list of celebrities goes on and on. Among the big wigs that were an important part of our generation also made a mockery of the life expectancy table:

- Zsa Zsa Gabor, age 93;
- Lena Horne, age 92;
- Jean Stapleton, age 90;
- Shirley Temple, age 85;
- Jonathan Winters, age 87.
- Maureen O'Hara, age 95.

> "OLD AGE IS ALWAYS 15 YEARS OLDER THAN I AM."
>
> Bernard Baruch
>
> "I LIVE IN THAT SOLITUDE WHICH IS PAINFUL IN YOUTH BUT DELICIOUS IN THE YEARS OF MATURITY."
>
> Albert Einstein

Let me now introduce you to seasoned citizens that may be unknown, but can well serve as models for the rest of us as we age.

1. George Dawson of Dallas, Texas, learned to read and write at 98. He learned his ABC's in only two days skipped printing the letters and went straight to writing in cursive. After all he was in a hurry to replace his official "X" with a perfect signature so he could autograph his first book, Life is so good which was published at age 102. He started to work full time at the age of eight that deprived him of the opportunity to get an education, He died at age 103.

2. Beatrice Wood from Ojai, California, at age 100 plus, was still creating works of art that are displayed in art galleries around the world. She said, "Choosing

to live in the timeless, I am now at the easiest and happiest time of my life." She died at age 105.

3. Audrey Stubbart worked a 40 hour week as a proofreader and newspaper columnist at the Examiner in Independence, Missouri, until age 105. Prior to her death she was the oldest verified newspaper columnist. "I think I can deal with anything," she said, "I more or less have."

4. James Wiggens until his death at age 94 served as editor of a weekly newspaper in the coastal town of Ellsworth, Maine. He has held this position since 1922. He had a booming career at the Washington Post and later as Ambassador with the United Nation. Instead of going into retirement, he purchased a weekly newspaper in 1966 in Ellsworth, Maine, which soon received national attention. "Working takes some of the curse off old age," he said.

5. Edith Polese, at 102, was still operating a cigar stand in the Cosmopolitan Hotel in Denver.

6. Jack Christal, a flagpole painter of Reno, Nevada, was still active in his late 70's, when he inched his way 100 feet above a pavement to put a new coat of gold paint at the top of the Riverside Hotel in Reno.

7. Han Way Chin, a Chinese immigrant who worked as a grocery clerk at stores in Sacramento, died a month short of his 112th birthday. Mr. Chin never took vacations and worked until he was 76; saving his money and providing financial help to family members. Until he was in his 80's, Mr. Chin took

long walks -- sometimes five miles or more almost every day, which most likely contributed to his longevity.

8. Eiji Toyoda, known as Toyota's global helmsman, lived to age 100. In 2013 he was awarded the Grand Cordon of the Order of the Rising Sun, one of Japan's highest honors for his role in Japan's rise in the global auto industry.

9. Iva Wood Blake, at 100, spoke about the day in 1895 when she met Cary Nation in the small town of Canadian, Texas. She watched her take a hatchet and attack the main saloon in town for serving alcohol to the residents.

10. Maude Pratt Managan, at age 100 loved to share with her friends in Hot Springs, Montana, how her parents traveled in a Conestoga wagon from South Dakota to western Montana.

11. Frank Buckles, until he died at age 110, had the distinction of being the last Doughboy from World War I. He fudged about his age, enlisted in the army at 16, and soon found himself in France. After the war, the veteran soldier was a farmer in West Virginia for over 50 years. He was actively involved in fighting for a national World War I Memorial on the Mall in Washington D.C. The veteran soldier, who served his nation 93 years ago, had strong passion to fulfill his mission.

12. Richard Overton, at age 107, has the distinction of being the oldest living veteran of World War II. He

still drives a car, and walks faster than many who are quite younger.

13. Nelson Mandala was the first black chief executive of South Africa. He lived an active life on his long and difficult walk to freedom, and died in December, 2013, at the age of 95.

14. George Francis was very excited to see Obama's victory. He lived through 19 presidents and saw Babe Ruth bat a home run. He was born in 1897 in New Orleans, and lived 112 years and 240 days. At one time he had the distinction of being the oldest living American.

15. Vito Vergathompson, who lived to 105, was the oldest licensed driver in California. At age 100, he renewed his license which then expired at age 105. He was part of a family of restaurateurs, judges, lawyers and other professionals. Their hard working "Uncle Vito," who took life in stride was their hero.

16. Edna Parker, at her 115th birthday, was considered the oldest person in the world and attracted the attention of researchers who took a blood sample for the groups DNA database of super-centenarians. Don Parker, her 59 year old grandson, said, "She's never been a worrier and she's always been a thin person so maybe that has something to do with it."

17. Elsie Calvert Thompson, America's oldest person, died just a few weeks before her 114th birthday. She was known for her happy personality and loved to be around people. She enjoyed ballroom dancing and

playing the piano. As most centenarians she was optimistic, happy, and laughed a lot.

18. Alice Hertz-Sommer, believed to be the oldest Holocaust survivor, died February 23, 2014, at age 110. She was an accomplished pianist and claims music kept her alive.

19. Mieczyslaw Horszowski played his final concert at age 99, and taught a lesson the week before he died, just one month before his 101st birthday.

20. Peter Arthur Rubinstein retired from the stage after his 89th birthday.

21. Benzion Netanyanu was the father of the Prime Minister of Israel. He was a prominent historian and became the editor of Encyclopedia Hebraica. He recently dead at age 102.

The centenarians I have met are fascinating people who love to share their action packed lives, which in some ways influenced the destiny of our nation. Most of us read about these events in history books, but the elderly experienced them when America was a young nation. They are truly the gems among us.

They certainly are living proof that the greatest classroom is at the foot of the elderly.

Historians are very interested in centenarians for the light that they shed on the past. Doctors and psychologists feel strongly that this group is very important to our future. Already research has shaken up some long held beliefs.

"Centenarians are a pretty diverse group," explains John Thompson, a physician and researcher at Sanders-Brown Research Center on Aging at the University of Kentucky, in Lexington. "They don't exhibit as uniform a physical or emotional profile as some investigators had expected."

According to the Journal of Longevity, "Those who make it close to the 100 mark, and beyond, are the type who avoids hospitals and doctors whenever possible."

When ill, they tend to be optimistic about recovery. This optimism accompanies an inclination, even passion, toward good health habits. They watch their weight, exercise, and do not smoke. Their most common characteristic is a feisty spirit and a sense of independence.[2] How fortunate our country is that the number of people living to over l00 is steadily increasing. The main objective of this book is helping others to join that group and to enjoy the journey.

The author has a strong passion to take the reader by the hand and prove to you, based on scientific research, that it is possible to make it well beyond the 100 year mark, while growing not older, but younger.

However, there is no such thing as a "free lunch". You have to play by the rules. "Grand slam" aging starts with healthy living. Do not expect to find the Fountain of Youth in a pill box or a physician's office.

Aging with vitality and elegance, or going downhill fast, is first and foremost up to you. It is your personal choice, not fate.

---

[2] Journal of Longevity, Vol 6, No.3, 2000.

> "YOU ARE OLD, FATHER WILLIAM," THE YOUNG MAN CRIED, "THE FEW LOCKS WHICH ARE LEFT ARE GRAY. YOU ARE HALE, FATHER WILLIAM, A HEARTY OLD MAN. NOW TELL ME THE REASON, I PRAY."
>
> "IN THE DAYS OF MY YOUTH," FATHER WILLIAM REPLIED,
>
> "I REMEMBER THAT YOUTH COULD NOT LAST. I THOUGHT OF THE FUTURE; WHAT I DID THAT I NEVER MIGHT GRIEVE FOR THE PAST."
>
> **Poem by Robert Southey**
> **Poet Laureate, England**

Many believe that longevity depends mostly on the genes. If genes were the total answer, I would not be here today. My father had his second and fatal heart attack during my wedding at age 59. Needless to say, it was a traumatic event that caused a lot of grief at what should have been a joyous occasion. Now 63 years later I still remember the advice his physician gave to him after he was diagnosed as having coronary artery disease. "Joe, if you feel like running, walk, if you feel like walking, sit down, or better, lie down. Most important, take it easy and be as inactive as possible." That is certainly not the type of advice that would be given today. Sadly, he was not advised to stop smoking which most likely had more to do with his poor health than his genes.

His brother, my Uncle Barney, lived in the same apartment, ate the same food, had the same job, and visited us in his 80's. He was not a smoker.

In no way should this occurrence suggest that genes are not important. Of course genes count. Those you get from your parents can bolster or reduce your chances of living a long and healthy life by making you more resistant or susceptible to major diseases. For example, research has uncovered specific genes that seem to protect or contribute to age-related illnesses.

However, at a June, 1998, meeting in New York, fourteen national experts in gerontology, exercise, and nutrition, prepared a prescription for longevity. In it they noted that genetic factors account for only 30-35% of individual differences in longevity. The rest might be attributed to life style.

At my 80th birthday my granddaughter Sarah asked "Grandpa are you going to die?" I answered back, "No sweetheart, I have a formula to live forever; so far it is working."

Seniors with grandchildren love this one.

A little girl was sitting on her grandfather's lap as he read her a bedtime story.

From time to time, she would take her eyes off the book and reach up to touch his wrinkled cheek.

She was alternately stroking her smooth cheeks, than his again.

Finally, she spoke up, "Grandpa, did God make you?"

"Yes, sweetheart," he answered. "God made me a long time ago."

She then asked "Grandpa, did God make me too?"

"Yes sweetheart. God made you just a little while ago." Feeling their faces again, she said, "He's getting better at it, isn't he?"

Ronald M. Krauss, M.D., who chaired the Nutrition Committee of the American Heart Association stated, "Most genes make people susceptible to disease, but they rarely cause it."

We may have inherited a shaky family tree but whether or not you are going to join the army of centenarians is not solely dependent on the genes, but how you wear them. You may not be getting proper exercise, or you are eating an unhealthy diet. You may not have the ability to cope with your stress or as we now realize have not been laughing enough or perhaps you have been exposed to poor environmental factors.

Aging with youthful vigor or by sliding down a spiral of declining energy and health is mainly due to your personal choices and not fate.

The good news is that through healthy living and humor, you can compensate for your weak branches. For instance, half of all fatal cancers are linked to poor diet, smoking, and lack of exercise. These are all factors that individuals can control. Environmental pollution, on the other hand, is responsible for a mere 2% of all cancer death[3]. Would you like another opinion? According to William Haskell, M.D., cardiologist at Stanford University, the food we choose to eat can overshadow our genes. "It is something that we have control over. There is ample evidence that what we do for ourselves has a much bigger impact on our long-term risk than heredity."

As so well expressed by Thomas Perls, M.D., of the New England Centenarian Study—"Although genes play some role in age related decline, lifestyle choices appear to be far more significant." Some of us inherit Fords and some of us Volvos -- but you can still get more than the 100,000 miles out of the Ford if you treat it right.

Whenever there is a discussion of genes, I think of a friend of mine who was a doctor and admonished me when I was working on my book, Love Your Heart. "Lee, it all depends on your genes as how long you will live, and other factors as diet and exercise are inconsequential." Sadly, he had a fatal heart attack at age 52 while on a hunting trip. At his funeral were his older brother, and his parents who were in their 80's.

Gerald E. McLearn, PhD, also stated, "By the age of 80, for many, there are hardly any genetic characteristics left."

According to a study in Boston University, it's 70 to 80 percent environment and 20 to 50 percent genes.

---

[3] The Good News Book, Time, 12-2-96.

Studies have shown that the serious losses in physical and mental functioning commonly attributed to age are neither inevitable nor immutable. As Edmund A. Murphy, M.D., then at the John Hopkins School of Medicine, commented, "There is a tendency to fatalism where genetics is concerned. If we are convinced that this disorder originates in our genes, where we cannot get at it, we may abandon attempts to prevent arteriosclerosis, eating eggs for breakfast, drinking a fifth of bourbon after dinner, and allowing our muscles to waste from sloth. If we take the stand that we are masters of our fate perhaps we can achieve some success in combatting this worst of all curses from Pandora's Box".[4] You can stop smoking. You can cut down on foods rich in sugar, salt and saturated fat, and choose your diet from a variety of healthy foods.

You can take time to meditate. Enjoy a good laugh or participate in other activities that will help you cope with the stress in your life. And of course you can exercise. With few exceptions there should be a daily physical exercise program for everyone in the world.

As stated by Hippocrates, Father of Medicine, "Be thine own Physician."

Future chapters will help you to make the right choices so you will age with vigorous enthusiasm.

Yet, there are many seniors who when asked if they want to live to 100 still respond. "Thanks, but no thanks. Who needs longevity to sit in a rocking chair and

---

[4] E.A.Murphy, "Genetics and Atherosclerosis" Coronary Heart Disease. New York, Grune and Stratton, 1962.

stare at the TV or even worse, waste away in a nursing home draining the reminder of my assets? No, I don't want to live to be 100 or older."

This finding emerged in a wide ranging AARP survey on attitudes toward longevity. When asked how long they want to live, 63 percent of the 2,032 respondents opted for fewer than 100 years. Many people assume that with age their mind and memory will deteriorate. Thomas I. Peril, M.D., a geriatrician who was at the head of a New England study of centenarians at the time, disagrees. He estimates that 30 percent of America's oldest have acute minds while 20 percent or more have short term memory problems, but still are getting along just fine.

A group of 40 year old buddies discuss where they should meet for lunch. Finally it is agreed that that they should meet at the Prime restaurant because the waitresses are cute and wear low cut blouses.

Years later at age 50, the group meets again and discusses where they should meet for lunch. They decide to go to the Prime restaurant as the food is good and the wine selection is also good.

10 years later at age 60 the group meets again to discuss where they should go for lunch.

Finally they agree on the Prime restaurant as it is quiet and smoke free.

10 years later now at 70 years of age, the group meets again to discuss where to go for lunch.
Finally it is agreed they should meet at the Prime restaurant because the restaurant is wheel chair accessible and they even have an elevator.

10 years later at 80 years of age they meet and decide it would be a good idea to meet at the Prime restaurant for lunch as they have never been there before.

A priest is walking at the Mall and sees John, one of his parishioners. He walks over and says, "Hello, John, how are you doing? I haven't seen you for a long time." John responded, "I don't go to church anymore." The priest asked, "How old are you now?" "85", John answered. "Well, at that age don't you think of the hereafter?" "Yes," John answered. "All the time, when I go in the kitchen, I always think, what am I here after? When I go in the living room or garage I think, what am I here after?"

After a meeting at his church, a man headed for the parking lot to drive home. After a few minutes he could not find, his car, but he was not concerned. As most seniors, they get a bulk of their daily exercise looking for their vehicle whether a car.

But after checking the area several times and not locating it, he suspected that it was stolen. He was especially frantic because against the advice of his wife he always left his keys in the ignition as he thought that way he would not lose them.

He immediately called the police, confessed that he left his keys in the car, and it was stolen.

Then he made the most difficult call of all to his wife. "Honey," He always called her honey when he was in distress. "No lecture, please, I left my keys in the car and it was stolen."

There was a period of silence and she shouted "John, you did not take the car. I dropped you off."

I said, "Well please come and get me."

She retorted, "I will, as soon as I convince this policeman I have not stolen our car."

If you are of my age group you can relate to that and most likely have a big smile on your face.

Most seniors also can adjust and even find humor with memory as well as hearing problems.

There were three seniors out for their morning walk. One yelled out, "It's windy today." The other one said, "No, it's Thursday." The next one said, "Me too; let's get a drink."

A Doctor had just completed an examination on a woman 80 years old. He was so impressed with her good health he asked her, "I don't want to embarrass you but I am curious. Do you still have intercourse?" She said, "Wait, I will ask my husband." She opened the door to the waiting room which was full of other patients, and yelled out. "Honey, do we still have Intercourse?" He yelled back with anger "If I told you once I must have told you ten times. No, we have Blue Cross."

A doctor was shopping and he saw one of his patients, Abe, who was in his seventies, walking with his arm around a sensuous looking young woman who must have been in her thirties. He said, "Hi, Abe, How are you doing?" "Fine, Doc, just doing what you told me to do: 'To get a hot mama, and be cheerful.' " The doctor replied, "I did not say that. I said you have a heart murmur. Be careful."

Actually, only a small percentage of the elderly are warehoused in nursing homes. Ninety-five percent of those over 65 do not live in one. The number of those who choose to live in a nursing home is dwindling.

Be nice to your children. They will choose your nursing home.

A Harvard University study of centenarians led by Margery Silver, M.D., found that those who reach 100 usually have no dementia problem up through their mid-90s. Dr. Silver's colleague on the study, Thomas Perls, M.D., sums up their remarkable findings by stating, "Now, we know a substantial number of people can remain robust and healthy through their 90's. At least that should change our attitude about old age. It is no longer a curse but an opportunity." This study shattered the assumptions that the older you get the sicker you get.

A group of seniors were asked how they would like to live to be 125 years old. The expected response was "Are you kidding? No way." The question? "Would you like to live to 125, if you could hold on to most of your health and have your mind remain alert?" That received a more positive reply.

"With normal aging, not a heck of a lot changes," said Michael Freedman, M.D., a gerontologist at New York University Medical School. So, you might like to reconsider your response. At 84 years, George Burns was quoted as saying, "Young or old -- just words."

"Old age does not equal disease," said Cheryl Phillips Harris, M.D., Medical Director for Geriatric Services at Sutter Health in Sacramento, California. "If you are healthy in your 50's or 60's the chances are good that you can stay healthy into your 80's." This message comes through loud and clear from those who make it their mission to study how and why we age.

According to researchers at Loyola University's Stritch School of Medicine, Maywood, Illinois, the quality of life has generally improved for U.S. seniors who are 85 years of age.

But to live to 125, many would think impossible? Not as impossible as you may think; Incredible? Not as incredible as you may believe; Farfetched? Not as farfetched as you may imagine.

Today's demographers proclaim that we are just beginning to see that the real limits of the human life find no limit. Living to 100 years or more and being in good health is far from the impossible dream. In fact by 1985 over 25,000 people had reached the century mark, two-thirds more than just five years earlier. By the year 2000 over 50,000 had survived past the age of 100 -- almost double the 1990 total. The number of centenarians in the

U.S. has doubled every decade since 1960, and the majority is mentally and physically in good health.

In 2010 the U.S. was number one with estimates of 53,324. Japan was second with about 30,000, but rising at a faster rate than other countries.

In 2011, the oldest living American was Walter Breuning, a Montana resident, who lived 114 years and 205 days, until he died in 2011.

Arnold Goldstein, a demographic statistician for the U.S. Census Bureau in Maryland which generally has been conservative, now predicts that there will be an astonishing one million American centenarians by the year 2050 and close to two million of them by 2090.

The chance of a human surviving to be 80 years old has increased 21-fold since the beginning of civilization, and the chance of surviving to 100 has increased 3000-fold. In theory even the centenarians have a quarter of a century or more to go because of the biologic upper limits of the life span[5]. The idea is futuristic, but it is not beyond the realistic imagination that once the mechanism of the aging process is known, it would be possible to change the process through bioengineering or some other technology so we could live longer. Says Vincent J. Cristofalo, PhD, a cell biologist and director of the Center for Study of Aging at the University of Pennsylvania: "I am not saying it's going to happen soon, but it's no longer a crazy idea."

---

[5] The Patient: A Systematic Approach to Maintain Health Jan 15, 2000 Vol.6 No.4.

"There appears to be no absolute limit, which is contrary to what I thought ten years ago," says Michael Rose, Professor of Ecology and Evolutionary Biology at the University of California, Irvine. He made the following prediction, "Mankind will postpone human aging substantially in the future, doubling the human life span at least. When we have accomplished this, we will be ashamed that we did not work on it sooner." Remember it wasn't so long ago we considered a person 39 years of age over the hill. That is why Jack Benny stopped counting his age at 39. He, as many other comedians far exceeded their life expectancy and contributed to our health by keeping us laughing as he did until age 80. The number of super-centenarians those living beyond 100 is also increasing so rapidly that 125 seems a reasonable number.

But reaching 125 years? Are you serious, you might ask? Yes, I would answer definitely! We are currently heading in that direction.

According to the Gerontology Research Group (GRP), there have been over 600 verified American super-centenarians (people from the United States who have attained the age of 110 or more). [1] As of December 22, 2013, the GRG lists 20 verified living super-centenarians. The GRG lists people as living super-centenarians if their age has been "validated" and they have been confirmed to be alive within the past year. [2] In addition, 23 Americans listed are considered "pending" and 23 "unverified." The oldest living verified super-centenarian from the United States is Jeralean Talley, aged 114 years, 213 days. [3] The oldest person ever from the United States was Sarah Knauss, who died on December 30, 1999, at age 119 years 97 days.

With the death in June 2012 of Jerroemon Kimura of Japan, the title of the oldest living human being was handed to another Japanese citizen Misao Okawa born on March 5, 1898. An Osaka resident that just passed her 115th birthday when Mr. Kimura was interviewed in 2009 and asked his secret for living so long, he answered "that he exercised daily, ate small portions of food, and read the newspapers two hours a day so he would keep up with the times."

Similarities that are shared by other super-centenarians are that they have parents that also had long lives. They are females and have a strong social network. This includes lots of visitors and friends to see that they are highly motivated and have a reason to get up in the morning. Wow! Doesn't this information put you in a younger mood?

As gerontologists amass information on the aging process and understand more about the life span, they think that 125 years appears to be a realistic figure.

A study that should help unlock the unrevealed secrets of the centenarians is now underway. Most centenarians are stumped by their longevity. This is so well expressed by Bernice Madigan a super-centenarian "Honey I don't know myself how I do it."

The answer may soon be disclosed as the DNA of 100 centenarians are being examined to see if they have a protective gene which markedly increases their resistance to age related diseases as heart disease and Alzheimer s.

The goal of the study is according to Thomas Peris, M.D., "not to increase the life span but the health span". [6]

Longevity is a global sleeping giant, not only in this country but also in Japan and many other countries as Europe as well. Quite a few gerontologists when asked about the limit to the human life span respond that no one really knows. Theoretically there might not be a limit.

The United States still has a long way to go. According to a recent report by the Institute of Medicine and the National Research Council, "The tragedy is not that The United States is losing a contest with other countries, but that Americans are dying and suffering from illness and injury at rates that are demonstrably unnecessary."

This is not a laughing matter and could, and should, be changed. The following chapters will provide the latest information to keep you in the best of health regardless of your age.

---

[6] "contestants race   to map DNA   of 100 centenarians": Thomas Peris, M.D., Wall   Street Journal, September 20 2012 ,

EXERCISE TODAY FOR A ROBUST TOMORROW

BETTER TO HUNT IN FIELDS FOR HEALTH UN BOUGHT THAN FEE THE DOCTOR FOR A NAUSEOUS DRAUGHT.

THE WISE FOR CURE ON EXERCISE DEPEND.

GOD NEVER MADE HIS WORK FOR MAN TO MEND.

John Dryden Poet.

17th Century

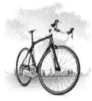 I have been asked the question numerous times: "Lee, you have been active in the field of health for over 60 years. What is the most important thing that I can do to cinch a place in the growing army of centenarians? Is it exercise, diet, or perhaps, controlling the stress in my life?"

There is no one item or magic switch for you to turn on that will be the ticket to carry out that wish. However, for myself, I would have to put exercise at the top of my list. As Tom Spector a professor of genetic epidemiology has stated, "The act of exercising may actually protect against the aging process."

Sharing this belief are many gerontologists who agree that exercise is the closest thing to an "anti-aging pill" now available. Senior citizens, who exercise regularly, certainly do not show the typical symptoms of aging such as slow reflexes, reduced muscle tone, or bone brittleness. Indeed many of them claim that they feel fitter than they did at a much younger age when they were physically inactive.

This is a not a new theory. It was reported at a meeting of 1200 sports physicians from 46 nations. M. Waldo Hollman, M.D., Professor of Sports Medicine and Cardiology at the Cologne University of Sports Medicine sounded the alarm that technical advances reduce the need for physical exercise. The minimum requirement is becoming increasingly difficult to fulfill in industrial societies.

Exercise and periods of rest are the most important measure against diseases of the heart which is the number one killer of Americans. So to beef up the odds of becoming a centenarian you have to get moving.

If we total all the people who die each year from accidents, criminal acts, AIDS, cancer, and all other diseases, it still does not total up to the lives taken each year from the failure of this vital muscle. Your lifetime depends to a great extent on how you treat this vital organ -- your heart.

When you think about it, the heart is truly an amazing organ. It begins to beat months before you are born, and continues to beat at least once every second, every day, every year of your life, propelling oxygen and other nutrients to every one of the many billions of cells in the body. This through a blood vessel network whose length is more than four times the circumference of the earth.

Your heart is an untiring organ, beating about 100,000 times daily, 40 million times a year. Unlike a clock, the heart, with only a fraction of a second of rest between beats, does not need rewinding. It continues to pump for a lifetime. Of course that lifetime depends, to a great extent, on how we treat this vital organ. This tiny organ, about the size of a clenched fist, moves more than 4,000 gallons, or ten tons, of blood each day and every night, a task equivalent to carrying a 39 pound pack to the top of the Empire State Building.

Is it too much to ask that we give our heart enough exercise to keep it fit, and us alive? The answer is, of course, no! Yet sadly, only a small percentage of seniors exercise often enough.

Exercise is currently considered an essential tool for anyone on a cardiac defense disease prevention program. Numerous research studies now provide evidence that exercise strengthens the heart.

Inactivity is one of the main reasons that 1.2 million Americans have a heart attack each year. The couch potatoes and inert seniors are most visible in this group.

To stir you to put exercise at the top of the list and challenge the actuarial tables, hear what some prominent physicians have to say about the power of regular workouts.

Structurally as one ages between 30 and 70, muscle deterioration results in a loss of from 30 to 40 percent of muscle mass. Functionally, there is even a greater decline in endurance and strength as we grow older. While muscle weakness and fatigue occur superficially at any age, the rate of change speeds up when aging is combined with decreasing physical activity -- a dangerous duo.

Keep in mind, oldsters do not have to be super athletes, and stress themselves in physical activities they do not enjoy. Exercise is currently considered an essential tool for anyone on a cardiac prevention program. Numerous research studies now provide evidence that exercise strengthens the heart. J. Naughton, M.D., and J. Brughn, M.D., of the Division of Cardiology, George Washington University, reports that men who do not exercise have twice as many heart attacks as those who are physically active. They suggest that if suitable exercise programs are started early in life, these heart attacks should be prevented.[7]

Similar studies show the value of exercise for patients with heart problems.

Wilhelm Raab, M.D., of the University of Vermont, College of Medicine, serving on an international team of scientists studying the problem of heart disease, pointed

---

[7] j. Naughton, M.D., and J Bruhn, M.D., Emotional Stress, Physical Activity and Ischemic Heart Disease," Disease a Month, July 1980, 1-34

out that lack of exercise is a serious threat to western civilization. It is not the so called "athlete's heart" which should be considered abnormal, he says, "but rather the degenerating inadequate loafer's heart."

The Institute of Health Research, San Francisco, states, "Instead of concentrating on cures, the medical professional should spend a lot more on prevention, and one of the best ways to prevent a lot of disorders of modern society is by regular vigorous exercise, and I mean vigorous, in terms of what it does for the heart and lungs."

David B. Rutstein, M.D, who, at the Harvard Medical School, spoke of the heart's fragility as a myth. Since the heart is chiefly muscle, it should be apparent that the constant exercise makes it extremely tough. Joseph Wolfe, M.D., head of the Valley Forge Heart Hospital, explains, "It is important to note that the heart gains strength through work which produces an extra blood supply with better nourishment. Regular exercise with periods of rest is the most important measure against disease of the heart."

Thomas Perls, M. D., of Beth Israel Medical Center and of Harvard Medical School states, "Exercise is like putting gold in the bank."

Ralph P. Paffenbarger, M.D., of Stanford, a pioneer in the epidemiology of life style diseases, studied students after graduation for a quarter century, and concluded that every hour spent in vigorous exercise as adults will be repaid with two hours of additional life span. To put it another way, if you worked out 12 hours every day, statistically you'd never die. At least, you probably wouldn't die of cardiovascular disease. The most obvious and significant effect of aerobic exercise is that by raising cardiac output, it strengthens the heart muscle and improves the blood flow.

But there are numerous other benefits of exercise that seniors are unaware. The 1996 Surgeon General's report on physical activity and health concluded that exercise is beneficial to almost every organ and system in the body.

Studying the records of 5,000 men who died in British hospitals, J.N. Morris, M.D., of the British Medical Research Council found that those who had been in active jobs had a significant lower incidence of coronary heart disease than those in sedentary jobs, and the disease they had was less severe and developed later.

London bus drivers who sat down with little movement all day had a much higher rate of coronary disease than the conductors, who walked up and down the double decker vehicles punching tickets.[8]

H.A. Kahn, M.D., found that post office clerks who sit all day sorting mail had a much higher rate of coronary disease than carriers who are constantly on the move. Physically active farmers and laborers in Georgia presented a significantly lower rate of coronary disease than the less active farm owners.[9]

---

[8] J.N. Morris, Coronary Heart Disease and Physical Activity Work: Evidence of a National Necropsy Survey,   British Medical Journal 2 (19580 1485-96.

[9] C.G. Hames, J.C. Stule, et al., Coronary Heart Disease among Negroes and Whites in Evans County Georgia. Journal of Chronic Disease

In Israel, a study of 9,000 inhabitants found that over half of the cases of coronary disease were in the inactive group, and the death rate for sedentary workers were three to four times that for active workers. Both the immediate death rate, and the six-year death rate from heart attack, was much lower for the active group. Since the members of these settlements eat the same diets in communal dining rooms, the effect of exercise is clear.[10] An earlier Surgeon General report by Dave Satcher, M.D., states, "We could reduce deaths from CVD (Cardiovascular Disease) in America by 50% if everyone would incorporate moderate physical activity like (walking, gardening, swimming, washing the car, jogging, and bicycle riding) into their daily schedules. He recommends 30 minutes a day, three times a week of moderate exercise.

I have exercised for 30 minutes a day for six days a week without fail for the past 60 years. Now at age 88, I am reaping the benefits of this sagacious investment of time.

The author fears at this point if he presents anymore studies to motivate you to get you moving that you the reader may feel I am over doing it. But the studies are so revealing and so important that I want to make the sale to you.

"As much as 50 percent of the decline in physiological functioning, weak muscles, stiff joints, low

---

18 (1965)1443.

[10] D.Brunner and G.Manelis, "Myocardial Infarction among Members of Communal Settlements in Israel," Lancet 2 (1960} 1049.

energy levels is actually not due to disease and normal consequence of age," said Ann O'Hanlon, assistant professor in the University of New Orleans and active in gerontology programs.

Paul Dudley White, M.D., the world famous heart specialist who cared for former President Dwight Eisenhower after his heart attack stated, "Death from a heart attack before 80 is not God's will. It is man's will."

An articles in Jan 23, 2012 issue of Archives of Internal Medicine adds to the mountain of research that finds physical activity can be a major contributor to healthy aging. It concluded, "Older women who lived the longest, exercised. That middle age exercise helped cognitive skills and it added to bone density."

All of these conditions threaten older adults' ability to function independently and handle tasks of daily living.

Recent studies in physiology also show that properly prescribed exercise in middle to old age can actually turn back the clock physiologically l0 to 25 years. Roy J. Shephard, M.D., an expert on exercise and aging from the University of Toronto, summed it up by saying, "It now appears, after all, that exercise may well turn out to be the long elusive Fountain of Youth."

Regular physical activity has also been associated with greater longevity as well as reduced risk of physical disability and dependence.

In this chapter I will also show how exercise will help to prevent other serious health problems that "rough up" the senior years. There are numerous other benefits of exercise that most seniors are unaware. The 1996 Surgeon General's report on physical activity and health concluded that exercise is beneficial to almost every organ and system in the body.

It looks as if exercise may truly be one of the main ingredients within the Fountain of Youth. It will not only make you healthier, but look and feel younger.

A University of North Carolina at Chapel Hill study will surely lead you to believe so. After a study of 3,100 men, it concluded cardiovascular exercise offers more heart protection then pushing back the clock 19 years. And conversely, lack of fitness is even riskier than smoking.

Having been an exerciser for many years now, I believe that I am far more "heart fit" today than when I started many years ago. My feelings are the same as those of Per-Olaf Astrand, M.D.,[11] world-renowned exercise physiologist and physician, who declared, "It will take 100 years to determine the exact relationship between physical activity and premature death from coronary heart disease. But personally, I can't afford to wait that long to find out, so I elect to exercise now."

I would like to think that by now I have buttoned up your enthusiasm for physical activity and motivated you to find time to get moving in a 24 hour day. You can surely allocate 30 minutes to exercise and to help to fight against heart disease and other chronic problems. And

---

[11] "I elect to exercise now" P.O. Astrand, presentation at the national Convention of the American Association of Health, Physical Education and Recreation, April 1970,Seattle Washington.

most importantly, exercise does not have to be unpleasant.

The old adage "no pain no gain" has proven to be not words of wisdom, but discouraging and misleading. Physical activity can be a lot of fun. The options are many and will be discussed in this chapter. But most importantly, don't listen to the skeptics.

I don't exercise at all. If God wanted us to touch our toes, he would have put them further up on our body."

"I have to exercise early in the morning before my brain figures out what I am doing."

Studies have shown loud and clear, if seniors got off the couch and exercised, many lives would be saved each year. So, if you love your heart, **EXERCISE**.

> SPEAKING GENERALLY ALL PARTS OF THE BODY WHICH HAVE A FUNCTION, IF USED IN MODERATION AND EXERCISED IN LABORS IN WHICH EACH IS ACCUSTOMED, THEREBY BECOMES HEALTHY, WELL DEVELOPED,AND AGE MORE SLOWLY. BUT IF BRUISED AND LEFT IDLE THEY BECOME LIABLE TO DISEASE DEFECTIVE IN GROWTH, AND AGE MORE QUICKLY.
>
> **HIPPOCRATES 400 B.C.**

I know many of you are thinking, "I just do not have the time to exercise, between shopping, attending meetings, keeping in touch with the grandchildren, and other activities. I am overloaded as it is." Excuses -- that is the most common one.

I immediately think of Thomas Jefferson. He was Secretary of State twice, President, and wrote the Declaration of Independence at age 32. Yet, he had the time to exercise two hours every day. He lived to be 83. He was a firm advocate of walking, and shunned the use of the horse for transportation.

Exercise changes attitude and the outlook on life. Seniors should look to Thomas Jefferson as a role model and plan to exercise daily.

Keep in mind that if you do not find time for exercise now, you will have a lot of time for illness later. As stated so well by Thomas Fuller, M.D, in 1732, "Health is not valued until sickness comes."

Man is by nature a lazy animal inclined to put out the minimum energy necessary for survival. It is a sign of our affluence that special exercise programs are needed to compensate for our daily inactivity. No longer do we have to cut wood to cook food or to provide warmth for the family. All we have to do is strike a match or push a button. It is rare to see someone washing or polishing his car; it's easier to drive to a car wash. How about the mail carriers: they now drive instead of walk to deliver the mail, which deprives them of healthy exercise.

Engineers have been very successful in contributing to our lazy preferences. Lawn mowers are now available so that you can sit on them as you cut the grass. Elevators carry you up and down the stairs. TV sets lure you to sit down and watch a variety of programs (of course you do get exercise looking for the remote control). Video players and computers are taking us off our feet to sit or lie down. Being sedentary is the name of the game, and too many seniors are playing it on a daily basis.

Before the industrial revolution, we were much more active and human muscle provided most of the energy used in agriculture and in factories; no, more! We no longer have to be active. This gives us more time to be physically inactive. Sadly, the average American adult spends their extra time the wrong way: 170 minutes a day watching television and movies, and if that isn't bad enough, they use up another 101 minutes driving the car, but less than 19 minutes exercising. Add up the time spent sitting in the car, watching television, and on the computer which you can find time to do, and certainly that raises questions about excuse "**No.1**".

Also, keep in mind that sitting can kill you. "People who sit for the majority of their day have much higher mortality rates than people who don't, even if they're physically active during another part of the day," says Peter Katzmarzyk", who is an epidemiologist at the Pennington Biomedical Center in Baton Rouge, Louisiana.

According to a 2010 report on a study by the American Cancer Society that tracked roughly 53,000 men and 70,000 women for 14 years, the longer you sit the greater the risk of dying.

Women who did the least exercise (like brisk walking), and who sat for at least six hour a day during their leisure time, were almost twice as likely to die as those who did the most exercise and who sat for less than three hours a day.

Men who did the least exercise also placed themselves in the danger zone, and by sitting for at least six hours a day were one-and-a-half times more likely to die.

Unfortunately, too many graying seniors have all kinds of excuses to avoid putting on their athletic shoes.

Another common excuse "**No.2**" is: "I am too old to exercise."

Let us now look at some senior men and women who would question that attitude.

American Masters participants, aged 40 to 70, both men and women, compete regularly in track and field events conceding nothing to age. Their amazing feats in the last decade are changing many former ideas about aging, and have suggested that previous standards for human potential at any age may have been far too low. Recent university studies have shown that people in their 60's and 70's can reduce blood pressure, weight, and nervous tension while increasing body strength by exercising.

Ask any of them why they do it, and their answers will show their enthusiasm for exercise.

"Health and fun," were the reasons given by 67-year-old Bud Deason, of Hawaii, holder of some old age group world records. Kelly, a 64-year-old consulting engineer from Eugene, Oregon, and a runner specializing in the 5,000 and 10,000 meter races, firmly believes everyone should keep active. "I run to live; to better enjoy my life." he declared.

Norm Bright, a 68 year old Seattle marathoner and steeple chaser said that when he was young he had wanted to be an explorer. "Now, I am one," he explained. "I'm exploring myself, discovering what I'm capable of." He broke three hours in the Boston Marathon, finishing first in his age group. He has beaten European runners on their own tracks, has run to the top of Pike's Peak, and has set numerous age group records.

The hero of the 1981 Boston Marathon was Johnny Kelley, the 73 year old legend of Cape Cod. Finishing his 50th Boston Marathon in four hours. He received, "the greatest reception I ever had. It made me cry -- almost."

Eula Weaver of Santa Monica, California jogged two miles every day around her high school track at the age of 88.

Adolph Hoffman, at 87, holds the record for pole vaulting in his age group.

Ted Hatlen, at age 90, held the world records for his age group in the high jump. At age 85, Clara Tovey, had an exercise routine that points out dramatically that age is no criterion of one's ability to continue a physical activity program. Four times a week, she rises out of bed at 5 a.m. and begins with 30 minutes of aerobic exercise. She then dives into a pool for a few laps, rides an exercise bicycle, and moves to the weight machine where she pumps iron. "Because it gives me energy, I wish more older people would exercise like this." she says. "I feel differently altogether; because I exercise I have a different attitude."

Cleo Christiansen logged 2,200 miles walking at shopping malls. She saw an advertisement suggesting walking around the malls as a way to get your daily exercise, and decided to go for it. She walked an average of 6-8 miles a day and, now in her late 80's, is still walking daily. She also enjoys ballroom dancing.

Suzi MacLeod, of Bend, Oregon, at age 75, set a new world mile record in the women's 75-79 class with a time of 8:16:3.

Talking about world records set by a senior, this one is a shocker. Tom Lacey, at age 89, and recently widowed, took up a new sport, wind walking. He holds the world record for crossing the English Channel at 160 miles per hour with only goggles and layers of clothes to fight the wind chill, as he stood on the wings of a biplane.

An inspiration for many older people was Larry Lewis, who lived to be 106, and ran consistently for 94 years. The star of the film, "Run Dick, Run Jane," Lewis declared, "The minute I hear a man say he's going to lie in the sun and enjoy his retirement; I know he's about to meet his maker."

I often have thought what a dramatic impact could be made if runners like Larry Lewis, in their senior years, could run down the beach where many oldsters bask in the son and demonstrate that wrinkles and white hair don't necessarily mean one is "over the hill."

Excuse "**No.3**": Another common excuse is: "I hate to admit it but I have been motionless most of my life, and worked hard to avoid any type of exercise. So, it is probably too late to start." This would be a perilous and self-defeating attitude. A negative view, which according to a Yale led research team has shown what older individuals believe about aging can have a direct impact on their health. The study suggests that negative beliefs or stereotypes about aging that many elderly Americans encounter in their daily lives can increase their cardiovascular stress.[12]   For those who were active throughout their life, there is no question about it. You are much better prepared to continue on an exercise program. But for the rest of you: better later than never. Yes, you can catch up.

Johnnye Valien, age 76, is a grandmother of seven who started exercising in her 50's. Now she throws the javelin and runs the 80 meter hurdles, among other events.

Marge Anderson started swimming at 84, and in her 90's, won an award.

Not many would accept excuse "**No.3**" as they watched Helen Klein of California carry the Olympic torch its way toward Salt Lake City for the Olympic Winter Games. She thanks her exercise program for helping her setting an American record in the 75-79 age group at the California International Marathon. She also set a record in running 100 miles in less than 24 hours.

Research has shown that even people who began exercising in their 90's and 100's realize gains in their cardiovascular and muscular fitness. Investigations of men and women in their 90's demonstrated the benefits of strength training and emphasized that it is never too late to begin an exercise program.[13]

---

[12] Negative review of aging increases cardiovascular stress in older persons. Yale scientist finds Release of Gerontological Society of America, June 27, 2000.

[13] Wayne T. Phillips, PhD, Strength training not only for the young Men's Health   April 16,1996 pg.5

A study at the University of California, at Davis confirmed the urgency for seniors to get going regardless of age. It compared exercisers under 65 to those over 65 and found that age is not a limiting factor in improving overall fitness. Although the older group started out at a slower pace, both groups met personal fitness goals at the same rate.

The British Heart Study at the Royal Free Hospital School of Medicine in London also reported that it is never too late to get started. Over 1000 men (ages 52-72) had filled out questionnaires about their exercise activities in 1978 and again in 1992. If they had a history of poor health, they were excluded.[14] Men who walked at least an hour a day in 1992 had a 38 percent lower risk of dying during the study than men who were sedentary. And, men who were sedentary in 1978 and began at least "light" activity by 1992 had a 45 percent lower risk of dying than men who remained inactive.[15]

An Israeli study noted that previously sedentary 85 year olds reaped benefits from exercise, and that even people who began exercising in their 90's and 100's realize gains in both musculoskeletal and cardiovascular fitness. Active octogenarians also had less depression and loneliness.

It supports the findings of other investigators reporting in the Archives of Internal Medicine that continued physical activity, even among the oldest old

---

[14] Lancet 351 1603 1998.

[15] U.C. Davis Health System, Vol.6, No.2, July 2000.

who led sedentary lives, should be encouraged to exercise. Indeed it is never too late to start.

Laura Thorpe, PhD, a researcher at Chicago's Rush University Medical Center, advised old patients who want to increase their physical activity to do so under a doctor's supervision. Still, Thorpe said, "Even those who are not exercisers or athletes can start and see substantial benefit."

According to Tufts University expert Marian Nelson, PhD, "It is never too late to start moving, even well into your 90's all of these systems can be stimulated."

So, to turn back the clock on the aging process no matter the age, or the wrinkles, or gray hair take that first step even though it's taken you a long time to do so. Exercise may very well be the body's best friend. It is a natural and safer way to ameliorate many chronic health problems and, of course, less expensive.[16]

Excuse "**No.4**": Many survivors are fearful of physical activity, which is understandable but, for most, a dangerous point of view.

Not too long ago, doctors would tell people who had heart attacks that they would have to take it easier the rest of their lives. Now most cardiologists feel that recovery really is complete when the patient gives up living in fear and resumes his normal life. Thanks to major breakthroughs in the area of heart disease, many of you who have had a heart attack or stroke and were

---

[16] J. Amer, Med.Assoc.272; 1994.

fortunate enough to survive can look forward to a long and healthy life.

That is, if you accept Mother Nature's warning that you better sit up and notice: you were not taking good care of your circulatory system, not exercising or relaxing enough, not eating properly, and not listening to that cigarette cough.

If you do accept the warning, you will look back one day and realize that your attack was a blessing in disguise, for you survived the first, and prevented a recurrence. Remember, if you want to play the health game, you have to follow the rules. Repeating an unhealthy life style will most likely precipitate another heart attack. To prevent this, there is a lot you can do. I would, also, recommend very strongly that you enroll in a cardiac rehabilitation program.

If you have had an encounter with heart disease, as millions do each year, talk to your body. It will listen. Tell it this is not the final chapter, but the opening of a new life that could be even healthier and happier than before. Prominent cardiologists and Industrial leaders will support you in your adoption of this attitude. As Harvey Wolinsky of the Mount Sinai Hospital and Medical Center states, "large numbers of Americans have taken responsibility for their health habits and, in a short time, achieved major stunning relief from an epidemic disease that had for decades been an increasing scourge."[17]

---

[17] "Americans have taken responsibility," Harvey Wolinsky, "Taking Heart" The Sciences (February 1981).

A cardiac rehabilitation program will be a great member on your team to help you stay on track. This program has helped show many seniors that a person's active days are not over.

William Haskell, M.D., Co-Director, Stanford Cardiac Rehabilitation program, who states, "Selected patients after acute myocardial infarction have benefited from appropriate increases in physical activity. They have had fewer complications associated with bed rest, made a more successful adjustment to their disease, shown improved cardiovascular function, and physical working capacity, returned to gainful employment earlier and more frequently, and had fewer and less severe re-infractions."

That statement alone should be enough to motivate heart patients to seek out such activity.

If you have had a heart attack, you should contact your local hospitals and other sources to find a nearby cardiac rehabilitation program. Make certain that in addition to exercise they offer nutritional counseling and, most importantly, counseling to modify Type A behavior which most likely contributed to your coronary incident.

The program at Mt. Zion UCSF Medical Center developed by Diane Ulmer and Meyer Friedman, M.D., produced a dramatic reduction in the rate of cardiac problems recurring. No drug, food, or exercise program ever devised, not even coronary bypass surgery, has matched the protection against recurrent heart attacks that this behavioral counseling program has achieved.

While serving as President of The American Heart Association, Golden Empire Chapter, and chairman of a cardiac rehabilitation committee, I observed several meetings at the Mt. Zion Hospital and Medical Center in San Francisco. I was very impressed by its spectacular results. Dr. Friedman has been a major inspiration to me and most gracious in sharing his studies of the type A personality, which will be discussed in the chapter on stress.

For those who are still giving excuses, there is a Chinese proverb, "The person who says it cannot be done should not interrupt the person doing it."

"WE WERE MEANT TO BE FIELD ANIMALS :TO RISE WITH THE SUN, TO BE IN THE OPEN AIR, TO BE PHYSICALLY VIGOROUS, AND TO EAT ONLY WHEN HUNGER DICTATES."

PAUL DUDLEY WHITE, M.D.

The reader should realize by now that **exercise strengthens the heart**, which is a muscle, and physical

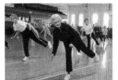

activities make the blood flow faster through it, and helps to keeping it in good shape through the senior years.

Following chapters will point out how exercise increases the good kind of cholesterol. It appears to make blood less sticky so there is less chance of blockage. This increases the flow of life-sustaining oxygen in the blood.

This chapter will bring out the value of exercise to prevent other bad situations that plague the senior citizen. Why it may even be the best prescription to guarantee the senior a place in the lineup of centenarians.

Many gerontologists feel that exercise is the closest thing to an anti-aging pill now available. Senior Citizens who exercise regularly certainly do not show the typical symptoms of aging; such as slowed reflex times, reduced muscle tone, or bone brittleness. Indeed, many of them claim that they feel more fit than they did at a much younger age when they were physically inactive.

If protecting the senior from heart problems as atherosclerosis (commonly referred to as hardening of the arteries) was exercises only claim to fame, it should be enough to get us up and going. Especially now, for the first time medical studies have demonstrated that we cannot only prevent atherosclerosis, but can even reverse serious damage to our arteries, letting the blood continue to flow bringing oxygen to nourish the heart.

The hidden benefits of exercise can only be described as super human. And inactivity by seniors can blot out the golden years.

The 1996, Surgeon General's report on physical activity and health concluded that exercise is beneficial to almost every organ and system in the body.

Now let us look at the incredible and far reaching role of exercise in protecting the senior citizen against the variety of problems that disrupt the quality of their life.

For example -- **exercise is a natural remedy to lower** **high blood pressure** and improve fitness in seniors well into their later years.

The older you are the more likely you are at risk of having hypertension. It takes its toll of seniors, and it often gives no warning.

According to the National Health Lung and Blood Institute, one out of four adults has high blood pressure. For adults ages 70 and older it rises dramatically; two out of three have high blood pressure.

Hypertension triggers a third of heart attacks and is the leading cause of stroke and kidney failure. Many physicians now believe it is possible to lower high blood pressure a moderate amount through regular physical activity.

"Physical Activity can help control blood pressure, and that's the leading risk factor for stroke," notes Edgar J. Kenton, M.D, Professor of Clinical Neurology at Theodore Jefferson University in Philadelphia. He is also an active member of the American Heart Association Stroke Council.

Kenneth Cooper, M.D., and Associates at the Cooper Clinic in Dallas found in a study of 3,000 men that there was a difference of four to eight points in blood pressure between separate groups of men and women who were in excellent physical shape, and similar groups of men and woman in poor physical shape.

Testing results can be misleading since many tense up when the cuffs are put on and the number shoots up. This is referred to as the "white coat syndrome." Resting awhile and repeating the test will often provide a more reliable diagnosis to see, "if your number is up."

Your risk of stroke and heart disease starts to climb as your blood pressure rises above normal (normal means below 120 (systolic) over 80 (diastolic)).

Systolic measures the pressure that the blood exerts on the arteries and vessels when the heart beats. Diastolic is the pressure that is exerted on the walls of the arteries around the body in between heart beats, when the heart is resting. The new hypertension recommendations say doctors should consider prescribing drugs to patients age 60 and over whose levels are 150/90 or higher. The previous threshold was 140/90.

If your blood pressure is up, before you get started on a program of taking pills, ask your physician if a change in your diet along with managing stress and exercise may clear up the problem.

> **F**ace Dropping: Does one side of the face droop or is it numb? Ask the person to smile.

> **A**rm Weakness: Is one arm weak or numb? Ask the person to raise both arms. Does one arm drift downward?

> **S**peech Difficulty: Is speech slurred, are they unable to speak, or are they hard to understand? Ask the person to repeat a simple sentence like, "The sky is blue." Is the sentence repeated correctly?

> **T**ime to call 911: if the person shows any of these symptoms, even if the symptoms go away, call 9-1-1 and get them to the hospital immediately.

Just as regular exercise can reduce the risk of heart attack, physical activity may also help prevent brain attack, also more commonly known as stroke. In released guidelines, the Prevention Advisory Board of the National Stroke Association recommends "taking a brisk walk for as little as 30 minutes a day" as one of 10 strategies to help prevent stroke, America's leading cause of adult disability.

According to I. Min Lee, M.D., assistant professor of epidemiology at the Harvard School of Public Health, "Walking, stair climbing, and participating in moderately intense activities as -- dancing, bicycling and gardening were shown to reduce the risk of stroke."

Many do not realize that stroke is the third leading cause of death in both men and women in the United States.

Annually, 700,000 suffer from stroke. Over one third have recurrent incidents. High percentages are seniors.

Nine out of ten strokes are like a heart attack, but in the brain. The human and economic toll is overwhelming.

People who are active are 25 percent less likely to have a stroke than a sedentary counterpart. "Physical inactivity is associated with an increased risk of stroke, according to a study that tracked 72,000 nurses for eight years. Those who were active for at least four hours a week had a 54 percent lower risk of ischemic stroke (the most common kind of stroke caused by an interruption in the flow of blood to the brain) than those who were sedentary."

"Exercise is so important to cardiovascular health in general and in reducing the risk of coronary heart damage that we have long suspected it might protect against stroke as well," according to Phillip B. Gorelick, M.D., professor of neurology at Chicago's Rush Medical College and Chairman of the NSA panel. Now we have the evidence to say that physical activity is an exceedingly important factor.

For the seniors who suffer from a stroke; a rehabilitation program including physical activity should be started under the supervision of your doctor.

Most of us get fatter as we age; there is a reason for 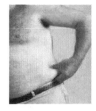 that. It just doesn't happen. It is because most of us exercise less and thus have a lower metabolic rate, caused by a loss of muscle. Eating too much of the wrong foods, of course, also contributes to this problem.

William B. Kannel, M.D., who directed the Framingham Study (to be discussed later), has stated that if everyone were of optimal weight, there would be 25% less coronary heart disease, and 35% less congestive failure and brain infarction.[18] Once again, exercise to the rescue.

Exercise can increase the body's metabolism and make it more efficient in burning calories. It also makes respiration more efficient. Dieters who exercise on a regular basis also lost less muscle than those who just cut down their calorie intake. Exercise turns fat to muscle; it also helps to keep the weight off and the bulge from returning. It certainly cuts down on the expense of altering clothes.

Many worry about how excess weight diminishes the appearances, but a more legitimate concern is that being overweight may increase your risk of high blood pressure, high cholesterol, and a multiplicity of problems.

---

[18]Dr. Kannel who directed Bray, G.A., Gray. D.S., Obesity Part 1 Pathogenesis Western Journal of Medicine(October 1988)149;429-441 Part 2 Leitz Mann   MF et al., M.D., Recreational Physical Activity and the risk of Cholecystectomy in Women New England Journal of Medicine   1999 341 :777, (PubMed.}.

Obesity, which affects one out of three Americans, is now considered by the American Medical Association as a disease. [19]

Name an herb, a pill, or drug that can accomplish as much to keep your weight down without side effects as exercise does. There isn't any!

---

[19] Kelly Fitzgerald "Obesity is now a disease, American Medical Association Decides" Medical News Today 8-17-2013

Diverticular Disease

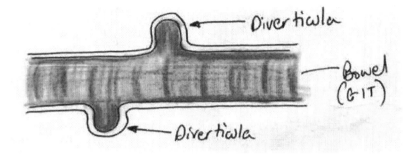

Diverticulitis disease is **very common in western countries**. It is present in nearly half of Americans by age 60 and over two thirds at age 80.

Exercise is important to help prevent diverticulosis. It promotes normal bowel movements and puts less pressure on the colon. In one of the few studies that have been done, the most active men had a 37 percent lower risk of symptomatic diverticular disease than the least active men.

It is interesting that diverticulitis is rare in countries where diets typically are high in fiber.

Gallstones

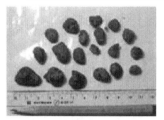

Physical activity appears to play an important role in the prevention of gallstone, which occur in up to 20% of American women and 10% of American men by age 60. The Harvard researchers made the finding when they studied almost 46,000 men ages 40 to 75 for eight years. Those who exercised the most had the least risk for gallstones.

Active women are 30 percent less likely to have gallstone surgery than sedentary women. In one study, women who spent more than 60 hours a week sitting at work or driving were twice as likely to have gall stone surgery as did women who sat for less than 40 hours a week.

Prostate Cancer

A study by I.M. Lee, M.D., showed that men who burned

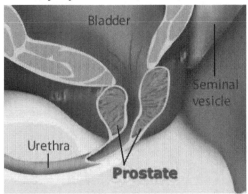

4,000 calories per week or more (the equivalent of an hour's active workout) had a much lower incidence of prostate cancer than did men who burned fewer than 1,000 calories per week. Investigators theorized that increased physical activity produced lower levels of prostate-stimulating androgens.

Researchers in Dallas assessed the physical fitness of 13,334 initially healthy men and women, and then followed them for an average of eight years. They found that even mild exercise postpones death and regular exercise may help to prevent cancer.[20] Men diagnosed with prostate cancer that did vigorous exercise as biking, jogging, swimming or playing tennis for at least three hours a week had a 61 percent lower risk of dying from their cancer than men who exercised vigorously for less than one hour a week.[21]

---

[20] Lee, I.M., Physical activity and risk among college alumni, American Journal of Epidemiology {vol.135, no}.

[21] J. Clin. On Col 29:726, 2011.

I can vouch for the fact that it **is no fun to have an enlarged prostate.** Benign prostatic hyperplasia (BPH) is a common problem for senior men.

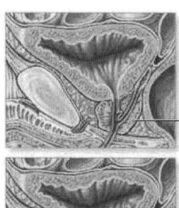

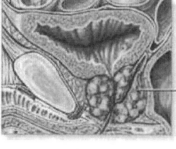

Normal prostate

Prostate cancer

It is probably safe to say that there are no other annoyances that cause more fear or anxiety for men. It often presents the same symptoms as prostate cancer, but, fortunately, it is not malignant and does not always develop into a cancerous condition. It is treatable. I will never forget when my urologist told me, after an extensive exam, that I had one of the largest prostates that he ever examined. I would have preferred that he said that about the adjacent organ.

In one study, men who walked two to three hours a week had 25 percent lower risk of an enlarged prostate than men who seldom walked.

Colon Cancer

The Surgeon General's report concluded that **activity protects against colon cancer**.

The evidence pertaining to the role of exercise and its effect on colon cancer is documented. Studies indicate that even light to moderate regular activity is associated with lower risk than inactivity.

A study at the Washington School of Medicine in St. Louis reviewed 52 studies of exercise and colon cancer. The most active people were about 23 percent less likely to be diagnosed with the disease than their counterparts. The evidence is fairly clear, according to Harvard's I. Lee, M. D., who examined dozens of studies, that men and women who are physically active have a 30 to 40 percent lower risk of colon cancer compared to individuals who are not active. Other studies back up this, Michael Thun, M.D., vice president emeritus for epidemiology and surveillance at the American Cancer Society states "Physical activity is central to reduce your risk of cancer, and with respect to colon cancer, the direct effect is well documented. Studies show even light to moderate regular activity is associated with lower risk compared to inactivity." Perhaps by speeding food with its potential carcinogens through the intestine, exercise may curb the risk of colon and rectal cancer. Exercise may also augment immune defenses.

Colonoscopies and other screening tests are helping seniors to fight against colon and rectal cancer but the diseases still claim more lives than any other cancer except lung cancer. This is another highly motivating reason to exercise.

Breast Cancer

With breast cancer, there's fairly consistent evidence that **reduced risk occurs only with greater moderate to vigorous activity.** Most encouraging is that it is never too late to start an exercise program to prevent cancer.

Although there may be some questions as to the exact amount of exercise required for maximum benefit, there is no doubt that Americans are not getting enough.

Exercise seemed to lower the risk of breast cancer in normal weight women, says a study of more than 74,000 postmenopausal women.

Normal weight women who did the equivalent of 1¼ to 2½ hours a week of brisk walking had a 30 percent lower risk of breast cancer than sedentary women. Those women who did the equivalent of at least 10 hours a week had a 37 percent lower risk.

The study also revealed that the impact of exercise on overweight women was weaker and disappeared if they were obese. Overweight and obese women have a higher risk of breast cancer whether they exercise or not.

Researchers at the National Cancer Institute which reviewed 23 studies that tracked 37,500 breast cancer patients and 4,000 colon cancer patients for 3 to 13 years revealed that those who got regular exercise were less likely to die, even if they didn't start to exercise until they were made aware that they had the disease. Edward Giovannucci, M.D., of the Harvard School of Public Health stated in an editorial published with the study that, "Adequate physical activity should be a standard part of cancer care."[22]

A good reason why this book is not on exercise alone is because diet, stress, and other exercise certainly stand out as one of our best support systems to enjoy the golden years.

---

[22] Nat'l Cancer Inst.104:797, 815, 2012

Lung Cancer

Lung cancer **kills more Americans than breast, colon, and prostate cancers combined**.

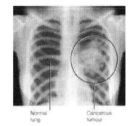

Normal lung   Cancerous tumour

Needless to say, smokers account for this frightening statistic. Nonsmokers and seniors that have been exposed to asbestos, diesel exhaust, air pollution or second-hand smoke can still get lung cancer, so they should also look forward to a daily workout.

Arthritis

If you have arthritis, moderate low-impact exercise will reduce this disabling problem.

The ability to have comfortable movement is something that healthy senior citizens take for granted and assume that it will always be there. But increasing age brings unwelcome changes. Unpleasant musculoskeletal weakness, stiffness and pain are among the most frequent complaints physicians hear from middle aged men and women.[23]

---

[23] Bourse American Osteoporosis foundation.

Osteoporosis

Osteoporosis is **well known to oldsters**. The older you 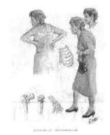 are the weaker your bones. By age 75 more than a third of all women have osteoporosis, and by age 85 more than half do. Rates for men are lower at every age. Bones are like any other part of the body; if you stress it, it responds.

For two decades, researches followed a group of 3,262 Finnish men aged 44 and older. They found that those who were more active suffered fewer osteoporosis related hip fractures than those who were sedentary. Men who described their physical activity as "vigorous" had the lowest fracture rate of all.

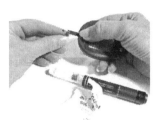

Diabetes is a **disease of the human immune system** that makes it difficult for the body to produce insulin. Without this insulin, the body cannot convert sugar from foods into nutrients for cells. When an excess of sugar builds up in the blood, serious damage may eventually occur to the organs. It affects about 26 million Americans and is increasing rapidly. Twenty seven percent of Americans who have it do not know it.

The main types of diabetes are as Type 1 and Type 2.

The main cause of Type 1 is that the pancreas, the organ that secretes insulin, is destroyed by autoantibodies. They are antibodies (immune protein) that mistakenly target and damage specific tissues or organs of the body. That is why people with this type always need insulin either through injection or a pump.

Type 1 is an autoimmune disease. Your body's immune system protects you from diseases and infections, but if you have an autoimmune disease your immune system attacks health cells in your body by mistake. It is often diagnosed in childhood.

Type 2 is the most common type for seniors. The cause is primarily a complicated medical condition known as insulin resistance. In the early stage, although there is plenty of insulin, it doesn't work well. A change to a healthier lifestyle will often help, but some will eventually need insulin either with or without medication.

The disease raises the risk of heart attacks, strokes, kidney disease, blindness, amputations, and nerve damage. It is often associated with weight gain and older ages.

Once again, as you have heard frequently in this book, exercise as well as diet can often solve this problem.

Falling

Falling is a **major hazard to older people** that causes 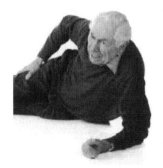 the death of over 9,000 in the United States each year. It can be dangerous to anyone, but according to the National Safety Council, it is the leading cause of accidental death and disability in the 65 plus age group. It keeps a lot of orthopedic surgeons and nursing homes in business, for an estimated 30 percent to 50 percent of older adults fall each year. More than 200,000 break a hip. Many become disabled for an extended period of time, sometimes permanently. In fact, falls contribute to 40 percent of nursing home admissions annually, the National Institute on Aging reports.

According to a British study, older women assigned to a home-based (strength and balance training) exercise program had fewer falls than women who didn't exercise. There is another major impact to falls. If a person falls often it is so scary that they reduce their activities such as shopping, gardening, and working in the house. The cutting back on physical activity is in itself, dangerous.

Muscle Problems

Remember those Charles Atlas ads showing a man with bulging muscles kicking sand in the face of a meek-looking individual at the beach. It was very effective and many enrolled in gym classes, so they could resemble Charles Atlas.

Muscle building for seniors is very important for muscles wither away if they are not used. For every decade after about age 50, you lose some 6 percent of your muscle mass, which comes with a 10 to 15 percent loss of your strength. But anyone can build muscle strength back up with exercise. Even seniors over 100 years old can partially reverse some of the loss that occurs with aging.

A combination of aerobics and strengthening exercise is the best defense against falls and disabling fractures.

Sleep

A study at Stanford University School of Medicine showed that people over 50, a group most likely to have trouble sleeping, **will do fine if they exercise daily**.

The men and women, who were healthy, but sedentary, were put on 30-40 minute exercise sessions at least 4 times a week. It included brisk walking or cycling on a stationary bicycle. They slept almost an hour longer and fell asleep in half the time. "Sleeping like a rock" is not a common expression among many exercise seniors, but other studies show regardless of your age insomnia can be treated.

Just as reading a good book, exercise can also help to relax the mind -- no pill, just the will to exercise.

Nervous Tension

> "A man too busy to take care of his health is like a mechanic too busy to take care of his tools."
>
> **A Spanish Proverb**

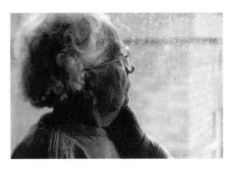 As I wrote in the previous chapter, I felt confident that many of the readers were well aware that exercise was important for a healthy heart. Was I preaching to the choir? But I doubt whether many of **you were aware of how vital a role physical activity plays** in preventing numerous other health problems that plague seniors.

The first systematic study of the effects of exercise on nervous tension was started in 1953 by Thomas Cureton, M.S., and a strong proponent of physical fitness. Studying 2,500 adults over a 10 year period he became convinced that physical exercise helps alleviate nervous tension. Until then, however, there had been no controlled studies of this observation. That was soon to change. Researchers have found that physical exercise can help keep your mind to stay as fit and youthful as your body. It is known that a sedentary lifestyle is accompanied by electrical and chemical changes in the brain -- a gradual winding down of brainwave frequency and decreased levels of two neurotransmitters, dopamine and norepinephrine (noradrenaline).

Anxiety and Depression

People with anxiety or depression who do aerobic 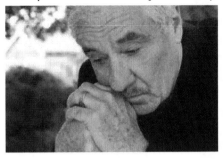 exercises like brisk walking or running, curb their symptoms, possibly by releasing natural opiates.[24] **"People who are active are less likely to develop depression,"** says researcher Steven Blair in a study of approximately 2,000 residents of Alameda County, California. People who were more active were nearly 20 percent less likely to be diagnosed with depression over the next five years than less active residents. In addition, to helping blood circulate, exercise can prevent heart disease by reducing stress. Kenneth Cooper states that, "Real physical exercise erases mental fatigue." Dr. Paul Dudley White said, "Exercise is the greatest tranquilizer."

---

[24] K.H. Cooper. The new Aerobics {New York: Bantam Books, 1970.

Mental Fitness

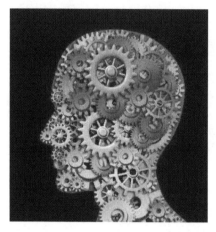

To keep your mind fit as you grow older -- **keep your body fit**. Long term aerobic exercise such as walking may help older people keep mentally sharp, according to the Medical College of Pennsylvania. A preliminary study there found that men age 60 and older who exercised regularly for five or more years scored significantly higher than non-exercisers of the same age and intelligence on tests measuring mental quickness and recall. "There is only one quality worse than hardness of heart and that is softness of head."

Enhance Memory and Thinking

Can't find your keys, the remote control, your glasses or 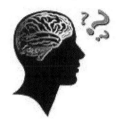 where you parked your car? Sound familiar? Could be that looking for them almost daily provides some exercise but not enough to keep you out of the danger zone. There is growing evidence that **exercise can enhance memory** and thinking as people age. In a study published recently, Kristine Yaffe, M.D., a neurologist at the University of California, San Francisco, administered a standard test of mental function to nearly 6,000 women, 65 or older, tracked their physical activity over the next six to eight years, and then tested them again. Those who walked the most were least likely to show a cognitive decline over the period.

Most of us, as we age, are concerned of becoming a victim of Alzheimer's disease. **This is a legitimate worry** since according to a 2012 report of the Alzheimer Association on disease facts and figures; 5.4 million Americans have Alzheimer's. The costs for care in the United States are 200 billion dollars a year.

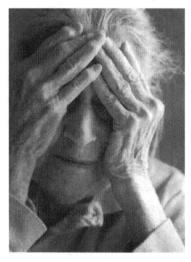

Guess what? You should know this is coming. The brain likes exercise. It is bad enough that inactivity of the senior reduces your muscles to mush, but can it affect your brain?

According to the Alzheimer's Research and Prevention Foundation, regular physical activity is probably the best way to shield your brain against aging. It reduces your risk of developing Alzheimer's disease by 50%.

"The evidence is fairly solid that people who are more physically active are at lower risk of cognitive decline and dementia," says Constantine Lyketsos, M.D., director of the Division of Geriatric Psychiatry and Neuropsychiatry at John Hopkins School of Medicine in Baltimore.

Ongoing research indicates like your muscles, your brain needs regular workouts to stay healthy and fit as you age. It also requires a well-balanced diet, low in fat and cholesterol and high in anti-oxidants. Sounds familiar doesn't it?

Quality sleep, an active social life, puzzles and riddles also help seniors prevent this disabling disease.

A cleaning woman was applying for a new job.

When asked why she left her last employment, she replied, "Yes, Sir, they paid good wages, but it was the most ridiculous place I ever worked. They played a game called bridge and last night a lot of folks were there."

"As I was about to bring in refreshments, I heard a man say, 'Lie down and let's see what you got.' "

"Another man says to the lady, 'I've got strength but no length.' "

"Another man says to the lady, 'Take your hand off my trick.' "

"I pretty near dropped dead just then, when the lady answered, 'You jumped me twice when you didn't have the strength for one raise.' "

"Another lady was talking about protecting her honor, and two other ladies were talking and one said, 'Now it is time for me to play with your husband, and you can play with mine.' "

"Well, I was putting on my hat and as I was leaving, I hope to die if one of them didn't say.

'We may as well go home now as this is the last rubber.' "

A little silver haired lady calls her new neighbor and says, "Will you come over here and help me. I have a jig saw puzzle, and it is driving me out of my mind. I can't figure out how to get started."

Her neighbor asks, "What is it supposed to be?"

"According to the picture on the box, it's a rooster."

She lets him in and shows him where the pieces are spread all over the dining table. He studies the pieces a moment, then looks at the box, then turns to her and says, "First of all, no matter how hard we try we are not going to assemble these pieces to anything resembling a rooster."

He takes her hand and says, "Secondly, I want you to relax. Let's have a cup of tea." and then, he said with a deep sigh, "Let's put all the Corn Flakes back in the box."

Nobody believes old people. Most think we are senile.

An elderly couple who were sweethearts and celebrating their 60th anniversary revisited their old school. They found the old desk that they shared, and he had carved, "I love Mary."

On the way home, a bag of money fell out of an armored car and rolled over to where they were walking. She picked it up and quickly took it home and counted it, and yelled out to her husband. "Wow, we found over $50,000."

He said, "We have to give it back". "No way," she replied, "finders' keepers," and hid it in the attic.

The next day two F.B.I. agents went door to door looking for the money.

They asked her, "Did you find any money that fell out of an armored car yesterday?"

"No," she answered. The husband said, "She's lying; she hid it in the attic." "Don't believe him; he's getting senile," she yelled out.

The senior agent looked at his assistant and whispered, "Who do we believe?"

He decided to sit the man down and question him. Tell us the story from the beginning. "Well, when Sally and I were walking home from school yesterday."

The agent looks at his partner and says, "We're out of here."

Exercise will give you, according to several studies, **vigor and a more active sex life**. It will make you look better, and psychologists will say that self-image may be one of the most important sex components of all. It aids the circulation and reduces stress, both important for sex. It may not convert you into a passionate lover, but it will give you more energy. Rather than make you tired, it will give you, according to several studies, vigor and a more active sex life,

By getting into shape you improve your self-confidence as well as your energy levels. You develop a positive outlook on life which contributes to your ability to perform regardless of age.

The next time your husband has a headache tell him to run around the block.

An 87 year old man asked the Doctor to lower his sex drive. He responded by saying:
"Don't be ridiculous. At your age, it's all in your head."
"I know that," he responded…"I want you to lower it."

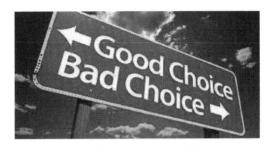

"LACK OF ACTIVITY DESTROYS THE GOOD CONDITION OF EVERY HUMAN BEING,

WHILE MOVEMENT AND METHODICAL PHYSICAL EXERCISE SAVE IT AND PRESERVE IT"

PLATO

Hopefully by now you are excited about getting started on an exercise program.

The question I have to ask the reader is, "How can you not be excited since studies show that exercise lowers the risk of stroke by 27%, incidence of diabetes by approximately 50%, incidence of high blood pressure by approximately 40%, can reduce mortality and the risk of recurrent breast cancer by approximately 50%, can lower the risk of colon cancer by over 60%, can reduce the risk of developing Alzheimer's disease by approximately 40%, can decrease depression as effectively as Prozac or behavioral therapy."

There are most likely other hidden benefits that will surface later as future studies are made regarding health for seniors.

If only watching television several hours a day would provide the same benefits -- Oh what a healthy nation we would be.

The good news is that we can rejoice in the awareness that there are so many choices for a form of exercise that will not only increase longevity, but will provide a high quality of life for the seasoned citizen.

Other good news is if your life style up to now has not been the healthiest one, you can have another go at it and, yes, with "enthusiasm".

But before you start any exercise program, you should get a complete physical, especially, if you have led an inactive life style. This will alert the doctor to any physical problems that might be exacerbated by your shifting gear and suddenly becoming active. Another good reason for you to discuss an exercise program with your physician is that if you are taking prescription drugs, they may affect your body's response to exercise. Hopefully, you have a doctor who believes in exercise. Unfortunately, there are still many that are not excited about physical workouts.

Even if you are in good physical condition, regardless of your activity, it's vital to avoid sudden bursts of energy. It is equally important not to stop abruptly after any physical exercise, but to take the time to cool down the system, to adjust to the change of pace.

You also should be aware of signs that could put you in the danger zone. If you are or someone else has one or more of these warning signs, don't wait. Call 911 immediately even if the signs go away.

I went to the doctor for my yearly physical.
 The nurse starts with certain basics.
"How much do you weigh?" she asks.
"140," I say.
The nurse puts me on the scale. It turns out my
 weight is 150.
The nurse asks my height?
"Five foot eight," I say.
She says that I only measure "5'7."
She then takes my blood pressure and tells me
 that it is high.
"Of course it's high!" I scream. "When I came in
 here I was tall and slender! Now I'm short
 and fat!"
She put me on Prozac.

I don't like to go for a physical exam, for as soon as the doctor observes that you are a senior with white or gray hair, they assume that you are not in good health.

After I had my complete physical at age 65, the doctor commented, "It is amazing at your age. It appears that you are in excellent health. It must be the genes."

"How old was your father when he died?"

I responded, "Who said that he was dead? He is 82 and plays tennis twice a week and golf on Sunday," I said.

The doctor commented, "That is incredible. Well how old was your grandfather when he died."

"Who said he is dead", I answered. "In fact his birthday is next week. He is going to be 102 years old and is getting married."

"That is amazing, but why would anyone want to get married at that age?"

"Did I say he wanted too?"

SIGNS OF A STROKE

1. **Sudden numbness** or weakness of the face, arm or leg, especially on one side of the body.
2. **Sudden confusion**, trouble speaking, or understanding speech.
3. **Sudden dimness** or loss of vision, particularly in one eye.
4. **Sudden trouble** while walking, dizziness, loss of balance or coordination.
5. **Sudden severe** headaches with no known causes.
6. **Other less common signs** may be: double vision, drowsiness, nausea, or vomiting.
7. Does one side of the **face drop**, or is it numb? Ask the person to smile.

1. **Discomfort in the chest**. Most heart attacks 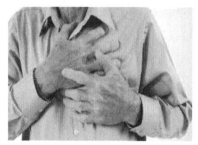 involve discomfort in the center of the chest that stays with you more than a few minutes or goes away and then returns. It can feel like uncomfortable pressure, squeezing, fullness or pain.

2. **Discomfort in other areas of the upper body**: symptoms can include pain or discomfort in one or both arms, the back, neck, jaw or stomach.

3. **Shortness of breath**: this feeling often comes along with chest discomfort but it may occur without it.

4. **Other signs**: one may break out in a cold sweat, nausea or lightheadedness.

If you or anyone has any of these signs immediately call 911.

Some heart attacks come on suddenly and are intense, but most start slowly with mild pain or discomfort. Fifty years ago the chances of dying in the hospital from a heart attack were one in four for men under 65. Now because of new types of treatment, 97 percent of these patients survive, especially those who recognize the signs and respond with haste.

Heart disease is the biggest killer of women. It kills more women than breast cancer and cervical cancer combined. What makes this scary is that 64% of the women who die from a heart attack or stroke do not have any previous symptoms that men often have to alert them.

Warning signs can occur while you are watching a TV program, eating a high fat meal, resting or being under stress. If you follow the rules, the chances will be less likely that you will experience serious problems while exercising.

Rejoice in the awareness that you have many choices so you can pick your way to good health with exercises that will be safe and healthful.

You can step outside your door and walk, run, go cycling or swim. You can stay inside and let a video guide you into an exercise program that will lead you to a long and pleasant journey.

You will be sending a message to your heart and other vital parts that, "I may have led a lazy life up to now, avoided physical activity and put out the minimum amount of energy daily, but that is in the past. Watch me now."

By joining the ranks of senior citizens who exercise regularly, you will not show the typical symptoms of aging such as slowed reflex times, reduced muscle type, and bone brittleness.

You will feel more fit than you did when you were many years younger, but physically inactive.

Unfortunately, the word exercise often flashes a picture of someone toiling, or doing a laborious task, struggling or plodding along. But exercise is movement: dancing, walking in the park, swimming, gardening, bowling, tennis, golf. The list is endless. But one thing they all have in common is that using the body as it should be used will make a dent in degenerative diseases that plague the senior and improve the quality of your life.

A prescription for older people is certainly different than that of a teenager, and there is still a multiplicity of choices.

A consumer report on health shows that over 60% of Americans complain that there are too many choices, and they don't have a single source they can trust to help them make a decision. No wonder -- they are bombarded almost daily with testimonials that are motivational but questionable. So which program or type of equipment do you pick? As you make this decision, you are not a young stud anymore and you want to strive to be fit, not the fittest.

You may be tempted to make up for years of being inactive and overdo it.

Just as not exercising enough can be dangerous, too much can damage your heart and shorten your life expectancy.

You probably know that old Chinese saying "A journey of a thousand miles must begin with a single step." So ready, step -- GO!

That single step which is a giant step forward for good health could very well be in the form of walking. This is a favorite form of exercise for older people. It is a low impact aerobic activity that will improve cardiovascular fitness and muscle tone, as well as other health benefits with the lowest risk of injury or sudden heart failure.

WALKING

Walking is **the most physical form of exercise for the** 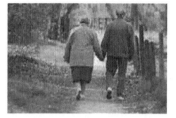 **majority of seniors**. And a sagacious choice it is.

You will not need to go to a specific place or purchase expensive equipment.

A vigorous walk will do more for the mind and body than many of the medicine and drugs touted daily over radio and television.

Walking is now coming into its own. A recent poll indicates that two out of three active American adults obtain their exercise by walking. Sixty-eight percent of exercising men now include walking in their workouts. Surprisingly, 25% of these exercisers added walking to their routine within the last few years.

Walking is wonderful because it is an exercise that doesn't feel like exercise. Slow walkers should not be discouraged. If you are not able to partake of a faster pace, every step is a step toward better health.

Most people know that it is good for them and that it burns calories, but many walkers do not realize that it strengthens the heart and can add years to one's life in terms of heart health.

The Journal of American Medicine reports that walking has been shown to reduce anxiety and tension and aid in weight loss. Regular walking may also help improve one's cholesterol profile, help control hypertension, and discourage osteoporosis. Physicians also generally agree that walking is the safest, most efficient exercise for the aged.

Researchers in Seattle wondered whether exercise was beneficial or detrimental to senior citizens. To find out, they evaluated 1,645 randomly selected members of an HMO. All the participants were over 65 years of age and all were free of diagnosed heart disease at the start of the study. The data collected included age, health, physical activity, blood pressure, smoking, alcohol use, body mass index (a measure of body fat), education, and income. The subjects were followed for four to five years to see if physical activity affected the rate of hospitalizations for heart disease for the overall mortality rate.

The results were very revealing. People who walked more than four hours in an average week were 31 percent less likely to require hospitalization for heart disease than those who walked less than one hour per week. Exercise was protective in people 65-74 years old, but was even more helpful for people older than 75.

The walkers also enjoyed a 27 percent lower mortality rate than their sedentary peers. The Journal of American Medicine reports that walking has been shown to reduce anxiety and tension and aid in weight loss. Regular walking may also help improve one's cholesterol profile, help control hypertension, and discourage osteoporosis.

Walking helps the circulation of blood throughout the body. As the muscles in the legs move they squeeze the nearby veins, forcing the blood back to the heart giving a feel of well-being.

Physicians also generally agree that walking is the safest most efficient exercise for the aged.

Further proof that should motivate you to put on your walking shoes was one of the largest studies of 70,000 nurses who were studied over a period of 15 plus years by The Harvard School of Public Health. It reported that nurses that walked the most -- 20 or more hours per week -- reversed up to 40% of their risk of strokes caused by a clot.

Walking most likely contributed to the health of former President Harry Truman who lived to be 88. He often complained that he had to slow his walking pace for the much younger reporters who interviewed him during his daily walks.

Rose Kennedy walked four to five miles every day until her ninetieth birthday.

Dr. Paul Dudley White used to park his car at least six blocks from his office so he would be assured of some form of exercise daily, regardless of his hectic schedule.

When I delivered mail during the cold winter days in Boston as a substitute carrier, I used to marvel at the elderly carriers who would trek through the streets and up and down the stairs all day. They looked so hardy and robust.

Unfortunately, the new generation of carriers have been provided vehicles to deliver the mail, which deprives them of the benefits of walking.

Thomas Parr of England, reputedly the longest-lived man in recorded medical history (1483-1635), was still actively threshing grain at the age of 130, and continued to take long walks until his death at 152. He lived under nine British kings. There is a monument in his memory in Westminster Abbey. Even before his time, walking was recognized as a healthful activity. Hippocrates prescribed walks to prevent mental disturbance and control expanding waistlines.

> *Reminds me of my grandmother. She started to walk five miles a day at age 70. Now she is age 90 and we don't know where the hell she is.*

> *I enjoy long walks, especially when they are taken by people who annoy me.*

Emphasizing the value of walking, the Jewish physician Maimonides, (1135-1204), who rose to become the doctor of Saladin, advised that even a person who eats good food and follows sound medical principles can't be healthy if he doesn't exercise.

Other More strenuous exercises as jogging and running

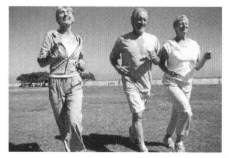

that were the favorite activity of my generation **may strengthen the heart to a greater level, but are not as practical for seniors.**

Yet many seniors share enthusiasm for running. You can always observe many gray-haired women and men participating in marathons.

Among the 181,000 runners in a recent New York, marathon, 4,719 were in their fifties, 1,217 were in their sixties, 19 were in their seventies, and one was over 80.

Fauja Singh, 100 year old, the world's oldest marathon runner, may have come in last with the time of 8 hours, 25 minutes, 17 seconds in a 2011 marathon in Scotiabank, Toronto. But, it is still quite an achievement for the oldster who did not start running until he was 89.

You can walk away from poor health. You should not be discouraged if you are not able to partake of a faster pace or more strenuous activities.

Regardless of the pace every step is increasing your chances of reaching that 100 plus mark.

I ran in several marathons and enjoyed running, but I realize now in my senior years (with aching knees), I would have been better off if I swam or biked more instead. However, I am confident that running contributed keeping my heart healthy.

In the water **may be just where the senior exerciser** 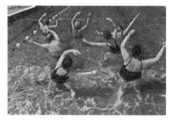 **wants to be.** The buoyancy of the water supports the body so you can move around without pain. It is recommended for anyone over 50 who wants to maintain aerobics fitness.

According to a February, 2012 study, reported by the American Journal of Cardiology, swimming reduces blood pressure and improves artery health in elderly adults. This was the first study to demonstrate swimming's vascular health benefits for older sedentary seniors. "Because swimming puts less stress on joints and the body's cooling mechanisms than many other exercises, it is an ideal form of activity for older adults," the study's authors noted.

Professor Paul Hutinger, a research specialist in physiology of exercise at Western Illinois University calls swimming the Fountain of Youth because unlike many forms of exercise it easily becomes a lifetime activity.[25] Herbert DeVries, professor of kinesiology, of the University of Southern California's Andrus Gerontology Center found dramatic confirmation of the anti-aging effects of swimming. Swimmers, aged 50 to 87, given hour-long workouts three times a week, showed profound changes after six weeks. Many of those in their

---

[25] Jane Brody, "Exercise is the Fountain of Youth," New York Times, 10 June 1986.

seventies regained the strength and vitality they had in their fifties.

A report by the President's Council on Physical Fitness and Sports compared the advantages of swimming to those of other sports ranging from bowling to bicycling. It rated swimming as best for building the body's stamina. Swimming equals jogging's ability to improve muscular endurance and is second only to calisthenics for increasing suppleness and flexibility. It is also superior to jogging and bicycling for developing overall body strength.

Studies show no difference in the cardiorespiratory efficiency of swimmers and joggers, and that either activity could improve the cardiorespiratory systems of middle-aged men and women. A study at the University of Texas Health Science Center in Dallas showed that swimming can significantly improve cardiovascular function.

Simeon Margolis, M.D., PhD, professor of Medicine and Biology at John Hopkins suggested in a 2010 report that aquatic exercises can be helpful in reducing low back pain.

Look at Roy Webster, who at age 75 found the 62-degree water "the coldest ever," but as the oldest of 159 participants still managed to finish the mile long swim across the Columbia River. Two other senior swimmers are Lloyd and Joan Osborne of Kailua, Hawaii. Lloyd, at 71, could swim 50 yards freestyle in under 30 seconds, while Joan, at 63, held several national records in her age group. Thomas Lane, a California Lawyer who participates in a Master's

Swimming Program (a program developed in the early 1960s to promote physical fitness through continued exercise), stated, "I've really felt terrific since I've been involved in Master's swimming, and when I get up in the morning and look in the mirror, I think, 'my goodness, that's young Tom Lane there!' "

Many seniors are attending aquatic exercise groups on a regular basis and rave about the programs. In addition to the health benefits, they enjoy meeting other people in their age group that are also interested in living a healthy life style.

A woman swam in a local 100 breast stroke contest and came in last. She later complained that the other women used their hands.

Why do squirrels swim on their back? They want to keep their nuts dry.

If swimming doesn't appeal to you and you want to avoid the pitfalls of running, yet be healthy and slim, how about bicycling?

Bicycling **gets your heart and lungs into the cardio respiratory zone** while enjoying the fresh air. It improves your overall muscle function, helps to keep the weight down, and combats stress. It provides these benefits with a small risk of over exertion or strain. Of course, you should wear a helmet.

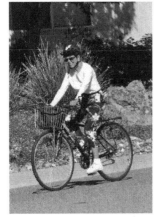

Clifford Graves, M.D., a California physician and founder of one of the nation's first cycling clubs, recommends cycling as a sport you can have fun with while you strengthen your heart.

Dr. Jack Wilmore, former physiologist at the University of California at Davis, recommends cycling for people who want to get in shape but finds jogging hurts their feet, leaves them gasping, or just bores them to tears. He conducted a study that found that cycling presented fewer problems than jogging or tennis. "It's a much more fluid movement," he said. "You don't have the continual pounding, so there's far less problems with aches and pains, and, of course, it can be used as a mode of transportation." He summed it up so well when he said, "If you have hurt on your feet, try your seat."

More and more seniors are bypassing their car and mounting their bicycles to do a variety of errands, an ideal way to have a fitness workout. It is an inexpensive means of transportation.

You are in charge so you can adjust the pace to your individual level of fitness.

Thirty minutes a day, for five days a week, should provide an adequate amount of exercise to put you in the healthy zone.

Paul Dudley White, M.D., a strong advocate of walking and cycling, regularly used to pedal many miles a day over the roads of Martha's Vineyard, continuing well into his senior years. "People hold up their hands in horror that I do it," he remarked, "But I hold up mine in horror that they don't."

Alexander, a 70 year old former pro wrestler, pedaled his way across the country from Los Angeles to Weymouth, Massachusetts, to attend his granddaughter's high school graduation.

Recently, my wife and I joined several other seniors and biked the highways of old Route 66 from Arizona to the California border. We averaged 35 miles a day. Yes, there were many hills, but we were all able to do it as we were active oldsters.

Cyclists, who compete on a professional level, are considered among the fittest athletes.

Spinning, a new form of exercise on a stationary bicycle, is becoming very popular. It gives an intense cardiac workout. The hardest part of learning to ride a bicycle is the pavement.

Tennis

Tennis **has long been a popular sport**. The televising of tennis matches between well-known players has added to its popularity.

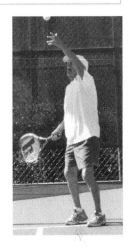

If you visit a country club, you will observe many gray-haired players in their 60's to their 80's participating in doubles matches. They certainly look especially fit compared to other seniors in their age group that are physically inactive.

Rarely do they have to pause to rest except to question line calls. They may have trouble keeping score, but are able to keep up with many players that are as much as thirty years younger.

At age 86, the author still plays tennis 2-3 times a week.

Ira Percy celebrated his 90th birthday and 68th year of playing tennis in a smashing way. He demonstrated how vigorous activity had kept him spry and strong enough to play a junior-senior tournament named in his honor.

Peg Smith, another senior citizen, "just didn't want to be a tea and toast lady playing bridge and putting on weight." The prospect of a life of idleness after retirement held no fascination for her. At the age of 78, she entered an International Senior Olympics Tennis

Tournament which she won that year, and has won every year. At 83 she was the oldest participant in these Olympics.

Peg is known to practice five times a week. She plays two or three sets a day with players aged 25 to 45. Her shelves display the many trophies she has won. Peg's biggest problem is finding partners in her age group. But, since she has beaten competitors as young as 60, she finds plenty of people with whom to play. She urges women to take up tennis at any age, with a physician's approval.

A middle management executive has to take on some sport, by his doctor's orders, so he decides to play tennis. After a couple of weeks his secretary asks him how he's doing. "It's going fine," the manager says. "When I'm on the court and I see the ball speeding towards me, my brain immediately says, 'To the corner! Back hand! To the net! Smash! Go back!'." "Really? What happens then?" the secretary asks. "Then my body says, 'Who? Me? You must be kidding!'"

Where is the first tennis match mentioned in the bible? Answer: When Joseph served in the Pharaoh's court.

Pickleball

Pickleball is **a sport that is gaining popularity among seniors**, especially former tennis players. The smaller size of the court and the speed of the pickle ball (which moves at one third average speed of the tennis ball) makes it a more ideal sport for the senior.

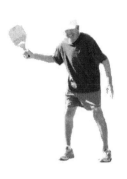

As yet, I haven't mentioned one activity that is **very popular with seniors**, golf. I often think of how Paul

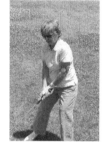

Harvey described this activity. "It's a crazy game; you yell out four, get a six, and put down a five."

Dr. Paul Dudley White refers to golf as, "Nothing more than spoiling a good walk." He most likely was referring to the many golfers who rely on the golf cart to transport them around the course; another example of a modern convenience that deprives us of physical activity.

Another disadvantage of golf is that the exercise it provides is not continuous. You pause repeatedly to look for the ball, or wait for the foursome in front of you to move on.

Yet, when I observe how physically and mentally fit, Bob Hope and many other older golfers were, it must provide substantial healthy benefits, especially for those who walk the course.

A big plus is that it is also a social game. Many seniors have met people on the golf course that share the passion for the game and become longtime friends. Most important is that golfers relax with their game, and not expect to be another Tiger Woods.

Another big plus for this game is that you can continue playing this game for many senior years. Helen Goldberg of Sacramento played well into her 90's. She hit a hole in one at age 82, and her best score for 9 holes at age 95 was 30.

An interesting thing about golf is that no matter how badly you play, it is always possible to get worse.

Long ago when men cursed and beat the ground with sticks it was called witchcraft. Today it's called golf.

I play in the 80's. If it's any hotter than that, I won't play.

A man and his wife were celebrating their 50th wedding anniversary on a trip. While having breakfast, the wife saw her husband staring out the window and said in a harsh voice, "John, I hope you are not thinking that if you were home now you would be playing golf. You spoil so many of our vacations thinking of how much you miss your golf games." He responded, "Now stop nagging I am not thinking of golf. Will you please pass the bread and putter?"

The other day I came home from work and was greeted by my wife wearing a very sexy outfit holding a rope in her hand. She said, "Tie me up and do whatever you want." I tied her up and went to play golf.

Several men are in the locker room of a golf club. A cell phone on a bench rings and a man engages the hands free speaker function and begins to talk. Everyone else in the room stops to listen.

Man: "Hello"

Woman: "Honey, it's me. Are you at the club?"

Man: "Yes"

Woman: "I am at the mall now and found this beautiful leather coat. It's only $1,000. Is it OK if I buy it?"

Man: "Sure, if you like it."

Woman: "I also stopped by the Mercedes dealership and saw the new 2012 models. I saw one with my favorite color."

Man: "How much?"

Woman: "$65,000"

Man: "OK, but for that price I want it with all the options."

Woman: "Great! Oh, one more thing while I have you on the phone. The house we wanted last year is back on the market. They are asking $900,000."

Man: "Well, OK, but go ahead and make them an offer for $850,000"

Woman: "OK. I'll see you later. I love you!"

Man: "Bye, I love you too." *The man hangs up.*

The other men in the locker room are looking at him in astonishment.

Then he asks: "Anyone know who this phone belongs to?"

A man and a woman were aboard a cruise ship and became quite close, going to cocktail parties and dances together. One evening he said, "I feel it's only fair to warn you that I am a real golf nut. I live, eat, sleep, and breathe the game". "Well since you're being honest, so will I. I'm a hooker." He responded "That's not a problem; it's possibly because you're not holding your wrists straight when you're hitting the ball."

After a two year study, the National Science Foundation announced the following results on America's recreational preferences.

The sport of choice for unemployed or incarcerated people is basketball.

The sport of choice for maintenance level employees is football.

The sport of choice for blue collar workers is bowling.

The sport of choice for supervisors is baseball.

The sport of choice for middle management is tennis.

The sport of choice for corporate officers is golf.

Conclusion: The higher you rise in the corporate structure, the smaller your balls become.

If I haven't whetted your appetite for exercise by now, you still have many choices. They may not be as valuable as the ones we have discussed, but as Lawrence Morehouse, PhD, of the U.C.L.A. Human Laboratory stated, "Even an exercise such as toe wiggling is better than nothing."

I can just see a big smile on the reader's face thinking, now I've found the exercise I've been looking for. But remember, we're striving for maximum benefit, not for something that is better than nothing. So just keep moving and consider other healthy choices.

Let it snow! Let it snow! Let it snow!

When the snow falls, the opportunity for fun exercise is 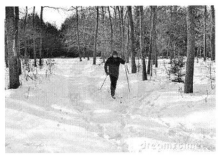 endless. Snow shoeing is **fast becoming a popular sport** for the graying. You can enjoy the beauty of the countryside as painted over by the snowflakes as you plod along getting a good cardiac workout. It is a less intense activity and very popular among seniors whose hair matches the color of the snow.

Cross country skiing is also popular among seniors who can handle and crave vigorous activity that moves both the arms and legs and burns off 700 calories an hour.

If you are going cross country skiing. Pick a small country.

Many of the elderly can also be seen skiing down the slopes. It is gratifying to see that many once considered over the hill are now skiing down the hill. They are also no stranger to the skating rinks where you can often see them gliding along with their grandchildren.

Stair Climbing

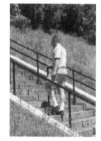

Whenever I am on a vacation staying at a hotel that does not have an exercise room and the weather is miserable, I climb the stairs located at the fire exits for my workouts.

Stair climbing is **an aerobic exercise**. In a study by Stanford University, Professor of Epidemiology, Ralph S. Paffenbarger, M.D., 16,936 Harvard alumni, who attended college between 1915 and 1950, were asked what condition their heart was in, how many flights of steps they climbed, how many blocks they walked, and what type of sports they participated in. The study found that men who climbed fewer than five flights a day had a 25 percent greater chance of a heart attack than those who climbed more than five a day.[26]

A consistent stair climbing program develops the strength and firmness of leg and buttock muscles. As you walk up and down stairs the quadriceps (muscles on the front thighs) are continuously contracted.

---

[26] R.S M Paffenbenbarger Jr. "Men Who Climbed Fewer": Lancet 17 F1953.

Stretching

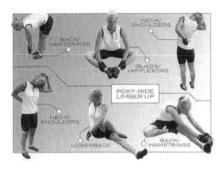

Another **inexpensive exercise** is stretching. This will help to prevent stiffness that can lead to falls. They are performed slowly and gently, more similar to meditating than exercising. But they are very helpful in limbering the body as well as the mind. There are many classes available throughout the schools, country clubs, or other locations that add yoga, which will also teach you a breathing technique.

Quieting the mind and body can only generate healthy results for the seniors.

Strength Training

According to Michael Flynn, professor in the department 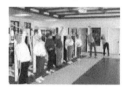 of Health, Kinesiology and Leisure studies and director of the Max E. Waste and Human Performance Laboratory at Purdue, "Our research, and that of others, has shown that strength training **can have a remarkable impact** on the lives of seniors."

For every decade after about age 50, you lose about 6 percent of your muscle mass which comes with a 15 percent loss of your strength. Even people over 100 years old can partially reverse some of the loss that occurs with aging.

Personnel at a health club or gym can get you started. Studies have shown that seniors, including 90 year olds, are less likely to fall or injure themselves after they begin a health training program.

It's never too late to rebuild lost muscles. A study of nursing home residents, ages 72 to 98, found that 10 weeks of progressive strength training for thigh and lower leg muscles increased muscle strength an average of 113 percent.

Unfortunately, strength training as an exercise activity declines steadily through adulthood, and by the age 75 few people are involved in resistance exercises.

Be sure to have a qualified person help you get started or read a book that will guide you so the workout will be healthful not harmful.

A senior man was working out in the weight room and he noticed a very attractive younger woman. He asked the trainer "Is there a machine I could use to impress her?" After looking at him up and down, he suggested, "Try the ATM in the lobby."

Dancing

According to a 21 year study of seniors 75 and older by

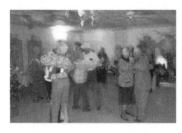 the Albert Einstein College of Medicine, dancing improves mental capabilities -- yes, makes us smarter. **May be not healthier, depending on the type of dance**, but typical of any kind of physical activity, it improves the quality of life.

The fresh air, the bending, the squatting, and the 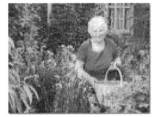 variety of movements will help to keep seniors, as with all forms of exercise, to thrive until age 125.

If the weather is bad -- no excuses, you have many options. You can, as many seniors do, join a club that most likely will have a variety of machines like tread mills, rowing, stationary bikes, strength training, stretching, stair climbing, and others to help you stay in good health and be a happy senior.

It will not only be a sound investment for good health, but save you a considerable amount of money in medical bills. However, keep in mind it is very unwise and even dangerous to your health, if you become a weekend warrior. That is, you are inactive every day except Saturday and Sunday and then go out for a fast pace activity.

The 12-year study of thousands of male physicians showed that men who exercised at least five times a week had a much lower risk of sudden death -- about sevenfold less -- than those who only exercised once a week, according to Christine M. Albert , M.D., a cardiologist and a researcher at Brigham and Women's Hospital.

So once again, let me remind the reader there is no magic panacea for a long happy and healthy life, but exercise provides almost everything that you would look for at the Fountain of Youth. So, get up and go for it.

I felt that my body was totally out of shape so my doctor suggested that I joined a fitness club. I took an aerobics class for seniors. I bent, twisted, gyrated, jumped up and down, and perspired for an hour. By the time I got my leotards on the class was over.

CHAPTER 3 **DIET**

EAT THESE FOODS TO YOUR HEARTS CONTENT

> **WELL NOURISHED CELLS ARE RELATIVELY RESISTANT TO OUTSIDE ATTACKS. THE STRONGEST HOPES FOR PREVENTION OF CANCER LIES IN THE FIELD OF SPECIALIZED NUTRITION.**

If exercise and humor were the whole answer, all the seniors would have to do to ensure a long and healthy 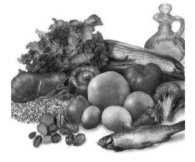 life would be to walk, swim, or cycle and exercise enough to increase the oxygen intake to the heart and lung and have several belly laughs a day. Exercise and humor, although vital for the elderly, will not do it alone.

There are many heartbreaking examples of persons who are very fit, muscular, even world-class athletes and yet died of a heart attack. e.g. French athlete, Jacques Busseau, who died while running in the New York Marathon. Jim Fixx, who wrote The Complete Book of Running, had a fatal heart attack while jogging. And Pete Maravich, the former basketball star, died while playing basketball with some friends.

These unfortunate incidents provide grim testimony that we cannot solve all our health problems through physical activity alone. The athletes most likely had numerous blood clots in their coronary arteries and were running around with a time bomb ticking away.

Mr. Fixx was a former smoker and had a family history of coronary artery disease. He also was known to eat a poor diet that was loaded with saturated fat. His running may possibly have prolonged his life, but could not overcome the effects of a poor diet and genes.

Seniors have special needs and, according to the National Elder Care Institute, have diets that are so bad that they are at risk for serious health problems. Part of the problem could be that they are bombarded daily by self-appointed health mavens who fire upon them misinformation as to what we should eat and drink. "You are never too old to enjoy eating," says Jeanne P. Goldberg PhD, R.D. Associate Professor of Nutrition and Director of the Center on Nutrition Communication at Tufts University in Medford, Massachusetts at an AMA media briefing on nutrition.

According to Jeffrey Blumberg (PhD of Nutrition and Senior Scientist at USDA, Human Research Center on Aging at Tufts University) an inadequate diet makes older adults with less effective immune systems more at risk for short term health problems. These older adults also tend to have more chronic illnesses such as hypertension, heart disease, and osteoporosis.

Research now shows that many of the signs of growing older that we used to attribute to age are actually due to diet.

Scientific evidence increasingly supports that good nutrition is essential to health, self-sufficiency, and quality of life of older adults.

Americans, that are older than 65 and have at least two serious chronic health problems, can most likely link them to poor nutrition. Among these health problems are heart disease, arthritis, diabetes, high blood pressure, and cancer.

If a senior eats unhealthy foods that are high in saturated fat, cholesterol and sugar, drinks a lot of alcohol, is unable to handle stress, and has not chosen their ancestors wisely, it will take more than exercise to protect them.

We are all familiar with the phrase, "you are what you eat." A more appropriate one would be, "you are what you do not eat." Americans have a greater variety of foods to choose from than any other nation. It is not difficult to choose wisely and to stoke the body with healthy foods. Too many seniors reach for the bad guys that are advertised daily to tempt us to make wrong selections that contribute to the demise of millions of Americans each year.

Food can be healing or destructive, and for the older person, making the right selection is even more important. Older people should especially be particular about what they eat if they want to enjoy a long and healthy life.

According to a position statement of the American Dietetic Association, "Scientific evidence increasingly supports that good nutrition is essential to the health, self-sufficiency, and quality of life for older adults."

Many problems that trouble the elderly are the result of eating the wrong foods. This chapter will provide you with guidelines to help you select foods wisely, and to avoid the high cholesterol laden products and the exotic desserts that are very tempting, but dangerous to your health.

This chapter will unlock for you the correct information so you will know what to include in your shopping cart. As seniors age their health needs change. Their metabolism slows down. This happens naturally, but becomes more pronounced if we don't eat smart or exercise. As your metabolism slows down, the body does not burn as many calories. You have to eat more of the good foods and less of the bad, and exercise more to avoid gaining weight.

Your digestive system changes; the body produces less of the fluids that it needs to process foods. As a result it is more difficult for your body to absorb important nutrients like folic acid and vitamins B6 and B12. If you, like many seniors, take one or more medications for health conditions, side effects such as loss of appetite or an upset stomach may occur.

This information may upset the reader, but the good news is we can manage the majority of problems that face the aged.

You can control how you age if you exercise, eat smart, hold the reins on your weight, and handle stress. It takes teamwork.

Now if you have wisely taken that first giant step to become a healthy senior by exercising, you are ready for step number two that should increase your chances for a sound mind in a sound body. This of course assumes that you have had at least one good belly laugh each day.

Skeptics will ask, "Is worth the effort." They will ask, "Am I going to have to give up all of my favorite foods?" Probably not. What you will accomplish with good nutrition, is to reduce the risk of problems that plague the elderly:

- Anemia
- Infections
- Hip fractures
- High blood pressure
- Osteoporosis
- Type 2 diabetes
- High cholesterol levels
- Heart disease
- Stroke
- Many forms of cancer.

Yes, without question, it is worth it. You have many healthy and happy golden years ahead of you. The U.S. Administration of Aging shows that 87 percent of older Americans have a chronic disease that can be improved through good nutrition.

Emerging scientific evidence about the burgeoning older adult population and dramatic changes in health care delivery, all accentuate the importance of food and nutrition or health, disease prevention and management.

George Christakis, M.D., former head of the nutrition program at the Sinai School of Medicine in New York claims that two thirds of our nation's public health and chronic disease problems are related to our diet.

The cost due to obesity is about 168 billion dollars, according to a study by the National Bureau of Economic Research which is a nonprofit and nonpartisan organization.

Needless to say, the cost to our nation is staggering and posing enormous financial problems. We should educate the citizens to eat wisely. It should be considered a patriotic act to do so. It would certainly help to solve the enormous fiscal problems facing our nation.

The relationship between diet and poor health of the senior has been well established, but sadly many are not listening. Americans spend more to stay healthy than any other country, yet heart disease and cancer (related to eating the wrong foods) are still the two main killers of seniors.

It is not that complicated to eat wisely if you follow, as I do, the recommendations of the Mediterranean diet. One that is heavy on fruits, vegetables, fish, and lots of nuts, olive oil, and beans.

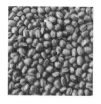 Beans are special food that are an excellent source of fiber. (Wipe that smile off your face.) Consumption of one dish provides about one-third of the fiber you should be eating each day. In addition to fiber, they're rich in protein, magnesium, potassium, iron, copper, and folate. Another plus is they're low in

saturated fat and sodium. However, it is advisable to rinse them to cut down on the sodium.

Although fiber is safe to eat, if you consume excessive amounts of fiber in a short time it can result in intestinal gas, bloating and cramps caused by fermentation of fiber and indigestible sugars in the colon. Most likely, it is not serious (maybe embarrassing) and subsides as soon as the bacteria in your system adjust to the increase of fiber. Add foods rich in fiber gradually to your system and it will reduce the chances of gas or diarrhea.

Foods that are mentioned in this chapter are known to be the best choice for healthy aging and disease prevention according to a large body of research.

A recent study in Spain that followed 7,447 people almost five years and was reported in the February 25, 2013 issue of the New England Journal of Medicine is considered historic. Steven Nissen, chairman of the Department of Cardiovascular Medicine at the Cleveland Clinic, was not involved with the study but notes that the preventive effect of the Mediterranean diet is similar to the effect of taking satins, the cholesterol lowering drugs. Dr. Nissen was so impressed with the study results that he commented, "What we can say to patients is this very palatable Mediterranean diet looks to be the healthiest. I'm going to change my own diet; add some more olive oil and nuts."

The countries that follow the diet as France, Italy, Spain, and Israel can all boast of being a country with a longer life span. Not so for the U.S.

Japan and China also have a healthy diet which features many of the same foods as colorful fruits and vegetables, olive oil, fish, and whole grains with few processed, packaged or refined foods.

Garlic is a food that also could contribute to the health of the Italians and Greeks who consume it with a passion.[27] Many medical researchers say garlic ward off more than vampires. Many studies show it is an effective cancer fighter. Garlic's healing powers are legendary. Over the centuries, it's been hailed by the ancient Egyptians, Israelites and Chinese and praised by Mohammed, Charlemagne, and Hippocrates. Can they all be wrong?

Though clinical trials are lacking, population studies in China and Italy have found that people who regularly eat a lot of garlic have less risk of developing stomach cancer than those who eat little amounts. An Iowa study looked at the diets of over 40,000 women and found those who consumed the most garlic had the lowest risk of colon cancer. That should be enough to make you go to your supermarket and stock up on garlic as well as breath fresheners, but it is not a cure all -- and as in other studies it is under question.

Another food that is prevalent in the Asian diet, and could well be a magic bean, is Soy. It is low in saturated fat, is a complete protein, and contains minerals and fiber. In Asia where tofu and other soy foods are a regular part of the diet, prostate cancer rates

---

[27]A.K. Bordia, M.K. Joasil, et al., Effect of Essential Oil Of Garlic on Serum Fibrinolytic Activity in Patients with Coronary Artery Disease.," Atherosclerosis 128{1977}155-159.

are low. However, as with garlic, their link to cancer may be tenuous. Nevertheless, since I have not found a study where it poses a danger, I opt to do as the Italians, Greeks, and Asians do and add both to my diet.

And let us not forget another Asian favorite food that studies show is also associated with a decreased risk of prostate cancer -- rice.

Good rice advice is to eat a lot of it. It is virtually fat-free, easy to cook from scratch and inexpensive. Whole grains, like brown rice, include the bran and germ of the natural grain that are lost in processing to make white rice, which contains only the inner endosperm. A lot of good stuff gets lost in the bargain. Brown rice is certainly recommended over white rice to be put in your shopping cart as it has ten times as much phosphorus and potassium as white rice.

Patrick Quillen, PhD, vice president of the Cancer Treatment Center in N.Y. says the cure must come from changing the environment within the body. The healthy foods may very well do that and slow the process of aging as well as preventing the major causes of deaths in our senior population.

A good start is to follow the words of your grandmother. Remember her shouting **"EAT YOUR VEGETABLES"**. Add fruit to that command and you have taken a giant step forward to good health. Grandma was well ahead of the times. Now these foods are recognized by nutritionists as one of the best ways to reduce your risk of cancer, diabetes and heart disease. "If everyone ate at least five servings of fruits and vegetables a day, that alone would reduce cancer incidence by as much as 20 percent", says Melanie Polk, director of Nutrition at the American Institute for Cancer Research.

These foods are also valuable as they are rich in potassium which helps to keep blood pressure in check, a problem that affects more seniors as they age.

Be sure to include in that lifesaving list of colorful fruits and vegetables, apricots, prunes, bananas, cantaloupe, watermelon, apples, oranges, grapes, strawberries, and all kinds of berries. Blue berries are known as a super fruit as they are very high in anti-oxidants.

One juice that appears to have a medicinal benefit for combating urinary tract infection is cranberry juice, which is also very high in anti-oxidants.

Another juice to select is grape juice. Red grapes, as red tomatoes, have cancer fighting ingredients.

Frozen fruit juices are another way to obtain vitamins but it does not measure up to whole fruit. An orange for example supplies three times more fiber than six ounces of orange juice. A medium sized apple contains five times more fiber than six ounces of apple juice.

Fruit juice can pose a problem as it is high in calories. In fact, about the same as a serving of Pepsi or Coke.

Thanks to food freezing and canning techniques, many vitamin rich foods are now available all year round. Avoid the products that add heavy syrup which give you high amounts of calories without more vitamins, minerals, and fiber.

Vegetables to place in your shopping cart are potatoes, beans, brown rice, seeds, Brussels sprouts, corn, spinach, kale, broccoli, tomatoes, carrots, garlic, and onions. This book will refer to these vegetables, and others, for they are all-important for the senior to attain maximum health.

They may not prevent cancer, according to a recent study, but there are a few hints that some vegetables might protect against some cancers. For example, a recent study found a 13 percent lower risk of estrogen-negative breast cancers (tumors that do not respond to estrogen) among women who eat more red, yellow, orange, and dark green fruits and vegetables.[28] Estrogen is the main sex hormone in women and is essential for menstruation and reproduction.

A study by Doug Larson, known for his quotes, stated "Life expectancy would grow by leaps and bounds if green vegetables smelled like bacon."

Save room for nuts, whole wheat, whole grains, fish, all of which are some of the foods seniors should eat.

The foods will not only satisfy your appetite but stoke up your body with premium fuel. Plus, they are low in calories.

These heart-healthy foods claim to fame is that they are listed in the Mediterranean diet. A diet and it is

---

[28] Am. J. Clin.Nutr.95:713,2012

worth repeating, that reduces the risk of cardiovascular disease and other serious problems that torment the senior.

I was very pleased to see that my favorite fruits were rated among them. Cantaloupe is the highest rated of all the fresh fruits, with watermelon a close second.[29] That may soon change and push back watermelon into first place, as a new study suggests this fruit has Viagra like effects to the body's blood vessels and may even increase libido. Both these fruits are high in vitamin C, and watermelon also contains more iron than any other fruit. It also has lycopene, which is receiving a great deal of recognition for its role in fighting against cancer.

Nuts are very important to maintain a healthy diet. I was also pleased that the pistachio nut (which is another favorite of mine) contains a substance that blocks your body from absorbing cholesterol. The pistachio nut may help prevent your arteries from clogging, keeping your blood vessels and heart healthy and strong.

Walnuts, that I also enjoy, are also linked to healthier blood vessels.

Other seeds and nuts such as, sunflower seeds, pumpkin seeds, and flax seeds are highly recommended.

Apples too have a lot to brag about. Remember the saying, "An apple a day will keep the doctor away." They are inexpensive, high in vitamins, low in calories,

---

[29] M. Jacobson and W.W. Wilson   Food Scorecard   Washington D.C. Center for Science in the Public Interest 1974

and are available throughout the year. They also have pectin a soluble fiber that may help to lower cholesterol.[30] The American Cancer Society and the National Academy of Sciences tell us that an apple a day can also do more than keep the doctor away. It can help keep cancer away.

Bananas should get equal billing. Eating them, as part of the daily diet can cut the risk of death by strokes as much as 40%, according to the American Cancer Society and the National Academy of Sciences.

Several studies have reported that foods from this group have caused a fall in blood cholesterol levels,[31] possibly because they decrease the intake of saturated fatty acids or because they contain generous amounts of pectin and fiber. Some have found that pectin -- a carbohydrate found in the skins of many citrus and other fruits as well as in vegetables can lower cholesterol levels considerably.[32] A preliminary study concluded that strawberries have the potential to prevent esophageal cancer. About 16,000 cases are diagnosed each year according to the American Cancer Society.[33] With all the

---

[30] G,H, Palmer and D.G. Dixon, "Effect of Pectin Dose on Serum Cholesterol Levels" American Journal of Clinical Nutrition 18 {1966}437;and A. Keyes, J. Anderson, and F. Grande, "Diet -Type{ Fats Constant}and Blood Lipids in man," Journal of   Nutrition   70{1960}25

[31] M.G. Hardings, A.C. Chambers, H Crooks, et al., Nutrition Studies of Vegetarians at Dietary Levels of Fiber, "American Journal of Clinical Nutrition 6(1958): 523.

[32] A.G. Shaper and K,W, Jones "Serum Cholesterol Diet, and Coronary   Heart   Disease   in   Africans   and   Asians   in   Uganda," Lancet{1959}:534

[33] Jennifer Corbett Dooren "Strawberries Tight   Cancer, Study Shows " Wall Street   Journal April 7 2011

good press about fruits and vegetables it is important to wash and rinse them thoroughly to remove the pesticide residues.

You are advised to wash and scrub fresh produce, under cold running water. Although running water won't remove all pesticide residues, it does help wash away many of the chemicals, dirt and bacteria from the surface of fruits and vegetables. This is important because bacteria on produce have caused outbreaks of food-borne illness.

We use this disinfectant solution for fruits and vegetables

1)   1 cup water

2)   1 cup white wine vinegar

3)   1 tablespoon baking soda

4)   1/2 teaspoon lemon juice

Prepare by mixing the ingredients thoroughly in a glass and then putting the end results in a spray bottle. Shake before applying.

Spray the solution on fruits and vegetables. Rinse with water.

Some may say is it not worth the risk? I'll just get my vitamins in a pill. Pills will not provide the benefits that you will get from the fresh food group.

A study from a panel of experts from Canada and the U.S. were called upon to review more than 50 studies on pesticides. They concluded that the benefits of eating lots of fruits and vegetables far outweigh any potential risks from low-level pesticide residue found in produce. Also, the panel estimated that all sources of synthetic chemicals including pesticides are responsible for only 2% of cancer deaths. Tobacco on the other hand accounts for about 30%.

The panel called for constant reevaluation and close monitoring. Though eating fruits and vegetables are important, it believes it's still desirable to avoid pesticides whenever you can.

The elderly can also be at greater risk from pesticide exposure because their immune system and organ functions decline with age. Many seniors are buying organic foods which do not use synthetic chemicals or pesticides but it is still questionable if this is a well-judged move.

Many gerontologists believe that the symptom of aging is the accumulated result of unprepared oxidative damage which a healthy diet can help to counteract.

Researchers at the Jean Mayer Human Research Center Imaging at Tufts did a study of 36 men and women (20 to 40) and (60 to 80).[34] They were fed a diet that included 10 servings of fruit and vegetables a day. Then, they measured the "antioxidant capacity".

Oxidants, that are potentially harmful, are naturally occurring in the body[35]. Antioxidants can help protect against their toxic effects which are linked to many chronic diseases such as heart diseases, cancer,

---

[34] Amer. J. Glin. Nutr .68:1081, 1998 & Circulation 98:2390, 1998.

[35] J. Nat. Cancer Inst.91:3171999

diabetes and Alzheimer's. They have been shown to slow the aging process. They also protect against free radicals that are molecules responsible for aging tissue damage and possibly some diseases. After two weeks, the anti-oxidant capacity of the participant's blood rose in both groups, though more consistently in the older people. Among the foods with the highest antioxidant capacity were oranges, cauliflower and peas. In a separate study from the John Hopkins Medical Institutions in Baltimore, researchers found a high antioxidant capacity in 83 people who ate eight to ten servings of fruit and vegetables a day than in 40 others who ate fewer servings.

John D. Potter, M.D., of the Fred Hutchinson Cancer Research Center in Seattle, headed up an international panel of experts examining diet and cancer prevention. In a review of 206 studies the panel consistently found that vegetables help to reduce cancer risk. The powerhouse foods in these studies were carrots, green vegetables, tomatoes, broccoli and cabbage.

Asians wisely use a lot of broccoli or cabbage. In a study of nearly 48,000 men, those who reported consuming broccoli or cabbage at least once a week had a lower risk of bladder cancer over the next ten years, than those who ate less than once a week[36]. They also consume a lot of onions and garlic, two popular foods in the Mediterranean diet. The researchers found no link

---

[36] J. Nat. Cancer inst.91:605, 1995.

with coleslaw or sauerkraut, perhaps because people report their intake of those dishes less accurately.

Brussels sprouts, mustard, kale, and collard greens have an extraordinary power to fight cancer. This family of vegetables contain powerful chemicals called indoles that block harmful carcinogens (substances that cause or tend to cause cancer) before they do their dirty work. Brussels sprouts can also help us enhance the natural ability of our bodies to resist prostate cancer causing agents. This will not only help the prostate but all the vital body parts.

These foods and others such as eggs, spinach, kale, romaine lettuce, broccoli, corn, kiwi fruit, are rich in lutein and zeaxanthin. All are reported to protect against age related cataracts and macular degeneration, the leading causes of blindness.

Spaghetti sauce and pizza were big news in 1995. That's when Edward Giovannucci, M.D., and his team found that men who consumed tomato sauce two to four times a week had a 34 percent lower risk of prostate cancer than men who ate no tomato sauce[37].

In previous studies researchers Ronald L. Prior, PhD, and Guohua Li studied 40 fruits and vegetables to determine their antioxidant content. Blue berries came out on top.

However, there are numerous studies that sound the alarm against loading up with supplements to

---

[37] Giovannucci.E.at al, "A prospective cost study of vasectomy and prostate cancer in U.S. mfn. Journal of the American Medical Association. {Feb.}1993:873-8

provide more antioxidants. This could be dangerous to your health.

Beware of those who try and motivate you to stock up on a magic pill or potion that will provide all of your health needs. You would be wiser to spend the money on fruits and vegetables. They will provide vitamins and minerals that protect the body by neutralizing free radicals.[3]

Until there is more conclusive research, the best source of antioxidants is a diet rich in fruits, vegetables and whole grains. As expressed in this proverb, "He who takes medicine and neglects his diet wastes the skill of his doctors."

Dean Ornish, M.D., who has pioneered reversal of heart disease without drugs or surgery and proved widespread economic benefit for patients and insurance providers, espouses whole foods, plant-based diet.

According to Dr. Ornish, "We now know what is true, a whole foods, plant based diet can prevent and treat heart disease, saving hundreds and thousands of Americans each year."

When you purchase your fruits and vegetables go for the color. The tiny chemicals that give them most of their color may be the ingredient that provides the most effective weapons to fight cancer.

If you have a choice between white potatoes and sweet potatoes take the sweet potatoes. Their orange color indicates the presence of photo chemicals that disrupt the chemical wedding between two common molecules in cells, a dangerous union that could impact your health. Small purple potatoes are also a wise choice.

You might want to select red grapes over white; the reds have more cancer fighting ingredients. Also, the redder the tomato: the better they are for you.[38] Speaking of tomatoes they do deserve special recognition. A Harvard study of the eating habits of 47,000 men over a period of six years found that those who had at least ten servings of tomato-based foods a week were up to 45 percent less likely to develop prostate cancer.

Tomatoes are also the best source of a carotenoid called lycopene, which may also block the initiation of the cancerous process. "Lycopene scavenges and suppresses damage to oxidation in the tissues," explains Northwestern University's Peter Gann, M.D. "As an antioxidant, it's more potent than beta-carotene, and it's concentrated in the prostate."

In 1999, Gann, and their colleagues found a lower risk of prostate cancer in men who had higher blood lycopene levels 13 years earlier.

"Not every study shows a benefit, but the ones that were best able to detect an association found it," says Edward Giovannucci, M.D.,

It is not a difficult chore to eat healthy. The right food choices are not that complicated. In fact they are rather simple. Eat less of red meat, sweets, refined grains, salt, and sugar. Replace those choices with

---

[38] Eat to Beat Cancer, Meals Confidential, Nov.19, 1995, p.6.

fruits, vegetables, whole grains, poultry (breast), fish, and nonfat dairy foods.

Be creative. For example, whenever I eat one of my favorite foods, pizza, I order one with a small amount of cheese, lots of onions, garlic, tomatoes, red pepper, mushrooms, olives, and no meat. There you have it -- a healthy dish.

Those who taste my pizza comment that it is delicious and does not taste much different than the typical ones. Conspicuous in its absence is sausage, pepperoni and any other meat based product and with good reason.

CALORIES COUNT

Yes, calories do count, but it can sure enough diminish the joy for a senior as he sits down for a relaxing and enjoyable meal and has to worry about the amount of calories on the plate.   To keep the weight down and the health up, reach for the good guys that I mention in the book numerous times; fruits, veggies, and fish.   Avoid the bad and ugly ones; red meat, sugar, and caloric desserts.   By doing so, you will keep your weight down and out of harm's way.   So read on and enjoy the delicious foods that will tickle the palate and add many robust years to your life.   It's never too late to turn your nutritional practices around and to take the path to better health.   It's up to you, so go for it and leave your calculator at home.

> "HE WHO DOES NOT KNOW FOOD, HOW CAN HE UNDERSTAND THE DISEASES OF MAN?"
>
> **Hippocrates: father of medicine 400BC**

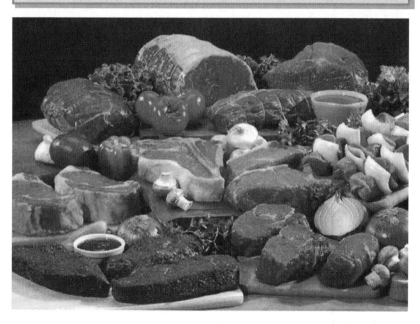

We often see pictures of **prehistoric man** with a club or spear in hand hunting for meat to feed his family; not true! The fruit and vegetable group is where they looked for nourishment; they **were mainly vegetarians**. Their intestinal tract is long which allows for the slow digestion of plant foods that are high in fiber, as opposed to the short digestive tract that is necessary to process meat and to get rid of the resulting toxic wastes hastily. Populations who eat plant based diets have a markedly reduced incidence of chronic health problems notably cancer and heart disease, says Claire Hassler of the University of Illinois.

Studies show that gastric cancer is more common among people who eat a lot of processed meat and red meats, smoked foods and salt cured or pickled foods.

On the other hand stomach cancer is less common among other people who consume a large amount of fruits and vegetables.

Yet in spite of the variety of choices available in this food group, sadly less than 22 percent of Americans eat the recommended five or more servings a day!

Populations who eat plant based diets have a markedly reduced incidence of chronic ills, most notably cancer and heart disease. The primitive tribes were unknowingly seeking out healthier foods.

Several studies have reported that foods from this group have caused a fall in blood cholesterol levels possibly because they decrease the intake of saturated fatty acids or because they contain generous amounts of pectin and fiber.

According to T.C. Campbell, PhD, a prominent authority in the field of nutrition, there are virtually no nutrients in animal based foods that are not better provided by plants.

Vegetarian food leaves a deep impression on our nature. "If the whole world adopts vegetarianism it can change the density of mankind", says Albert Einstein. His statement is backed up by many studies that confirm that red meat can be "a taste to die for".

I rarely eat red meat and do not feel that I am being deprived from enjoyable feasting. I select and enjoy the white meat from the breast of chicken and turkey, and eat a lot of fish. You can make a meat loaf from ground turkey that boasts on the label -- no skin and almost fat free.

If you have any doubts whether you should choose poultry or fish over red meat, researchers at the National Cancer Institute reported the results of the NIH-AARP Diet and Health Study of some 500,000, who participated in the study. Those who ate the most red meat, which was about 5 ounces a day, were 30 percent more likely to die of heart disease or cancer over the next ten years than those who ate the least red meat or about two-thirds of an ounce a day.

According to another recent study red meat (beef and pork) may harm the liver while white meat (poultry and fish) may protect it.

Researchers tracked 495,000 men and women for seven years. Those who ate the most red meat (about 4 ounces a day) were two and one half times more likely to die of chronic liver disease and about 75 percent   more likely to be diagnosed with liver cancer than those who ate the least red meat (about four ounces a week).

However in contrast the people who ate more white meat, as from the breast of turkey and chicken, had a lower risk of both illnesses.

Therefore, seniors should eat less beef, pork, and other foods that are rich in saturated fat such as egg yolk, cheese, ice cream, and other desserts as cakes, pies and cookies. Animal fats create excess cholesterol in the blood stream which is not friendly to the heart.

Research[39] tracked nearly 35,000 Swedish women for roughly ten years and concluded that red meat may raise the risk of stroke caused by blocked arteries in the brain. Those who ate an average of at least three ounces of red meat a day had a 22 percent higher risk of stroke caused by blocked arteries in the brain than those who averaged less than an ounce of red meat a day. Women who ate the most processed meat (at least one and one half ounces a day) had a 24 percent higher risk than those who ate little or none.

A 2012 study revealed that people who eat most red meat, (two servings a day), have a 40% higher risk of having a fatal heart attack, stroke or other cardiovascular disease than others that typically eat one serving every two to four days.[40]

A new health concern is Carnitine, which is a compound abundant in red meat and also found in some energy drinks. The new findings by a 2013 study led by Stanley Hazen, M.D., chief of cellular and molecular medicine at the Cleveland Clinic's Lerner's Research Institute, discuss the danger of a little studied chemical that is burped out by bacteria in the intestines after people eat red meat. It is quickly converted by the liver into yet another little studied chemical called

---

[39] Stroke 42:324, 2011.

[40] Arch,Intern.Med.172:555,2012

trimethyamine N-oxide (**TMAO**) that's gets into the blood and increases the risk of heart disease.

Meat eaters normally have more TMAO in their blood and unlike those who spurn meat, readily made TMAO after swallowing pills with Carnitine. So maybe the real danger to the heart is not just that thick fat on the steak.

Time will tell whether or not future research will back up these results. Studies often contradict other studies which baffle researchers. Nevertheless, I would encourage you, based on considerable research, to cut back on red meat to lower your risk of heart disease and cancer.

The skeptics will love this study:

The Japanese eat very little fat and suffer fewer heart attacks than the British or North Americans.

On the other hand the French eat a lot of fat and also suffer fewer heart attacks than the British or North Americans.

The Japanese drink very little red wine and suffer fewer heart attacks than the British or North Americans.

The French and Italians drink excessive amounts of red wine and also suffer fewer heart attacks than the British or North Americans.

The Germans drink a lot of beer and eat lots of sausages and fats, but suffer fewer heart attacks than Americans.

Conclusion:

"Eat and Drink what you like.

It's speaking English that kills you"

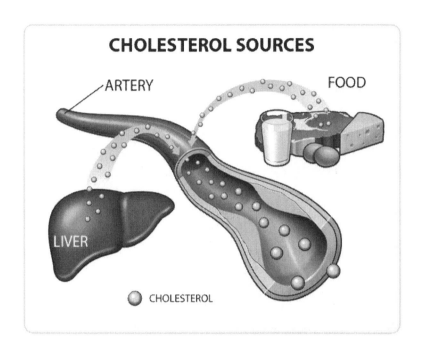

CHOLESTEROL SOURCES

ARTERY

FOOD

LIVER

○ CHOLESTEROL

Cholesterol is not all bad. It does contribute to the smooth functioning of the body otherwise it would not be put there. **The body uses cholesterol as the starting point to make estrogen and testosterone** (hormones made by the body which help to stimulate and maintain sexual function). Some people seem to have high levels of cholesterol because of inherited defects. For most of us, high cholesterol levels seem to come from a diet high in saturated fat.

Average American cholesterol counts are higher than those of the inhabitants of most non-Western countries, where fat consumption is lower. Your liver makes all the cholesterol you need, so you can't develop a deficiency. Whatever cholesterol you ingest is added to your overall cholesterol level. It generally becomes a problem when your diet leaves a cholesterol surplus in your bloodstream.

Unfortunately, you may not know that you have high cholesterol, as with hypertension, it does not always give warning and puts you at risk. Since, cholesterol is an integral part of every animal cell; you ingest it every time you eat foods of animal origin.

Although cholesterol is not a fat, it is fat like, in that it does not dissolve in water. It hitches itself to bundles of lipoproteins that transport it throughout the bloodstream. An excess of cholesterol may eventually be deposited on the walls of the arteries where it forms plaque.

In a few decades, enough of it can collect on the walls to slow or block the flow of blood through the arteries in a process called atherosclerosis, a form of arteriosclerosis, commonly called "hardening of the arteries". Often this narrows the coronary arteries which feed blood to the heart muscle. With flow slowed or blocked, heart pain could signal that the heart muscle itself lacks enough blood to provide oxygen and not enough energy to keep it pumping. Even a single meal that's high in saturated fat and cholesterol can cause your arteries to begin to constrict, and your blood to clot faster. Result a heart attack.

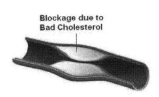

Blockage due to
Bad Cholesterol

If a blocked artery leads to a hemorrhage or to a lack of blood in part of the brain, a stroke -- with paralysis or loss of speech or other mental functions can result.

Fortunately, it is possible to partially reverse the effect of clogged arteries. Studies have shown that people who greatly reduce their cholesterol and fat intake and become more active can significantly improve this problem and in many cases without drugs.

According to a second National Cholesterol Education Program report in geriatric medicine, seniors should be aware that increases in cholesterol levels increase the risk of serious diseases that plague oldsters. A large body of evidence shows that lipid lowering can reduce the incidence of vascular related events. [41] Another good reason to monitor your cholesterol and to keep it within acceptable levels is that too much cholesterol in the blood may speed kidney failure.

According to the National Institutes of Health, patients with kidney problems who keep their cholesterol under control - either through diet or medicine are more likely to preserve their renal function.[42]

When I am shopping and I see a senior reaching for a cheese cake or steak, I am tempted to walk over and warn them of the danger of eating that food but fear the advice would not be appreciated and, perhaps, I would be barred from shopping in the store.

---

[41] Robert M. Mormando. Lipid levels: Applying the second National Cholesterol Education Program report to geriatric medicine. Geriatrics, August 2000, v55, i8, p.48.

[42] National Institute of Health, 3:00, 15-2001.

The intense controversy over the role of cholesterol in heart disease led to the famous 20 year Framingham study to determine the dangers of high blood cholesterol in over 5,000 Massachusetts residents. This was no minor undertaking. Thousands of volunteers free from heart disease were examined every two years to measure cholesterol level, blood pressure and other factors. After 10 years there was convincing evidence that blood cholesterol levels are definitely related to the presence and the development of coronary heart disease. A dramatic discovery indeed and also the study were able to relate blood cholesterol levels to heart attacks. The study was so impressive that the American Society for the study of Arteriosclerosis felt it could safely make the public statement, that high blood cholesterol was definitely a cause of coronary artery disease. It certainty convinced many Americans, including myself, to cut down on foods high on cholesterol. For those who still had doubts, the results of a follow-up study found that no one who had total blood cholesterol of less than 150 had a heart attack.

According to Alexander Leaf, M.D., chairman of the Department of Preventive Medicine at Harvard Medical School, "In societies where the mean cholesterol levels are 150 or lower without the use of drugs, coronary heart disease is essentially unknown as a public health problem."

Compared to other nations the American levels are too high.

The average middle aged American male has a level of about 250 milligrams of cholesterol in 100 millimeters of serum, although the average varies from one part of the country to another. Some physicians such as Daniel Steinberg M.D., professor of medicine at the University of California at San Diego, consider this average too high and the Japanese levels, for example 147 in men (45 to 49) years old are preferable. Claiming, that what we call a normal cholesterol level in the United States, is associated with a very high incidence of fatal heart attacks. Dr. Steinberg declares, "I see no reason to be self-congratulatory when a patient is treated and stabilized at the normal American level. His risk may be reduced, but it is reduced from an unacceptably astronomic value to a merely frightening high value"

Israel is an ideal country for medical research. Not only does it have the highest ratio in the world of physicians to patients but also it has had immigration from many countries.

One of the studies at the Hadassah Hospital that should shed light on the cholesterol question is that of Yemenite Jews who immigrated to Israel. In their homeland, they had lived on a frugal low calorie low animal fat diet. When they crossed the border doctors were amazed to find they had virtually no heart disease. Unfortunately, after 20 years in Israel, where most of them consumed a diet similar to ours in the United States, their cholesterol levels had risen from the 140 to 155 range to the 155 to 200 range and their incidence of heart disease was close to the same as that for other Israelis.

M. Toor, M.D., who studied atherosclerosis in Yemenites and Europeans, concluded that diet is positively related to the incidence of atherosclerosis.

These studies not only support the conclusions of the Framingham study but also add doubt that heart disease is strictly hereditary.

As Paul Harvey used to say, "Now, here's the rest of the story."

There are different kinds of cholesterol and fats. They can be friend or foe.

A senior should have their level checked every five years or more often if it is above the normal levels. Cholesterol levels tend to rise as you get older.

Below 200 is the recommended level to put you in the safety zone. For seniors many tables say 240 or less and the lower amount the better. A high percentage of seniors over 65 have high cholesterol.

The body packages the cholesterol in 3 different forms as HDL, LDL, and VLDL (high density, low density and very low density lipoproteins).

A desirable reading for low density lipoproteins (LDL) is below 130 and for high density lipoproteins (HDL) is above 40 and very low density lipoproteins (VLDL) below 40

Kenneth Cooper, M.D., M.P.H, founder and clinical director of Aerobics Center in Dallas, Texas, recommends that the average adult maintain a cholesterol level of 180 to 190. He also reports that 75%

of the patients he works with can control their cholesterol by dietary restriction, exercise and weight loss.

The Good the Bad and the Ugly

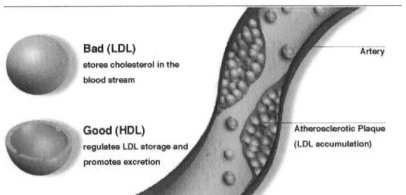

Bad (LDL)
stores cholesterol in the
blood stream

Good (HDL)
regulates LDL storage and
promotes excretion

Artery

Atherosclerotic Plaque
(LDL accumulation)

Now let us look at the whole story about cholesterol and fats. In the Framingham study, it was found that the **ratio of total cholesterol was a more reliable predictor of coronary artery disease than a reading on cholesterol alone**.

For example, if someone has a total cholesterol of 300(mg/dl) and a HDL (good kind of cholesterol) count of 75, that's a ratio of 4 to 1. That person is at some risk. But if another has total cholesterol of 250 and a HDL count of 25, that's a ratio of 10 to 1. That person is at higher risk even though he or she has a lower cholesterol count.

HDL carries excess amounts of cholesterol to the liver for recycling; helping to prevent the dangerous buildup of fatty deposits in the arteries and thus it is referred to as the "good cholesterol." The average ratio would be about 4. It would be more desirable it was closer to 2 or 3.

A good LDL to HDL ratio is 3.5 to 1 with an ideal ratio being 2.5 to 1.

High levels of HDL appear to be associated with reduced risk of Alzheimer's disease in older adults, according to a report in the December 1, 2010 issue archives of Neurology.

Swimmers and runners have high levels of HDL.

LDL and VLD, on the other hand, the "bad cholesterols", transport cholesterol and deposit it in the tissues, including the blood vessel walls, promoting atherosclerosis. VLDL carries a huge load of triglycerides and holds more total cholesterol than does LDL.

Triglycerides are molecules of ordinary fat that are circulating in the blood. They always travel in association with some cholesterol. Many diseases associated with high triglyceride levels such as diabetes, blood pressure and chronic kidney disease, are linked with an increased risk of heart disease.

A great body of evidence implicates triglycerides in the destructive process of arteriosclerosis.

High blood levels may signal an increased risk of stroke, at least in women. A growing body of research suggests that high levels are more dangerous for women than for men.[43]

If your exam shows that your triglycerides are over l00 mg/dl, lose weight, cut back on sugars, and replace saturated and trans-fats with unsaturated fats.

---

[43] Stroke 43: 958, 2012.

Triglycerides, which typically peak after a big meal, are present in the food and are also converted by the body from other nutrients, like carbohydrates.

"They are dangerous because they are so good at penetrating the arterial wall", states Borge Nodestgaard, M.D., chief physician in clinical biochemistry in Denmark's Copenhagen University Hospital.

Omega 3's in fish can also help in lowering levels.

Before you take your lipoprotein exam you should fast for 12 to 14 hours and some physicians suggest that you avoid strenuous exercise prior to the exam.

However, if you have a lipid panel reading that places you at a desirable range, it doesn't give you a license to not worry about eating foods that are high in saturated fats and cholesterol, and eat a cheeseburger and fries for lunch and cheesecake for dessert.

A new Strategy has developed where cardiologist are relying less on theses tables and more on the use of cholesterol lowering drugs. These drugs are known as satins, and are used to reduce the risk of heart disease and stroke. Satins are a popular choice but they may not be appropriate for everyone.

If you are taking drugs to lower your level, you still should eat a low-fat diet. Too often seniors have a false sense of security if their cholesterol is kept at an acceptable level through medication. Even if you are not taking drugs, normal cholesterol does not necessarily reflect a low risk.

How well I remember the results from my first exam, which indicated I was well over the 200 level. I was devastated.   I led a health style that I expected would show good results. In desperation I called a friend, Peter Wood, PhD, DSC, at the Stanford University of Medicine. Similar to me, he was an active runner and very interested in and well known for his research on the effects of diet, weight and exercise on the risk of heart disease. He retested me at his laboratory. The new results were considerably different and just about where they should be for someone who doesn't smoke, exercises daily, and eats a low fat diet.

My situation was not unusual. In 1985 the College of American Pathologists prepared a standardized blood sample with cholesterol of 263 milligrams per 100 millimeters, and sent it to 5,000 laboratories. The reports came back with values ranging from 197 to 397. The majority clustered in the range of 222 to 294. Even so, a value of 222 in a middle aged person would probably not be treated aggressively whereas a value of 263 might be and 294 should be.

If you get a high reading it makes good sense to repeat the test.

Your cholesterol level also varies from day to day and from season to season. Students show a rise during exam time. The cholesterol level of CPA's is higher during tax time.

As important as it is to have a normal cholesterol level, half of all heart attacks occur in people who do not have high cholesterol. Therefore, the full blame for bungling up the arteries cannot be blamed on high cholesterol alone. In fact risk factors such as genetics, cholesterol, blood pressure, obesity, age, gender, diabetes, stress, and a sedentary life style explain 50% of coronary artery disease.

FATS

Saturated Fat

Your body makes all the saturated fats it needs and 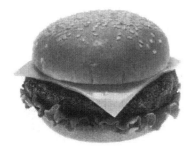 doesn't need any help from unhealthy fat laden foods which are the main dietary cause of high blood cholesterol and a very high danger to your health. High fat foods include animal products, salad dressings, gravies and processed foods. Dairy products, such as whole milk cheese and ice cream have a high fat content. Replace them with beans, nuts, poultry, and fish. Switch from whole milk to non-fat. Use nonfat yogurt, nonfat cottage cheese (watch the amount of salt), and other low fat products. There is little noticeable change, if any, in the taste, but there are much healthier ways to satisfy our needs through plant based food.

Red meat adds more saturated fat that clogs the arteries to the average American diet than any other food.

Studies show that a diet low in saturated fats cuts LDL (the bad one) about 20 percent more than one that is high in saturated fat.

Yet, fat is not all bad. Even carrots and lettuce contain small amounts. Fat helps to carry essential nutrients throughout your body and serves as a reserve for energy storage. But, there are much healthier ways to fulfill our needs through plant based foods.

New studies published in the March 2014 Journal Annals of Internal Medicine has sparked a debate: Are saturated fats the bad guys as expected?

However, the American Heart Association is steadfast in their guidelines. They continue to insist that you should avoid eating saturated fats if you, "love your heart."

The Association recommends a diet that is rich in fruit and vegetables, whole grains, fish, nuts, and unsaturated fat. They further state that less than six percent of the diet should include saturated fats and trans fats.

Trans Fat (the bad one)

Trans Fat is **another kind of saturated fat** found in the body fats of animals such as sheep and cattle that contains 2-5% of body fat. Trans-fats can also be made through the hydrogenation process. This process turns the liquid or unsaturated fat into a solid saturated fat.

Commercial food products as soups, baked and fast foods as well as chocolate, toppings with shortening and margarine are high in trans fats. The main reason manufactures are using hydrogenated oils in food production is to increase the shelf life of the products.

For the makers of partially hydrogenated oil, which is a source of artificial trans-fat, 2010 was not a happy year. Restaurants and food manufacturers continued to switch to healthier oils. On a gram for gram basis, trans-fats are definitely public health enemy number one. They are getting a lot of bad press lately for good reasons.

Trans-Fats are now listed on food labels so we can recognize and avoid them. This is another good reason why we should read labels. They usually are solid at room temperature and are derived from vegetable products. A diet high in these fats has been correlated with heart disease and other health problems.

Studies show that a diet low in saturated fats cuts LDL (bad cholesterol) about 20 percent more than one that is high in saturated fat.

Polyunsaturated Fat

Polyunsaturated Fat **promotes good health** as it helps

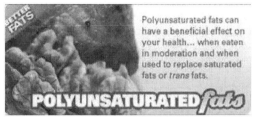

Polyunsaturated fats can have a beneficial effect on your health... when eaten in moderation and when used to replace saturated fats or *trans* fats.

lower cholesterol levels. They are found mostly in nuts, seeds, fish (especially wild salmon), algae, krill, plant oils, corn and flaxseed.

Monounsaturated Fat

Monounsaturated Fat **lowers LDL, the bad cholesterol**

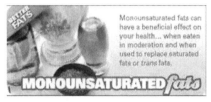

and leaves HDL the good kind alone. It is found in olive oil, peanut oil, avocado, seeds and most nuts.

Olive oil is used almost exclusively in Mediterranean cooking instead of butter, margarine and other fats. I use olive oils on salads, on my toast, corn on the cob, making popcorn, preparing vegetable dishes and stir frying fish. The data suggest that any oil that's high in unsaturated fats -- whether it's polyunsaturated or monounsaturated are associated with a decreased risk of cardiovascular disease, says Alice Liechtenstein, Dsc, of the U.S. Department of Agriculture, Jean Mayer Nutrition Research Center on Aging at Tufts University in Boston.

Seniors should put the right kind of oil on their shopping list for maximum health.

According to a position statement of the American Dietetic Association, "Scientific evidence increasingly supports that good nutrition is essential to the health, self-sufficiency, and quality of life of older adults."

Good health is increasingly difficult to obtain by Americans who are spending less time cooking at home. They are depending instead on others to prepare their meals. Americans get about one-third of their calories from restaurants which feature foods high in fat. This has undoubtedly contributed to the fact that, although

America is one of the richest nations, we score very low in overall health. The problem is not too little food but too much of the wrong kind.

Meat is not all bad, for it is a source of protein, which the body needs to replace dead cells and form new ones. Everyone needs an adequate intake of protein to maintain good health and to recover from illness and injury. However, there are many other healthy foods that will provide the body with protein without saturated fat.

For years, some of the most comprehensive health studies in the nation, including the Landmark Physicians Health Study, have linked nut consumption with lower risk of heart attack and other cardiovascular dangers. Nuts are an awesome form of vegetable protein and heart friendly. So valuable, that it deserves repeat recognition in this chapter as a good alternate for the heart unfriendly foods. But like fruit drinks they are high in calories.

The vegetable group can be used as a prudent substitute for red meat. It is not ranked high in protein, but if you combine them in a dish with brown rice, corn, and a little lean meat diced into small pieces you will provide the protein you need in a healthy and delicious manner. Yes, meat too can be served in a way to satisfy the palate and not clog the arteries, but a lot depends on the company it keeps.

If you are in the mood and just have to eat some type of meat, at least be sure to pick the leaner types as extra lean beef or turkey with as much as 99 percent of the fat removed. These low fat meats are now available at most grocery stores. Trim the skin and avoid all the processed meats such as luncheon meat, hot dogs, bacon, and bologna. These contain from 30 to 50 percent fat and enormous amounts of sodium, both of which threaten our hearts.

A typical two slices of bologna sandwich will be about 16 grams of fat. A much healthier choice for a sandwich, if you cut the mayonnaise, is turkey breast (without the skin) that is about one or two percent fat.

You will be doing your heart a favor that will be repaid in many joyous years.

Red meat can be "**a taste to die for**" as many studies have shown. Getting together with the family should be a cheerful not a dangerous experience.

Foods could offer pleasant and healthy meals but at the same time could set up the senior for a fatal heart attack. Even one meal of red meat that is high in saturated fat may release the hormone thromboxane. This hormone can cause the arteries to constrict and the blood to clot and prevent the heart from getting oxygen.

That is why emergency physicians are especially busy during the Thanksgiving and Christmas holidays. A very heavy meal can increase your risk about 4 times within the first few hours of eating it. Hence, a heart attack turns a festive event in to a disaster.

If the reader is somewhat discouraged by the results of these studies, keep in mind you do not have to give up all these goodies nor should I say bad ones. But if you are going to have a breakfast of bacon and eggs and for lunch a cheese burger and fries followed by a steak or ribs for dinner, you are putting yourself in harm's way.

Preparation of food is another way to fight back. Baking, boiling or steaming is much safer than frying. For example, look what we do to the potato. A popular American food, of which we consume an average of 85 pounds a year is changed by frying it in oil from a non-fat food of about 200 calories to a morsel of 450 calories with 22 grams of fat much of it trans-fat. Speaking of potatoes, studies have indicated that purple potatoes can help to fight against high blood pressure.

Many seniors eat regularly in restaurants and the food choices offered make it difficult to stay on a heart-healthy diet. Some chicken nuggets if cooked in fat have as much fat as a hamburger and even as much as one and a half pints of ice cream.

It is not only the fat that food is cooked in that we have to watch out for to enjoy a healthy meal. Salads present their own problems. If you load your plate with cheese, bacon and creamy dressings, your salad will have more fat than a quarter pound cheeseburger. A carrot and raisin salad or even an innocent looking tuna salad if loaded with mayonnaise can provide a large amount of calories and saturated fat.

Recently, I ate at a Greek restaurant and felt confident that the food would be healthy because as discussed earlier the Mediterranean diet is usually low fat and high in vegetables. Wisely, I ordered only the chicken kebabs but you still have to be cautious. The seemingly healthy gyro sandwich is a disaster, with 44 grams of fat, 20 grams of saturated fat, and 2300 mg. of sodium. That's all the saturated fat and sodium that the average consumer should eat in an entire day! The moussaka, with 48 grams of fat and 25 grams of saturated fat is even worse.

Greek food served in their native land is a much healthier fare. For example, Greek males who eat a low-fat diet have a very low rate of prostate cancer. Not the same for Greek males who immigrate to the US, and develop a taste for our fatty diet. This same peril develops for other immigrants who move to the United States.

Studies reveal that as immigrants from Japan adopt a westernized diet that their heart attack rate rises dramatically. It is much higher in Hawaii than in Japan and much higher in the Unites States than in Hawaii. Thus, the closer these people come to our shores and the more of our diet they adopt, the higher their risk of heart attack.

According to Ernst L. Wynder, M.D., president of the American Heart Foundation, Americans consume 42 to 44 percent of their calories in the form of animal fats while the average in Japan is 15 to 20 percent.

Some say heart attacks are God's revenge for eating his animals.

Try to limit the amount of meat you eat. The recommended size of one serving (about 3 ounces) of cooked meat is about the size of a deck of cards. Deal yourself that amount to stay in the healthy zone.

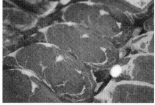 Red meat **may raise the risk of strokes** caused by artery blockages.

A Surgeon General's Report on Nutrition and Health which draws on 2000 studies states: "diet helped account for more than two-thirds of the 2.1 million deaths last year."

"Poor nutritional habits, besides the main cause of obesity, are strongly implicated in five of the nation top ten killers: coronary heart disease, stroke, atherosclerosis, diabetes and some cancers."

Ernst L. Wynder, M.D., President of the American Heart Foundation said that Americans consume 42 to 44 percent of their calories in the form of animal fats while the average in Japan is 15 to 20 percent.[44]

China is another country where coronary heart disease is rare and when it occurs it does so 20 years later in life than Westerners. Unfortunately, his difference does not hold for the Chinese who immigrate to the United States and adopt our high fat diet.[45] A study of

---

[44] For information on heart disease among the Japanese, see M.G. Marmot and S.L. Syme, "Acculturation and Coronary He art Disease in Japanese Americans. "American Journal of Epidemiology 104 {September 12 1976}:225-47; and T.L. Robertson, Hksto, J. Gordon et al., Epidemiology Studies of Coronary Heart Disease and Stroke in Japanese Men Living in Japan, Hawaii, and California. Coronary Heart Disease Risk Factors in Japan and Hawaii." American Journal of Cardiology 39{}; 244-p 1977.

[45] W.K, Ho and W.Y. Chan, "Evaluation of Serum Lipid and Lipoprotein Levels in Normal Chinese. The Influence of Dietary, Habit, Body Weight, Exercise, and a Familial Record of Coronary Heart Disease." Clim 61(1975); 19-25.

about 3,300 Chinese residents of North America and China show that people increase their risk of colon and rectal cancer when they eat a lot of saturated fat and fail to exercise. Thus, the closer they come to our shores and the more of our diet they adopt, the higher their risk of being stricken by the two highest causes of death.

The figures are startling: For example, the death rate from prostate cancer in the United States is 700% higher than in Hong Kong and 600% higher than that in Japan.

Populations that eat larger amounts of fat have strikingly higher rates of prostate cancer, according to Curtis Mettlin, PhD, Director of the Department of Cancer Control and Epidemiology in N.Y. Roswell Park Institute who participated in several studies related to cancer intervention.

According to Ernst Wynder, President of the American Health Foundation, differences in diet are the only way to explain why some countries have higher rates of prostate cancer. It is suspected that fat raises the levels of testosterone and other hormones (a chemical substance produced in the body that controls and regulates the activity of certain cells or organs), which could stimulate the prostate to grow along with any cancer cells that it may harbor.

This may explain why African-Americans have a 37 percent higher incidence of prostate cancer than Caucasians do according to the American Cancer Society. Studies have shown that African-Americans have higher levels of testosterone to begin with and a high fat diet could further elevate these levels. This is dramatic evidence that we should look for alternatives for red meat.

By now you must be at least be considering cutting down on your consumption of marbleized steaks, spare ribs, luncheon meats, and other popular American foods rich in saturated fats.

Here is another good reason to just say, "**no to meat**". We must feed animals several times as much protein as they ever yield. We are wastefully using grain that could be used to feed many starving people. Fertilizer and farming skills are being used to produce food for animals and not directly for people.

It is estimated that if Americans were to reduce their meat consumption by only 10 percent for one year, enough grain would be released to feed 60 million grain eaters for a year. Thus cutting down on these foods not only protects our own health but also increases the amount of food available for their consumption.

It also saves energy too. A Cornell researcher, David Pimental, PhD, told participants at a meeting of the American Association for the Advancement of Science that the energy required to produce a typical vegetarian dinner is less than a third of that used to prepare a beef dinner. He claimed that if Americans were to consume more energy-efficient beef substitutes such as chicken, as much as 75 percent of the energy used to produce food could be saved, that is up to 30 gallons of oil per person per year.

Seventh Day Adventists are one group of Americans who have said "NO" to meat, and they do not eat the typical American diet. They have a much lower death rate than other Americans.

Since 1954 more than 250 articles published on their life style in cooperation with the National Cancer Institute show they have 50% less risk of heart disease, certain types of cancer, strokes, and diabetes.

Vegetarian men can expect to live 8 years longer and women seven years longer than the general population.

A long term study of 47,000 Seventh Day Adventists revealed a much lower death rate than for the general population, and an even lower for those who were strict vegetarians. Seventh day Adventists also use whole grains and vegetables. They avoid alcohol, tobacco, coffee and other caffeine-containing beverages, hot condiments, spices, and highly refined food.

As George Ball, past president of the American Horticultural Society stated, "Let's make 2011 'The Year of the Vegetable'."

The reader may be thinking at this point that the author is a vegetarian.

"No way," as I always jokingly respond "I did not work myself up to the top of the food chain to become a vegetarian."

However, I am very close to being one. There are many substitutes for red meat that are both healthy and delicious.

For many that are vegetarians, the choice is a healthy one. Vegetarian diets may lower death risk from all causes -- including cancer. Results of a 12 year study of people who did not eat any meat had a 40 percent lower risk of dying from cancer and a 20 percent lower risk of dying from any cause that affects meat eaters. Researchers stopped short of recommending strict vegetarian diets. They suggested cutting down on fat and eating more vegetables, fruits and grains.[46] Unfortunately, many Americans still consume too much red meat. "Meat contributes to an extraordinarily significant percentage of the saturated fat in the American diet," says Marion Nestle, chair of the nutrition department at New York University.

However, the mad cow disease scare and E-coli outbreaks are converting more Americans to fish and poultry products. The average of over 100 pounds of meat a year that Americans are consuming is diminishing. Swimming to our rescue is the fast growing alternative to meat -- fish.

---

[46] Source: Margaret Thorogood, PhD, senior lecturer. Health Promotion Sciences Unit. London School of Hygiene, Keppel St. London 461E 7HT, and coauthor of a study of more than a 6000 vegetarians and more than 5,000 meat eaters in the United Kingdom.

These waterborne foods are **swimming their way to** 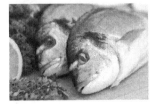 **the dining table and pushing meat off the plate at a rapid rate**. Many fast food restaurants are offering fish sandwiches perhaps due to a guilty conscious or pressure from health advocates. Chefs have known, for a long time, of gourmet meals that can be prepared with the focus on varieties of fish.

We've known for decades that eating fish helps one to stay in good health.

But only within the last 20 years have we been able to pinpoint the specific disease fighting agent in fish. Now that we know it, we should be hooked on fish.

Fish is a most special food because it contains two important varieties of long chain omega 3 fats that you will not find anywhere else in a conventional diet. They are just the sort of fat molecules that any healthy cell should gladly welcome.

The active agent is a pair of polyunsaturated fats. These omega oils are also called omega 3's fatty acids.

Essential fatty acids are the raw materials for several hormones that help to contain blood pressure, blood clotting, inflammation, and other important functions in building cells and keeping them that way. It also contains fiber and other nutrients essential for good health.

Omega-6 which is found in polyunsaturated fats also protects against coronary artery disease, promotes skin and hair growth, and makes tissues responsive to insulin. Insulin is a hormone that allows glucose, or blood sugar, to be taken up from the blood stream into muscle. There it's then burned for energy, and into fat, where it's stored and has other roles such as to protect reproductive functions.

Omega 3's are no longer new kids on the block. Pharmaceutical companies are now manufacturing it. Radio health shows are touting it daily as one of the greatest health gifts to mankind. Perhaps this is not too much of an exaggeration, for their contributions to the overall health of the senior is notable.

They help to lower triglycerides. Blood levels of these fatty substances tend to rise after meals thereby raising the risks for heart attacks and other serious diseases.

In addition Omega-3's help prevent arrhythmias, heart beat irregularities that can lead to sudden death. Research has shown that omega's fatty acids may reduce considerably the likelihood of the dangerous kind of irregular heartbeats.[47] Ventricular fibrillation is caused when the blood flow is suddenly reduced. It could be the result of blockage to the coronary arteries. Foods high in saturated fat are suspect in creating this problem. Keep this in mind as you scan the menu in your favorite

---

[47] Leaf A. Weber P.C. "Cardiovascular Effects of N-3 Fatty Acids Update, New England Journal of Medicine", 1988, 318 549-57.

restaurant and then without hesitation "order fish" as proof you love your heart.

A study of 20,000 physicians found that those who ate fish at least once a week had half the risk of sudden death than those who did not eat fish.

William Castelli, M.D., told his patients at the Framingham cardiovascular clinic, to eat fish a minimum of twice a week, preferably salmon. He was further quoted as saying "Whatever you do eat your salmon and lots of it." JoAnn Manson, M.D., Harvard Medical School professor states, "We found that eating fish at least twice a week could reduce the risk of heart disease by more than 30 percent."

Some studies show that fish eaters live longer and that they develop fewer age related diseases than non-fish eaters.[48] The oil in fish, omega 3 fatty acids, has been shown to protect your arteries by thinning the blood and lowering blood pressure. It also revs up your internal antioxidant defenses.

Several studies show that older people who eat plenty of fish have lower levels of beta-amyloid protein, associated with Alzheimer's, than those who eat less. Men who ate fish at least three times a day following a heart attack had 29% less mortality.

A significant benefit derived from omega-3 fatty acids is that they are believed to help prevent the blood

---

[48]W.S. Harris and W.E. Connor. "The Effects of Salmon Oil upon Plasma, Lipids Lipid s Lipoproteins and Triglyceride Clearance. {The transactions of the Association of American Physicians}" 1980: Vol. xc111. 148-155.

walls from the adverse effects of LDL cholesterol. As you remember, they are the bad guys.

The seniors who smoke, and I hope by now there are few oldsters who still puff away their senior years, should be sure to add salmon to their diet.

Scientists with the Center for Disease Control and Prevention discovered that Alaskan natives, whose chief form of protein was salmon, had less than a third of the heart attack rate of U.S. whites -- even though twice as many smoked cigarettes.

William Connor, M.D., a researcher at Oregon Health Sciences University who's been studying omega-3 for two decades contends that fish oil is more versatile than aspirin in combatting heart disease. While aspirin helps prevent dangerous blood clots and alleviates inflammation in the arteries, omega-3's do that and more.

It isn't just to protect the heart that should motivate you to head for the fish section when shopping. Studies indicate that men who consume more fish especially fatty fish three or four times a week had a lower risk of prostate cancer.[49] omega-3 have also been shown in laboratory studies to inhibit tumor growth and to keep cancer cells from spreading.

Something that should be of special interest to seniors is that the omega fats in fish may lower the risk of hearing loss. Most hearing loss in older adults occurs in the cochlea of the inner ear. Aging, genetics, noise

---

[49]Journal of Urology 165:2; 94 2001.

and some illnesses can harm the cochlea. Fish oils may aid blood flow to the cochlea just as they may prevent clogged arteries elsewhere in the body according to a recent Australian study.[50]

How about eating fish to protect the eyes? In a study of more than 70,000 men and women, those who ate canned tuna more than once a week had a 40 percent   lower risk of age-related macular degeneration than those who ate it less than once a month.

Degeneration of the macula (the center of the retina) is a leading cause of blindness in older people and unfortunately there are few treatments. Parts of the retina contain high levels of the omega-3 fatty acids that are found in fish.

It may be too early to say it protects the vision but given the growing evidence that it prevents heart attacks and strokes it makes sense to plan for several servings a week.[51]

Grandma was probably right when she said, "Eat fish, it will make you smarter". Studies indicate that it can play a positive role in mental health. The brain is largely composed of fat. Fats along with water are the chief components of brain cell membranes and the specialized tissues enclosing the nerves. The saturated fat that comes primarily from meat and full-fat products is not what the brain cells need. They do need polyunsaturated fats especially the long chain omega-3 fatty acids.

---

[50] Am. J. Clin.   Nutr.   92:416,2010.

[51] Am. J. Clin.   Nutr. 73::209, 2001.

Fish may also be helpful in reducing stress. Studies in Finland suggest that those who eat a lot of fish are less likely to be depressed or think of suicide. The Japanese eat the most fish and have the lowest rates of depression in the world.

Fish may well have been responsible for the building of our nation. Lewis and Clark feasted not on red meat but salmon during their exploration of the Pacific Northwest. William Clark described in his journal that salmon was a most delicious fish. They were wise to pick salmon which has the highest amount of omega-3's No wonder many nutritionists refer to it as the T-Bone of the deep.

The reason it is so special is that salmon search the water for small fish which have eaten smaller fish that consume a large amount of algae that has a lot of fatty omega 3. However, if you do not like salmon there are many other choices that are swimming up the rivers and oceans to be caught and served so we can have a healthy body. Sharing this wholesome list are sardines, trout snapper, halibut, scallops and shrimp.

Since the body cannot produce the fatty acids on its own, we should salute the fish. They swim on their challenging journey so we can be healthy.

Another big plus is that it so easy to prepare fish. You can boil it, poach it or broil it, but don't fry it.

Approximately, two servings of fatty fish a week is recommended. It is easy to prepare a delicious and healthy meal with fish. Be aware that some fish including swordfish, shark, and albacore have high mercury content and an excessive amount should be avoided especially by pregnant women.

It is debatable which salmon is best. I prefer wild salmon and shy away from the farm raised. You can also get wild salmon which is canned and reasonably priced.

The omega alpha linoleic (polyunsaturated fatty acid) acids in seeds, nuts, beans and whole grain may be as necessary as the omega in fish oils to prevent heart attacks.

There is clear evidence that populations who eat lots of fish and vegetables tend to have unusually low rates of heart disease, stroke, cancer, diabetes, and other disease, Perhaps, I should have encouraged fishing in my chapter on exercise.

As with many studies there are conflicting opinions as to the value of omega-3, but I tend to agree with the recommendation of the American Heart Association and eat at least two servings of fatty fish a week. Trying to get the benefits from the omega-3 capsules may not be the way to get the benefits and may even be dangerous.

Fresh wild salmon is my favorite. Expensive but after all, I fill my gas tank with premium fuel to keep my motor in good shape, so it makes good sense to stoke my body with the healthiest foods to keep it performing well at all speeds

---

As the senior embarks on a voyage to eat healthy and

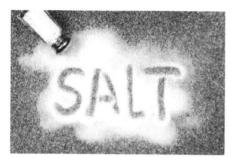

stay on course to become **a super-centurion they must avoid too much salt**.

Salt, sometimes called sodium, is also known as table salt or rock salt. It is a mineral that is composed primarily of sodium chloride.

It is found naturally in sea water and, unfortunately, in too many foods. It also does not fight fairly and is hidden in bread, chicken, soups, breakfast cereals and especially processed and pre-packaged foods. You can find it listed in small print among other ingredients but you will need your glasses and a well-lighted area to seek out the information making it more difficult for senior's health.

Unfortunately, Americans consume too much salt, by ensuring about 3400 milligrams a day and many as much as 4000, 5000 or even 6000 milligrams a day

The intake should be limited to no more than 2300 milligrams a day which is slightly more than a tea spoon. About three quarters of the salt we eat is already in the food.

According to a recent report published in the American Heart Association Journal. If the average daily sodium intake of Americans were to drop instantaneously to 1500 milligram, a day, which is a steep drop to a level considered ideal, as many as 1.2 million premature deaths could be averted over the course of a decade.

Nutritional anthropologists have deduced that our Paleolithic fore-bearers probably ate fewer than 1000 milligrams a day.

A high salt meal can stiffen your arteries within 30 minutes. Arteries that lose their ability to expand when they need to can increase the risk of high blood pressure, heart attack, stroke, and cognitive decline.

Studies have shown that reducing sodium levels in processed and restaurant foods by 50% would prevent more than 100,000 deaths per year from strokes and heart attacks. The expense of medical costs in our nation could be reduced as much as $18 billion annually by reducing sodium levels by one-third.

Perhaps we should put alarms on salt shakers to remind us of its danger.

Yet there are good things that one can say about salt even though it is posted on the hit list as foods that seniors should use with caution.

It helps control your fluid balance and the way your muscles and nerves work. The body automatically regulates how much salt or sodium is present. If the levels are too high we get thirsty and drink which speeds up the stimulation of salt through our kidneys.

Too much salt is linked to hypertension, high blood pressure and osteoporosis. If a senior has high blood pressure, it is advisable to become a label reader and cut down on their intake of salt.

Very elderly people as well as individuals with kidney disease are not able to excrete sodium and regulate body fluid efficiently. Salt (sodium chloride) is the main form of sodium added to foods and is probably its worst offender.

Ever since the U.S. Government first issued dietary guidelines in 1977 they have recommended a decrease in salt intake. It is believed to affect the risk of high blood pressure, which is a factor in coronary heart disease and stroke.

What is bad for blood pressure is SALT.

According to Norman Kaplan, M.D., professor of internal medicine at the University of Texas Southwestern, "Primarily the mechanism is that sodium will expand the volume of blood in the circulation and as volume increases pressure goes up. When we go on a lower sodium intake the overall volume goes down. He recommends fruits and vegetables and other potassium packed foods." He also states: "There are no natural foods that are high in sodium and to keep away from processed foods."

When I'm dining in a restaurant, I am always amazed by the number of people who reach for the salt shaker as soon as the meal is placed in front of them and pour liberal amounts on their plates before they even taste the food.

Many dental offices take the blood pressure of their patients when they are examined. Perhaps it would be a good idea to have the waiters do likewise before they place the salt shaker on the table.

It isn't only the salt from the shaker that causes the consumer to exceed the recommended amount of salt. It has a lot of help from many unsuspected sources.

Chicken parmesan sounds like a healthy choice on the menu of a restaurant but has over 3000 mg of sodium, more than two days of the suggested amount for a safe limit. Even worse is the senior who selects meat laden dishes that boast of it being free of trans-fats but also has over 3000 mg of salt.

You should of course cut back snack foods such as potato chips, pretzels, pickles, and popcorn, if it is as highly salted as they make in the theaters.

> *Recently I took three of my grandchildren to the theater; I was amazed how much it cost. But the real shocker was when I had to pay $5.00 for a box of popcorn I said to the young girl behind the counter; I remember when a box of popcorn was only 5 cents. She smiled and replied, "You will really enjoy the movie, and it has sound now."*

We unknowingly consume more salt than ever now because of our increased dependence on snacks and processed food. For example, a best-selling wiener has over twice the milligrams of salt compared to another. Likewise, a well-known brand of English-muffins also has twice as much salt with little difference in taste.

When you see the enormous amount of salt in soup, breakfast cereals, and other foods which have a reputation for being healthy, you realize how important it is to read labels. There are many of the same products with a much lower amount of sodium.

Fortunately, more seniors are concerned with this wide discrepancy among popular foods, and are reading labels and requesting that they not add salt to their order, when they eat out.

They should also request if dining in a Chinese restaurant, that the food does not have any MSG (monosodium glutamate). MSG can cause severe headaches or other discomfort. It is referred to in medical journals as "the Chinese restaurant syndrome."[52] Another suggestion is to ask them to stir fry the food in water rather than oil. That will cut down considerably on the calories without diminishing either the nutritious value or the taste with proper seasoning.

Those who doubt the relationship between salt and high blood pressure would do well to read the studies of L.B. Page M.D, who participated in Harvard

---

[52] H.H. Schaumberg, R. Byck, R. Gerstle et al., Monosodium Glutamate: Its Pharmacology and Role in the Chinese restaurant syndrome "Science 163 (1969).

University's Solomon Islands expedition in the late 1960,s and early 1970. Studies of eight tribal groups showed that blood pressure was more closely related to salt than to any other dietary factor.[53] In separate investigations, L.K. Dahl, M.D., E.D, Freis, M.D., and J.V. Joosens, M.D., established the influence of salt on blood pressure. Epidemiological studies in Polynesia, Micronesia, and South America have shown that people who eat relatively small amounts of salt (five grams or less a day and in some cases less than one gram) are remarkably free of hypertension.

Conversely, populations that consume large amounts of salt -- the northern Japanese farmers, for example, have a high incidence of hypertension.

If this evidence doesn't motivate you to avoid salt (as they say in the navy, "now hear this") studies conducted by T. Sata, M.D., have shown that a high salt intake is related to a high incidence of stomach cancer.[54] For a long time the association of salt to high blood pressure has been established. At an American Heart seminar based on considerable research. Dr. Page stated, "Salt intake should be limited from infancy and even adults should not exceed one-tenth of a teaspoon of salt a day. Athletes, nursing mothers, and people

---

[53] L.K. Dahl, "Salt and Hypertension.", American Journal of Clinical Nutrition 25(1972) 231 44.; E.D, Freis, "Salt," 53 (19760; 589,-95; and J.V. Joosens, "Trends in Cardiovascular Mortality Prevention and treatment of Coronary Heart Disease and its Complications," in Proceedings of the XV International congress of Therapeutics. edited by Jean Lelguime(Netherlands: Excerpta Medica.1979),pp18-21

[54] T. Sata et al, "The Relation Between Gastric, Cancer Mortality Rate and Salted Food Intake in Several Places in Japan, Bulletin of the Institute of Public Health (Japan) 8 (1959) 197-96.

working in hot, humid environments, he said do not need more than a teaspoon a day."

Excess salt is linked to a number of other conditions including stroke, cardiovascular disease, cardiac enlargement, daily per cap and osteoporosis. That should be enough of a list to motivate you to put down that salt shaker. If not here are other good reasons.

According to data available from the Korea Cancer Registry, a seven year study of 9,620 men and 2,773 women associated their stomach cancer with a high intake of salt.

Research from Leuvn University in Holland discovered that a high intake of salt can significantly increase the risk of stomach cancer.[55]

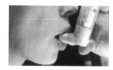 According to a study in England, a high sodium diet can aggravate asthma, at least in men. The chief investigator, Oliver J. Cary put 22 men with mild to moderate asthma on a low sodium diet. Because the improvements were modest he stated, "Sodium restrictions may only be of use in asthmatic patients with high sodium intakes." Nevertheless he adds, "Our results suggest that large increases in dietary sodium result in physiological deterioration in male asthmatic patients."

According to researchers in the University of Western Australia, lowering your sodium intake may also lower the risk of osteoporosis, or brittle bones. After two

---

[55] Thorax 48:714,1993

years researchers found no bone loss in the hips of women that consumed about 2,100 mg or less sodium a day. Above that amount, they found the more sodium, the greater the loss of bone. If the women lowered their sodium intake from 4,000 mg to 2,000 mg a day, she would protect her bones as much as if she consumed an extra 1,000 mg of calcium a day.

There are physicians that are of the opinion that not everyone has to be concerned with the amount of salt they consume unless it raises their blood pressure. However, a study of about 600 people concluded that those who were salt sensitive had a higher risk of dying over the next 30 years, even, if their blood pressure was normal at the beginning of the investigation. High blood pressure also put at risk of dying the individuals who were not salt sensitive.[56]

There is no practical way to see if you are among the 25 percent of people who are salt sensitive. But if you are, you had better stop shaking the salt on your food as you are more likely to develop high blood pressure and die prematurely. It is better to substitute a non-harmful ingredient to provide the taste you are looking for. The less salt the better. Keeping it below the typical average of 3,500 to 4,000 milligrams a day that Americans consume and closer to 1,000 will help you to stay out of the danger zone.

Stomach cancer is more common among people who eat a lot of processed meat, red meat salt cured or pickled foods. However, stomach cancer is less common

---

[56]Hypertension   37 429,2001

among people who consume a large amount of fresh fruit and vegetables. A very important food group as emphasized in prior chapters.

Patrick Quillen, PhD vice president of the Cancer Treatment Center of America says, "The cure must come from the environment within the body." This food group may very well do that and slow the process of aging as well as preventing the major causes of deaths of our senior population.

For some, salt may be considered the spice of life but if not used within bounds it could be a peril to life.

Yet there are studies in 2013 that also provide scientific evidence that doesn't support the 1500 mg recommendation for people who are 51 and older and those of any age who are African American and who have hypertension, diabetes, or chronic kidney failure. They also state low sodium intake may have adverse health effects and reducing the amount dramatically can increase health risks for some people.

However, the Heart Association after reviewing this research stands by their recommendation based on the strength of evidence relating excess sodium intake to high blood pressure, cardiovascular disease, and stroke. We have evidence that reduced intake of sodium can prevent and treat hypertension and can reduce the risk of adverse cardiovascular disease and stroke.

The government also stands by the recommendation that most adults reduce their daily sodium intake to less than 2,300 mg.

The World Health Organization concluded that elevated blood pressure is the leading cause of preventable death, and that suggests that staving off high blood pressure with low sodium diets is an important strategy.

After reviewing numerous studies it is apparent to me that sodium reduction remains critically important in preventing cardiovascular disease.

We should continue to reduce the amount of sodium in our diet especially in processed foods, read labels, and increase our potassium especially from fruits and vegetables.

> *Sugar is Dangerous*

Now that you have learned to be salt smart, let us look at

Sugar in the morning, sugar in the evening sugar at supper time.

Be my little sugar and love me all the time.

Charlie Philips-Odis Echols

"It was a song in 1958 well known as it was made popular by the McGuire sisters"

another food that affects the health of the Senior Citizen.

Sugar can be divided into two general categories. The first is the pure or refined form (sucrose and glucose) used in candies, pastries, and other unfortunately popular foods that are rich in calories and low in nutrients. The other category includes the form (fructose and lactose) that are present naturally in foods like milk and fruit, which also contain essential vitamins and minerals. Only the pure sugars are questioned. While honey, molasses, and brown sugar do contain small amounts of some vitamins and minerals, they contribute few nutrients and are no better for you than white sugar.

The Department of Agriculture recommends that you limit the amount of your sugar to the diet, but not many Americans are heeding this advice. They are eating more each year. In 1996 we averaged 25 more pounds of sugar per person than we did in 1986. That is over a 50 percent increase since 1900.

In 1999, Americans consumed an all-time high of 158 pounds of sugar per capita which most likely contributed to the soaring obesity rates in the United States. A more recent study states it is about 130 pounds. If that figure does not alarm you, picture yourself consuming five 22 pound bags of sugar during the year.

According to a study from the City University in New York[57] a third of Americans get almost half of their calories from foods like desserts, candy, soft drinks, chips and ice cream. These foods are low in nutrients and high in calories. It is difficult to avoid sugar. It is added into just about all the major brands of canned soup, including beef, consommé, cream of mushroom, and even cheddar cheese. Sugar also is listed among the ingredients of most cans of vegetables and sauces as well as jars of mustard, peanut butter, and ketchup. Even cough medicines, liquid antibiotics, and many children's vitamins contain sugar.

Another good reason to read labels is so that you can avoid high fructose corn syrup which is being added

---

[57] American Journal of Clinical Nutrition,72:929,2000

to a lot of foods, so much so that its use as a sweeter has increased 3.5 percent per year according to the World Health Organization.

Did you know that a major brand of ketchup tested by a food analysis laboratory was found to contain 29 percent sugar? That is more than you find in many brands of ice cream. When you pour dressing on a healthful salad you may be adding a product that is as much as 30 percent sugar. Substitutes for cream, which are popular among those of us who want to cut down on our intake of cholesterol, contain as much as 65 percent sugar, while a coating for chicken was found to have 51 percent sugar, the same amount as candy. They even added sugar to salt!

Look at the soft drinks often referred to as liquid sugar. Americans gulp twice as much soda as milk and six times more than fruit juice. There are sugary drinks out there wherever you go. They are located at most schools and hospitals (for shame).

Seniors should avoid the vending machines that offer a quick way to quench thirst. A 12 ounce can of non-diet cola which is the smallest size have about 10 teaspoons of sugar and 150 calories. Gulp it down with a cheeseburger and a sundae and you have the combination of a lot of cholesterol, fats, sugar, and salt. This is exactly what is contributing to the demise of one American every 39 seconds.

Six to eight glasses a day of water is a healthier way for seniors to satisfy their thirst. Water is essential for good health. The amount required depends on your climate and how often you exercise. However, drinking an excessive amount of water, and depending what medications you are taking, can be problem.

An occasional fruit drink would be a better choice than soft drinks which contain no nutrient value and an excess of sugar.

Throughout the Mediterranean many drink wine in moderation, and it is usually taken with meals. For men no more than two glasses a day, for women one glass per day is the recommended amount to avoid serious health problems.

There is a lot of hype about drinking red wine especially from vintners. There are doctors that also support the benefits of red wine since it contains flavonoids and resveratrol that are good for the seniors. The jury is still out to determine if you can derive the same, benefits from grape juice and avoid the health dangers of excessive alcohol. I personally look forward to an occasional glass of red wine with my wife before dinner as we find it relaxing while we discuss the day's events. Fortunately this has not created any weight problem.

Researchers, studying nearly 50,000 middle-aged men and women, found that light to moderate wine drinkers as opposed to teetotalers, or those who preferred beer or spirits, choose a diet that tends to be higher in fruits and vegetables, fish, salads and heart friendly olive oil. Unfortunately, this is not the choice of most Americans.

In less than a generation the lack of exercise and a diet full of fats and sugar have produced a rise in those who are dangerously overweight.

To help you make a healthy choice of what you put in your plate, McDonald's which is the largest chain and fast food company now posts the calorie counts on their menu boards in 14,000 U.S. outlets.

John Yudkin, M.D., recognized as an authority on nutrition, not only in his native England but also in the United States, feels strongly that sugar, not animal fat or cholesterol, is the big danger factor in heart disease. He states emphatically, "If only a fraction of what is already known about the effects of sugar were to be revealed in relation to any other material used as a food additive, that material could be promptly banned!" He observes, "That we have no physiological requirement for sugar and that our nutritional needs can be met in full without taking a single spoonful of white or brown or raw sugar on its own or in any food or drink."

Dr. Yudkin and his coworkers have conducted impressive laboratory tests on animals and human volunteers consuming a high-sugar diet. The diet produced many of the concomitants of heart disease, including increased cholesterol and triglyceride levels, decreased efficiency in dealing with high blood glucose, insulin, and other hormonal disturbances, and stickier blood platelets (part of the clotting process). If this is so, how did we ever get involved in consuming such a worthless food?

The United States has a daily per capita sugar consumption that is among the highest in the world. Dr.

Yudkin and others have found that when animals and humans are given sugar their triglyceride levels rise in proportion to the amount given. These researchers believe that triglycerides are more serious causative factors than cholesterol in atherosclerosis.

It is not only in the United States that sugar causes problems. Comparing diets and deaths from cardiovascular disease in various countries between 1955 and 1965, D.R. Maisroni, M.D., made a strong case against sugar. Finland, which showed a 30 percent increase in death rates during this period, had a 34 percent increase in saturated fat intake but a 123 percent increase in sucrose consumption. In Yugoslavia, where the death rate from heart disease increased three-to four-fold, the saturated fat intake fell by 26 percent but the intake of sucrose almost tripled. In Czechoslovakia, the consumption of sucrose was more closely related to deaths from heart disease than was high fat consumption. Obviously, in these areas at least, cholesterol was not the only factor contributing to heart disease. [58]

A. M. Cohen, M.D., of Jerusalem found that recently arrived immigrants to Israel from Yemen, who had consumed little sugar in their native land had little heart disease, while among Yemenites who had emigrated 20 or 30 years earlier and had adopted the high-sugar diet of their new country, heart disease was common and the incidence of diabetes was 50 times

---

[58] R. Maisroni, "Dietary Factors   and   Coronary Heart Disease ,"Bulletin of The World   Health Organization 42 (1970): 103-14

higher than for the new immigrants.[59] As we saw earlier, other researchers feel that an increase in saturated fats caused the Yemenite immigrants' heart problems. Similar studies of Australian aborigines, the primitive inhabitants of New Guinea, and the Polynesian inhabitants of Mabuig Island demonstrate that as the intake of sugar increases so does the incidence of diabetes.

Then there are the Masai tribes in East Africa who have little heart disease and live longer than other Africans. Their diet is almost only milk, a little cow's blood and a little beef. It's interesting to note that they eat virtually no sugar.

Another interesting group is the islanders of St. Helena, who have quite a lot of heart disease although they consume less fat than the Americans or the British. Since the area is extremely hilly and there is little mechanical transportation, they are physically active. Their cigarette consumption is less than that in most eastern countries. What is causing their high incidence of coronary disease? As you may have guessed, the major suspect is their consumption of about 100 pounds of sugar per person per year.

G. D. Campbell, M.D., of South Africa was amazed when he came to the University of Pennsylvania in 1953 and discovered that unlike the rural Zulus of Natal, the blacks of Philadelphia had the same high

---

[59] A.M. Cohen, S. Bavly and R. Pusnanski "Change of Diet of Yemenite Jews in Relation To Diabetes and Ischemic Heart Disease. Lancet 2 (1961):1399-1401
"

amount of heart disease as the whites in the city of Durban. However, Dr. Campbell and Surgeon Captain T. L. Cleave later observed that as the Zulus moved into Durban and adopted a modern diet high in refined carbohydrates, their incidence of heart disease rose.[60]Dr . Campbell was so distressed that he started a one-man campaign of radio programs and pamphlets in eight African languages to cut down sugar consumption among the Zulus and others.

Let's look at the Eskimos, who consumed a diet extremely high in saturated fat but had practically no heart disease until the American servicemen stationed in the north shared their candy bars with the Eskimo children and introduced their families to cookies, cakes, and other sugar-laden foods. Although previously foods gathered from hunting and fishing provided the Eskimos with their total diet and protein was exceptionally high, a new craving for sugar lowered their nutritional preferences.

Otto Schaeffer, M.D., a specialist in internal medicine, who practiced in the Arctic for two decades, reported that the Canadian Eskimos living near white settlements have adopted western diets, including a greatly increased consumption of sugar, and suggested that this change may be responsible for the increase in atherosclerosis and other diseases among them. Whereas the Eskimos previously were content

---

[60] T.I.Cleave The Saccharine Disease (Bristol: John Wright and Sons,) 1974and T.I.Cleave and G.D.Campbell. Diabetes Coronary Thrombosis, and the Saccharine Disease.(Bristol: John Wright and Sons,1966)

with berries to satisfy their sweet tooth, now they turned to the sugared soft drinks, candy bars, cookies, and other sweets they can buy in government-sponsored stores. Instead of chewing animal skins, they now chew chocolates. Among the remarkable changes in their health are earlier puberty and more rapid growth. Both changes are closely linked to diabetes, obesity, and heart disease. Since the change in diet among the Eskimos has been quite abrupt, it has been easier to recognize its effects on health than it has among the peoples of affluent western societies, where changes have been gradual.[61]

It's sad to think that as we prosper we use our money for foods that do not contribute to our good health. Aaron Altschul, M.D., an internationally known nutritionist at Georgetown University, called the phenomenon "affluent malnutrition."

As a society becomes affluent and changes its eating habits, he says, the incidence of obesity, coronary artery disease, hypertension, diabetes, and other diseases increases.

Unfortunately, sweets are on the table. In the United States, sweets used to be an expensive luxury. Now they have become a cheap staple that provides a fifth of our caloric intake. "Sugar is a new food." John Meyer, M.D., a distinguished nutritionist, told a Senate committee hearing. "It is one which the human system, at least in many people, is not equipped to live with."

---

[61] Otto Schaeffer, "When the Eskimo Comes to Town, Nutrition Today. November/December 1971, pp. '8-16

Some people feel that sugar can't be bad because it is found in natural foods. There's a vast difference, however, between getting sugar from an orange and getting it from a candy bar. When you eat an orange, you do get a little sugar but you also get the elements you need to metabolize it; when you dip into the sugar bowl, all you get is sugar. So, if you want to satisfy that craving for sugar (that started way back when your parents unknowingly gave it to you in your baby food), the best advice is to enjoy it as it occurs naturally in fruits and vegetables.

Other investigations suggest limiting its use. John Potter, M.D., states in a 1999 New England Journal of Medicine Editorial, that relatively high, "sugar consumption is consistently associated with the risk of colorectal cancer."

Sanjay Gupta, M.D., reported in April 1, 2012, on a CBS, news report that sugar can take a serious toll of your health worsening conditions ranging from heart disease to cancer.

It's been estimated that 50% to 90% of colon and rectal cancers are caused by diet. The links to increased risk include too much fat and too little fiber. Now, research suggests refined sugar may share in the blame, by causing high insulin levels, especially in those who are overweight. Elevated insulin, say some experts, can trigger the growth and development of tumor cells in the colon.

Researchers in Italy questioned more than 1,200 people with colon cancer, more than 700 with rectal cancer and more than 4,000 healthy controls about their eating habits. In keeping with the insulin theory, the more refined the sugar the subjects ate, the greater their risk for the two cancers.[62]

It is also implicated in the formation of gallstones. Instead of focusing on the association of sugar with dental problems we should look south for damage control. Gallstones are clumps or crystals of cholesterol that can send one to the hospital with considerable abdominal pain. Certainly severe enough to make you sorry you poured in that spoonful of sugar or reached for that extra piece of candy.

Researchers found that those who consumed at least 400 calories worth of sugar each day were three times as likely to develop gallstones as people who took in a maximum of 260 calories of refined sugar daily. Since Americans average over 300 calories of refined sugar a day they are at risk. Since Americans also consume too much saturated fat a day it puts them also at risk for developing gall stones. This is another good reason to cut down on both. Even if future studies attack the recent investigation, there is enough evidence to caution you to reduce your intake of sugar and the unhealthy company it keeps.

You may remember in the chapter on exercise that it helps prevent the formation of gallstones. It is interesting to see how a healthy life style combining exercise with a low fat diet, and one that uses less salt

---

[62] New Cancer Diet Link? Environmental nutrition, Nov.1997, Vol.20, No.11.

and sugar work in concert to protect you from so many ailments that are not only painful but life threatening.

For those who are proud that they are switching to fat free foods (like cookies, cake and ice cream) may be surprised that many of these foods are loaded with sugar.

The same problem occurs when they switch from high sugar foods and go into high fat ones, which is why you should always read the labels. It's a constant battle but will be well worth it for seniors and all segments of our society to be alert and avoid the bad guys.

Many seniors are also replacing sugar with low and no calorie sweeteners, but they are no magic bullets. They can be beneficial to a weight loss program. But they will not do it alone. Exercise and diet are most important to down load that bay window.

Another consideration is -- Are they safe? Although artificial sweets are regulated by the Food and Drug Administration, there are many studies that question their safety. Personally, I prefer to add fruits and other low calorie foods to satisfy my sweet tooth.

Since there is increasing evidence [63]that a high sugar diet is linked with serious diseases of the senior it makes good sense to remove those sweets from the table and replace them with nuts and other natural foods.

---

[63] David Kritchevsky,"An Update on Lipids, Lipoproteins and Fat Metabolism". in The Medicine   Called Nutrition see Note 2,pp.61-6 2007

A Doctor was addressing a large audience in Tampa:

"*The material we put into our stomachs is enough to have killed most of us sitting here years ago. Red meat is awful. Soft drinks corrode your stomach lining. Chinese food is loaded with MSG. High fat diets can be disastrous, and none of us realizes the long-term harm caused by the germs in our drinking water. But there is one thing that is the most disastrous of all, and we all have eaten or will eat. Would anyone care to guess what food causes the most grief and suffering for years after eating it?" After several seconds of quiet, a small 75 year old man sitting in the front row, raised his hand and said, "wedding cake".*

Breakfast

> ## "LET THY FOOD BE THY MEDICINE"
>
> ### Hippocrates

Breakfast **is a must**. You may not be a breakfast person but as a senior it is a good way to get the metabolism 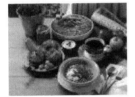 going and you as well. It is not only the most important meal of the day but the easiest to prepare.

Good health starts at the breakfast table. Just as you try to give your car quality fuel to keeps it running properly, so you should provide your body with the nutrients that enable your vital organs to function at their highest level of efficiency.

By now you are more aware of the foods to select and the ones to avoid. So let's get on to a healthy start by stoking your body with hearty foods.

When you think of breakfast you normally think of toast. What kind to choose may very well be the first question of the day. It is not an easy selection for the senior since you have a multiplicity of choices stacked side by side on the shelves with attractive and colorful packages beckoning you to take them home. Don't be enticed by the appearance and fresh odor. Take your time and read the labels. If you want the best bread, look for the words "100% whole wheat flour," on the label. It helps to guarantee that you're getting the nutrients and fiber that you need. If the label just says, wheat, it may contain refined flour. Reject all brands that have either preservatives or additives.

Yes, I have heard seniors say, "At my age I need all the preservatives I can get."

Next eliminate those from which the most nutritious parts of the wheat kernel have been removed. The kernel is made up of three parts. The first is the outer covering, a rough many layered shield rich in crude fiber. Next comes, the starchy mass called the endosperm and then deep inside the tiny embryo or wheat germ. Mother Nature has wisely provided nutrients needed to spark its growth into a new plant.

White bread is made from the endosperm, the least nutritious part of the kernel, with the bran and the wheat germ thrown away. White flour was being produced in Greece as early as 500 B.C. and by 50 A D. its production was widespread. Fortunately for the poor, it was a wealthy person's bread. By the 17th century practically everyone was eating it. Bakers now try to tempt us to eat bread made from this flour by claiming it is enriched. While it is true that several vitamins and minerals are added to it, they do not nearly make up for all the good that was taken out in the refining process. This is an additional good healthy reason to read labels.

Another good "shopping tip" is: With all the choices there is no reason to reach for the white. Whole wheat bread should be thought of as nutritional gold for many health reasons. It contains the nutrition of all parts of the flour. Removal of the brand and wheat germ may appeal to the American palate but it erodes the value of the meal.

Roger Bannister, M.D., ran the world's first sub-four minute mile. As a medical student, he ate wheat germ every day as part of his training. Swimmers and many other athletes also make wheat germ an important part of their diet. They feel that it helps provide fuel to the heart and keeps it running smoothly and efficiently.

This superb food provides high quality protein for building and repairing all vital organs and tissues. It contains polyunsaturated oils which as discussed in prior chapters are the good guys.

Compare it to a bad guy -- It contains more than 26 percent   protein, with no saturated fat while a T-bone steak contains 19 percent protein and lots of fat. The concentration of amino acids in wheat germ is twice that in steak, and wheat germ provides four times as much lysine (an essential amino acid). To think that wheat germ (this important source of nutrients vital to heart health) is purposely removed from flour before it reaches the table is illogical. Fight back and select the brands that proudly feature wheat germ in their bread.

It is even possible that wheat germ changed the course of history. During the siege of Stalingrad in the latter stages of World War II, it appeared that the Russians no longer could hold out against the Germans, who had swept across European borders conquering country after country. At one point it was impossible to get food to the front lines, and the Russian soldiers had to exist on bread and water. Stalin, who was the leader at the time, claimed that if it had not been for the whole wheat bread, they would not have been able to continue fighting through the bitterly cold days and nights.

We learned another valuable lesson during the same war when British children, evacuated to the countryside to escape air attacks, were fed whole wheat bread, in many cases for the first time in their lives. These children had good health forced upon them when they were deprived of the white bread to which they were accustomed.

When we eat white flour, we also are depriving ourselves of the wheat bran, which provides many valuable nutrients as well as fiber. If we ate the typical meal of the African villager, including cornmeal, beans, bananas, and potatoes, or if we ate a lot of fruit, vegetables and grains high in fiber, we would be protecting our bodies against a lot of health problems. Since most oldsters don't eat a well-balanced diet, eating bread with the bran intact will help us avoid the many problems that a diet low in fiber can cause. These problems include constipation, cancer of the colon and rectum (of which the United States has almost the highest rate in the world), appendicitis, hemorrhoids, varicose veins, diverticulosis, and coronary heart disease.

By forcing the liver to convert cholesterol into bile salts and subsequently excrete them, a high-fiber diet

3-231

reduces the amount of cholesterol in the bloodstream. Fiber also may be important in maintaining normal weight.

At the University of Bristol, Kenneth Heaton, M.D., a pioneer in fiber studies, noted that when he, his wife, and some of their colleagues increased the fiber content of their diets by using whole wheat instead of white bread, they lost weight gradually and smoothly. The losses went as high as 15 pounds without any attention to calories or any attempt to restrict the amounts eaten.

A Harvard School of Public Health study of 40,000 men concluded that if you have high blood pressure eating potassium, magnesium or fiber from breads, cereals and other grains may lower the level and cut the risk of stroke.

A 1986 study of more than 3,800 women aged 55-69 in Iowa concluded after nine years that women who averaged at least eight servings of whole grains a week had about a 15 percent lower risk of dying than women who consumed fewer servings. The link remained even after the researchers accounted for exercise, red meat consumption, smoking and many other factors.

Another important reason to read the labels and make a responsible choice is that it can help to prevent diverticulitis, a disease that former President Dwight Eisenhower called to the attention of the American public when he developed this problem. As you get older you are more at risk. It can feel like appendicitis and be as serious. With appendicitis the pain is usually on the right side. With diverticulitis the pain is usually on the left side caused by inflammation of a pocket on the large intestine. The good news is the problem can be resolved by surgery. An important way to prevent this disease is to consume 20 grams of fiber a day. This should take you out of the danger zone. Most Americans take about one-half that amount. It is a disease that should not affect Americans. It is rare in countries where fiber is high. It's more widely seen in Western societies where diets typically are lower in fiber and include more meats and refined grain products.

Doctors E. C. Toomey and Paul Dudley White found no cardiovascular disease symptoms among 25 Hunzas aged 90 to 100 years. Their blood pressures ranged from 120/70 to 150/90 and their cholesterol readings from 150 to 190, well below western rates, and their EKGs showed no evidence of heart disease[64] The spartan diet of these senior citizens included such fiber-containing foods as fruits, vegetables, nuts, and grains (wheat, barley, and millet) -- all foods that are readily available in our country at low cost. Most of our supermarkets now have a section where you can purchase the same foods that appear to have protected the Hanzas from the big killer of Americans.

S. L. Malhotra, M.D., chief medical officer and head of the medical department of the South Eastern Railway in India, claims that coronary heart disease is directly related to fiber and that one of the main protective features of the Indian diet is its fiber content.

---

[64] E.G. Toomey and P.D. White, "A Brief Survey of the Health of Aged Hunzas," American Heart Journal 68 (1964.): 841.

He feels that roughage is more significant than fats, cholesterol levels, and other factors we normally accept as being related to coronary heart disease.

It's ironic that poor rural African villagers have a much more nutritious diet than those of us who live in this wealthy modern society. We Americans seem to be consistent in doing things wrong. No wonder the World Health Organization ranks the United States 34th in overall health among nations. Despite strong evidence that fiber plays an important part in reducing cholesterol levels and protecting against atherosclerosis, our consumption of fiber-rich foods has been decreasing. For the sake of our nation's health, let's hope that this trend will be reversed.

By this time you should be furious with the food processing industry for refining flour, rice, potatoes, and other popular foods to make them whiter, softer, and smoother. By doing so, it has cheated us out of a most important nutritional ingredient: fiber.

At least we should require the processors to inform us of this injustice. Can't you picture a label reading: "Warning, the wheat germ has been taken from this product during its processing which might have protected you from heart disease and other fatal health problems." Then most likely you would see changes taking place in the food industry. Be sure to reject brands that list sugar first or second as well as ones that are loaded with additives no matter how many nutrients are added. It's wise to serve cereal made from whole grains, such as rolled oats and whole wheat. It isn't difficult to mix up a batch of good natural foods such as wheat germ, bran, rolled oats, nuts, and raisins to provide you with a nutritious breakfast.

Cereals

Another section in the market that takes up a lot of 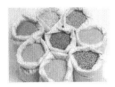 space and again presents a lot of choices is the cereals. Cereals **have long been very important in the diets of people throughout the world** and if we take the time to read labels and make a proper selection they can and should play an important role in our diets as well. In many parts of the world today cereals supply 80 percent or more of the total caloric intake as well as valuable amounts of nutrients. In addition to the foods discussed above, this group includes cornmeal, grits, rice, macaroni, and spaghetti.

Talk about choices, you could spend an hour looking at all the colorful cereals and breads that are tempting you to them in your grocery cart. It is really not that complicated. Eat whole grain wheat bread, cereals, and other products that contain bran. Have oatmeal, muesli, and other cereals made with whole oats. Read the labels and you can find many that are sodium free. Do so and you are that much closer to becoming a super healthy senior.

Dairy Products

This food group also **has an important impact on the** 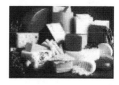 **senior's health.** Adults over 70 are advised to include low fat dairy products in their diet each day. A senior can fulfill this nutritional requirement from non-fat milk which has 0 grams of fat compared to whole milk that has 8 grams of fat. Except for those of us allergic to milk it should be considered a valuable source of nutrients. It's unfortunate that so many of us think of milk as a drink only for children. A single eight-ounce glass of low-fat milk provides about a fifth of our daily need for protein, a third of the necessary calcium, and a fourth of the vitamin, riboflavin. Calcium is particularly important because it helps in the normal clotting of blood.

Butter

Butter is **another popular food** in this group and the
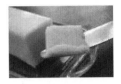 leading spread for over a half a century.
It's losing its popularity to margarine
and liquid vegetable oils. At one time,
the American Heart Association
recommended the switch because of its concern about
the relationship between saturated fat and cholesterol.
Many now are questioning this substitution. Some
margarine still contains trans-fats, and as discussed in a
prior chapter should be avoided. It is becoming easier to
do this. Many new brands are visible on the shelves at
super markets that proudly announce a butter substitute
with no trans-fats. Be sure to read the labels to see if
they harbor any other unhealthful contents.

In our household we use olive oil as a substitute
and enjoy the healthy change.

> "I Scream, You Scream, We All Scream for Ice Cream."

A much **too popular food in this group** is -- you probably guessed it, ice cream. Not only the grandchildren but the grandparents as well, scream for ice cream. Of course, it isn't as exciting or romantic as when we had to go to the drugstore or ice cream parlor to satisfy our craving. We can now store ice cream in the freezer section of our refrigerator and eat it as often as we crave it. This popular delight is undoubtedly adding to the problem of obesity as it is high in both saturated fat and sugar. There are even special brands that brag about their high fat content, 10-18 grams per serving.

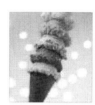

Ice cream is very low on the list of nutritional foods and is usually accompanied by another high calorie dessert. Meyer Friedman, M.D., feels that ice cream deserves special attention in the search for causes of heart disease. Perhaps we were wiser in our generation and only served it on special occasions such as birthdays.

A better choice than ice cream that is becoming very popular and is a good source of calcium is yogurt. There are a variety of non-fat flavors. But look at how we have taken this wholesome food and diminished its nutritional value by adding artificial flavoring and coloring, honey, sugar, and other additives. I often serve plain yogurt with fruit and nuts, a nutritious dessert that tastes as good as any syrupy sundae. Read the labels and you can find it without unwelcome additives. There are brands that are low in fat and sugar and high on taste.

G. V. Mann, M.D., has shown that yogurt lowers cholesterol in sedentary individuals and has suggested that it could be an important factor protecting the Masai against heart disease. "In countries where yogurt is a main source of fats, heart-disease is very rare."[65]

---

[65] G.V.Mann, "A Factor in Yogurt Which lowers Cholesterol in Man. Atherosclerosis 26(1977):335-40;" and G.V.Mann, "The Masai Milk and the Yogurt Factor: An Alternate Explanation," Arteriosclerosis 29 (February 1978:285

"Smile and say cheese" is an often repeated expression for seniors as they ask their grandchildren to pose for a picture, but **should we put it on our list of healthy foods for the senior**? Cheese, as all dairy products, is high in protein and calcium. That is the good news. But, as innocent as it looks it may put your health in the danger zone, unless you select the brand that is low in fat and sodium.

It depends on the brand. This is another good reason to take your eyeglasses when you shop and scan the labels. Two ounces of almost any brand has 6 grams of saturated fat. There are types of cheese with as low as 0.5 grams per serving, so you can enjoy your cheese without a feeling of guilt. If you do a little arithmetic you can see the big difference between various types. For example, every ounce of regular cheddar contains nine grams of fat, six of them saturated. Mozzarella cheese is a little lower, at seven grams of saturated fat. Part skim mozzarella, at five grams of fat and three grams of saturated fat, is just a touch better. An ounce represents a small amount of cheese, about a one inch cube.

Be thankful for the variety for choices for low-fat and non-fat cheeses. For every three grams of total fat a cheese loses, it drops about two grams of saturated fat. But, it keeps much of the calcium that makes cheese a great bone-builder. You can and should look for the softer type as they usually have fewer grams of fat.

However, I think the food industry has a lot of chutzpah charging more for brands with less sodium and less fat. If they give you a lower amount of something why do they charge you more for less? Since it will inevitably lower your medical bills it is still a good deal.

Americans are eating over 30 pounds of cheese a year. According to a 2011 study reported in the European Journal of Cancer, excessive amounts daily which is more than 53g (roughly the size of a small chocolate bar), raises the risk of bladder cancer by 50%. Researchers also noted that a daily portion of olive oil will lower the risk by one half. In addition to a healthy diet exercise is also recommended to lower the risk.

It's also not the cheese by itself that worries nutritionists but the company it keeps. Pizza, cheeseburgers, luncheon meats, and mayonnaise are high in saturated fat, and are typically found in sandwiches alongside a slice of cheese.

One slice of a meat covered pizza stuffed with cheese contains as much fat and calories as a hamburger (quarter pounder). Who eats just one slice at a time?

When you order a pizza, ask them to use very little cheese, and a variety of vegetables. That makes a high fat delicacy a healthy one.

Cream cheese is an innocent looking culprit. Yet, it is fattier than regular cheese. Each tablespoon has 5 grams of fat, three of them saturated. Better to ask for the fat free version before it is smeared on a bagel. With lox and onion and tomato you should hardly notice a difference in taste.

Americans consume over 243 egg yolks a year. They 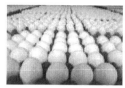 **add more cholesterol to the average American's diet than any single food**. It's too early to tell whether the modest increase since 1995 will continue.

The American Heart Association claims that, for most people, cholesterol intake should be limited to 300 milligrams a day and that since an egg yolk contains 350 milligrams we should eat no more than three a week, including those in cooking.

Even more cautious, Robert Levy, M.D., director of the National Heart, Lung and Blood Institute, says he hasn't touched an egg in years. According to a recent study, David Spence, M.D., a researcher at Western University in London said he found more evidence pointing to the harmful effects of egg yolks. He claims the cholesterol found in the yolk is almost as dangerous as smoking. However, Michael De Bakey, M.D., the eminent heart surgeon, ate eggs all the time and lived 99 productive years.

As in other areas of health there are often conflicting opinions.

The U.S. Department of Agriculture recommends that eggs be served regularly since it is one of the most nearly perfect foods. It is an inexpensive way to obtain a high quality of protein of approximately 6 grams in a large size. I think that I have found the perfect solution. I remove the yolk. It contains all of the fat and most of the calories. What is left is almost pure protein and rich in amino acids.

When I use eggs for cooking, baking or for sandwiches or salads, the yolks are discarded into the garbage disposal. So far, it hasn't clogged the linings of the sink pipes but if it does, better there than the inner lining of my arteries!

However, I make sure I eat at least one egg yolk a week as it has zeaxanthin, lutein, and choline that are good for eye health as well as other parts of the body. Whenever I eat out in a restaurant I request that the eggs be served without the yolk. Most are very willing to comply with this request.

Recently, on a cruise other seniors dining at the same table noticed that my scrambled eggs looked different, as they were white. When I explained that I had the yolks removed and the reason for this they decided to do the same. Several mentioned that it was an excellent idea since they had high cholesterol and were taking drugs to reduce the level.

Egg Substitutes

Egg substitutes are **becoming popular among the cholesterol conscious**. The substitutes range from about 15 to 60 calories compared to about 80 for an egg. Some brands however also have a high amount of grams of fat, another reason to be a label reader. You may also notice ingredients such as color additives. Therefore why not just remove the yolk and enjoy the rest of the egg in its natural state?

My wife has questioned my concern with eating whole eggs and reminds me of my grandmother who lived on a farm in Lexington, Massachusetts and always included eggs for breakfast. She lived far beyond her life expectancy.

Perhaps the foods we eat today are different from those consumed in the past. Animals now are raised in controlled environments, no longer able to get exercise by foraging for food. In an egg factory, for example, a moving belt carries feed to within the reach of every beak. If we penned up humans that way they would become very unhealthy, and the same could very well apply to animals.

We now have produced hens that give us eggs with much higher saturated fat content.

By adding chemicals to feed, we have produced animals with heavier weight and a larger proportion of fat that creates the marbleized steak demanded by meat-loving Americans. This development may make for higher profits, but it doesn't contribute to better health. No wonder the cardiologists are so busy! If we could inspire farmers to raise animals in open spaces, we might obtain fat that is soft and quite unsaturated. Experiments with different feeds also are attempting to achieve this goal.[66]You can now get eggs that are from range fed chickens.

Only as the public outcry mounts will changes take place in the market place so Americans can eat healthier meals.

---

[66] C.E. Allen, D.C. Bertz,D.A. Kramer,et al.Biology of Fat in Meat Animals {Madison.WJ College of Agriculture   and Life Sciences, University of Wisconsin,1976.

VITAMINS, PILLS, SUPPLEMENTS, HERBS

FRIENDS OR FOE

 All vitamins are important. They all have a vital role for normal metabolism and, the prevention of disease. What kind? How much? Are they necessary? Can too much be harmful?

The rapid graying of America has increased interest in exploring how to meet the needs of seniors. Healthy eating, as well as physical activity, is vital for people of all ages, but of special importance for the senior. A very high percentage of the elderly have diseases that can be improved by good nutrition. The elderly are more susceptible to diseases caused by the free radicals. Free radicals are molecules responsible for aging and tissue damage in the body. Antioxidants bond to free radicals rendering them harmless. The seniors naturally want their help and can find them in fruits and vegetables as well in vitamins.

Nutritional needs do change with age. "The diet and health link is particularly important as you grow older," said Jeffrey Blumberg, PhD, professor of nutrition at the Department of Agriculture's Human Nutrition Research Center on Aging. Many changes occur in the mind and body as the senior grows older. It is vital that the right selection and quantity of foods is made to remain active and disease free.

In general aging people need at least the same amounts of vitamins and minerals as they required when they were younger.[67]

Data from the Third National Health and Examination Study suggest that older people are at particular risk of inadequate diets because of the presence of chronic disease, physical disability, poor teeth, multiple medications, limited income, and social isolation. In addition, a decreased sensitivity of taste and smell and a sedentary lifestyle can adversely affect nutritional status.

Since aging slows the metabolic rate, older adults need as much as 600 calories fewer each day. However, many are adding too many calories, but too few nutrients. This contributes to the risk of obesity and poor health at the same time.

According to the National Elder Care Institute on Nutrition, one-quarter of older Americans have diets poor enough to put them at risk for malnutrition. Older people may also suffer from illnesses, or taking medication that can create difficulty in receiving the right amount of calories causing malnutrition.

Eating right after 50 requires the right choices to assure that all parts of the body will function properly. If the senior selects foods unwisely it can deprive them of

---

[67] Stephen Pratt Eating habits should be altered as you age nutritionists agree. The Sacramento Bee. November 11, 1998.

the nutrients required and they will die at a faster pace. Not a very pleasant thought at this stage in our lives. The proper diet is important at all ages but older people in particular develop many health problems as a result of poor nutrition.

The previous chapter has pointed out the significance of foods in the different groups that will provide the nutrients that the senior needs for maximum health. Foods, in their natural state, provide the vitamins without which we would not exist.

Vitamins are necessary for all parts of the body to act efficiently, to give us good vision, strong bones, good teeth, healthy blood cells, and a heart and nervous system that is in top condition. They are all organic nutrients that are necessary in small amounts for normal metabolism and good health.

Quite a responsibility – but, do we need additional support from a pill or powder or herb to accomplish the needs of the body? Many seniors must think so. Today 42 percent of U.S. adults report that they take vitamins every day.

Sales of vitamins, minerals, and supplements totaled nearly 23 billion dollars in the US (2012), according to Euromonitor International and were growing at a rate of five to seven percent annually. No wonder -- Senior citizens are bombarded daily by radios and TV commercials urging them to march down right away to the drug store, health store, or supermarket to stock up on a variety of vitamins, minerals and other supplements that will slow down the aging process, and keep them in good mental and physical health. They are told that their product will help them to prevent heart disease, cancer, and other serious problems that assault the older person. Former Senator John Breaux (D-LA), chairman of the Senate, stated, "Some of the promotional studies and advertisements simply prey on their fears."

This advice is often dispensed by individuals with an inadequate background in nutrition.

Enticing literature is mailed daily with claims that the Fountain of Youth may be found in a bottle or a pill that is yours for a reasonable price. Despite the exaggerated and in some cases deceptive advertising claims for many of these pills and potions and powders, the graying American is spending a fortune each year hoping to slow the ticking of the time clock, and perhaps reverse the aging process.

The advertisers who flood the seniors with false claims are even helped by our legislators. In 1994 Congress passed a law that permitted any product labeled a nutritional supplement to go to market without the Food and Drug Administration proving its safety or effectiveness. The result, as expected, was a rapid volume of products with varying combinations of vitamins, minerals, herbs and hormones, beckoning the seniors to present their credit card and stock their shelves to begin a journey toward good health.

But is this a prudent move for seniors to take to insure good health?

Not if you live in an area with abundant fresh food and clean air, you may in the words of Lawrence E. Morehouse, PhD, of U.C.L.A., "be doing little more than making very expensive urine". Many doctors feel that taking vitamin supplements will not reduce heart disease, lower blood pressure, prevent colds, provide extra energy, slowdown the aging process, or protect against air pollution.

A 2011 study finds little or no long lasting benefit for more than 182,000 middle aged and older women and men living in California and Hawaii, who were taking a multivitamin or mineral. They were just as likely to be diagnosed with cardiovascular disease or cancer as those in the group that did not.[68]

An earlier physicians study of more than 83,000 men aged 40 to 84 also questions the value of taking a multivitamin. One quarter that did was just as likely to die from coronary heart disease or stroke.[69]

A recent study published in the December, 2013, Annals of Internal Medicine showed that multivitamins had no effect on cognitive function or cardiovascular health and should be avoided.

On the other hand, many vitamin enthusiasts among them such well-known experts as Nobel Prize winner chemist Linus Pauling and Andrew Weil, M.D., feel that vitamin supplements can make an important contribution to physical and mental health. Obviously, when there are such pronounced differences of opinion among such creditable sources, more research is called for.

---

[68] Am.J. Epidemiol. 173: 90, .2011.

[69] Arch. Intern. Med, 169:294, 2009.

We must determine whether, as many say the need for supplements has increased because modern farming methods have depleted the soil to the point where food no longer provides us with the large quantities of nutrients that past generations enjoyed. Is this the case, or are others correct in saying that supplements are not needed because the plant's genetic structure, not the soil, determines the nutritional content of the plant?

These are important questions that urgently need answers. While awaiting these answers, what do you do if you want to provide your body with the best nutrition possible? Nutritionists, biochemists, and physicians at conferences I have attended seem to suggest that you should make every attempt to meet your nutritional needs through the basic food groups rather than through supplements.

The senior shopper does not have to go to a pharmacy or health food store to furnish the body with antioxidants. They can be found in any grocery store and reasonably priced.

Aware that these needs are not being met by the older person, the advertisers are promoting products to guarantee 100% plus of the required vitamins and minerals a day.

Many of the country's distinguished scientists produced a 500 page report that points out that most Americans get enough antioxidants through their foods and question claims that taking large doses is a wise move. Often the products, especially the ones with mega doses of vitamins, are not healthful but harmful.

If nutrients are to be used the person may think that increasing the intake will be beneficial, but according to D. George Blackburn, M.D, Associate Editor Health News, "it's tempting to think that more is better. But that's not always the case. A safe upper limit is especially important for healthy adults, who may have easy access to a plethora of vitamin and mineral supplements at any drugstore, but no guidance as to how much to take."

To assist the consumer, guidelines have been established by the National Academy of Sciences, the National Institute of Health, and the American Heart Association. Hopefully this should help you make the right choice. The Recommended Daily Allowance (RDA) for vitamins, set by the Food and Nutrition Board of the National Academy of Sciences-National Research Council, is gradually being enhanced using a new standard called the Dietary Reference Intake (**DRI**). The DRI is a general term for four different rating sets that will apply to vitamins, minerals, and proteins taken by men or women in specific age groups.

DEFINITIONS

(EAR)The Estimated Average Requirement

The Estimated Average Requirement (**EAR**) is the daily intake that meets the requirements of 50% of the population group.

If the EAR is unknown a rating called **Adequate Intake (AI)** is used, which is an estimate of average intake that seems to be healthy and not dangerous.

(RDA)Recommended Daily Allowance

The Recommended Daily Allowance (**RDA**) is the amount of selected nutrients considered adequate to meet nearly all the needs of healthy people. Since the need depends on the individual, I am reluctant to cite specific amounts but once again suggest the foods mentioned in prior chapters.

(IU)International Unit

It is a way to measure the amount of vitamins, hormones, and other biological substances. The definition of how much is in one **IU** varies from vitamin to vitamin and is set by international agreement.

(DV) Daily Value

The daily value for each vitamin or mineral is the Food and Drug Administration's (**FDA**) advice on how much it should receive each day from food and supplements.

(UL) Tolerable Upper Intake Level

These levels for the safe, upper daily limit is for adults only and will not always be cited. There is often inconclusive data as to the adverse effect.

It is important to know the difference between mg and mcg is a milligram or 1/1000th of a gram. For example: 5,000 mcg= 5mg.

Be sure you get the correct amount prescribed by the doctor as the difference of a few decimal points can mean a major over or under dose that could be harmful.

Since many health problems of the elderly are a result of poor nutrition, this chapter will help you to eat wisely and know how to safeguard your nutritional health. Wisely used, they can be a friend not foe. There is no substitute for a balanced diet.

Many of the country's nutritionists think that older Americans should use a multi-vitamin that provides 100 percent of the amount of the minimum daily requirement. Yet many of the country's distinguished scientists produced a report that most Americans get enough antioxidant vitamins from food. They question claims that taking large doses of vitamins is a wise move.

Not all multi-vitamins are the same and vary in quality. Look for a label that carries USP or National Sanitation Foundation (**NSF**) for more quality assurance. The label on the bottle should show you supplemental facts to guide you in making the right choice. This chapter will show you the foods to provide the vitamins which will assist you to stay healthy and enjoy the senior years.[70] Now, let's look at the vitamins from A to Z for the older adult.

---

[70] An author Richard A Maruttod, M.D., The Physicians Assessment of Elder Drivers. American Physician jan.2000,Vol.6 No.1

But first, a quick reminder that no amount of vitamins will compensate for a diet that is high in saturated fat, salt, sugar, and an excess of alcohol. Let the vitamins speak up and tell us why they are important. Keep in mind your individual needs can be different from dosages generally recommended. You should seek professional advice before you embark on a program of using vitamins and minerals as supplements in your diet.

Labels on bottles provide information on the daily suggested quantity of vitamins and minerals from food and supplements combined. The amounts have changed over the years, therefore, it is important that the requirements have been evaluated by legitimate sources like the National Academy of Sciences (**NAS**) or the Institute of Medicine (**IOM**).

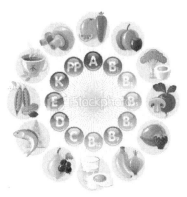

A nutrient is a chemical that the body needs to live and grow or a substance used in the body's metabolism which must be taken in from its environment. They are used to build and repair tissues, regulate body processes and are converted to and used as energy. Organic nutrients include carbohydrates, fats, proteins (or their building blocks, amino acids), and vitamins.

Vitamins are among the nutrients required for metabolism to supply energy and in some cases for growth itself. They are considered essential for good health, but are not synthesized by the body. The two major categories of Vitamins are: fat-soluble, and water-soluble ones. The fat-soluble ones are the vitamins A, D, E, and K. These vitamins are transported to the liver and stored in various body tissues. They are not normally excreted in the urine. These vitamins cause the greatest concern if taken in excessive dosages. The water-soluble vitamins (all members of the B complex and vitamin C) are excreted in the urine and are less likely to cause toxicity.

For many reasons vitamin-A may very well deserve to be at the top of the list. It is part of a group called retinoids and **is required for the growth and repair of body tissues, bone development, healthy skin, hair, teeth, nails and glands and vision acuity**. In seniors it is essential for those who want to drive in the evening and avoid accidents. It has been helpful in correcting night blindness.

> *Reminds me of the senior woman that introduced her friends to her new boyfriend who was most unattractive, disheveled and not easy to talk to.*
>
> *They asked her later, "Why Him?" She replied "He can drive at night."*

The importance of vitamins for eye health cannot be understated. Vision loss is a common manifestation of aging. Vitamin A, and many others also play an important role to give you good vision and protect you from the four most common eye diseases that stalk seniors: cataracts, glaucoma; age related macular degeneration; and diabetic retinopathy.. These ailments are often referred to as a silent stealer of sight because they unfairly progress, unnoticed by the senior until the problem causes severe vision loss.

But remember as stated by Elizabeth J. Johnson PhD. "It's always best to get the nutrients that help vision from foods." She also states, "Foods may contain many other helpful nutrients.

Sources: In suggesting foods that are rich in vitamins chicken liver will often be mentioned. I do so reluctantly, for one serving contains nearly twice the daily recommended maximum of dietary cholesterol and over four times the recommended daily intake of vitamin A. This would be toxic if consumed regularly. So although it is packed with protein and C vitamins, iron and zinc, it is better to eat chicken liver sparingly.

One of the major sources of vitamin A is the carrot. Mother Nature was considerate, for if you do not like carrots, you can fulfill your minimum needs of vitamin A elsewhere. There are other good sources. Better choices would be non-fat dairy foods such as skimmed milk fortified with vitamin A, low-fat cheese as well as paprika, red pepper, cayenne, chili powder, spinach, apricots, broccoli, cantaloupe, pink grapefruit, dark green and yellow vegetables, and butter nut squash. The greater the yellow or green color, the more beta carotene is provided.

Darkly colored fruits and vegetables are still good sources of vitamin A. However, according to Robert Russell, M.D., professor of Medicine and Nutrition at Tufts University, "It takes twice as much of them to yield the same amount of vitamin A in the body as we previously understood."

One and one half cups of cooked carrots meets the recommended daily allowance (**RDA**). It is still better to get vitamin A from food rather than a supplement. For example, lycopene which is the carotenoid in tomatoes may reduce the risk of cancer and may be missed in a supplement.

This is a larger group of about 600 nutrients known as carotenoids. Actually they are not vitamins. But since the most common is beta-Carotene and it is **converted in the body to vitamin A**, they are usually discussed as such.

According to American Institute for Cancer Research, carotenoids seem to prevent cancer by acting as antioxidants, that is, they scour potentially dangerous free radicals from the body before they can cause harm. There is also good news about their role in preventing several types of cancer, cardiovascular disease, and possibly dementia.

Although research to date support some of these claims, some warning lights have appeared recently to challenge this and suggest the need for investigations into the potential health hazards of excessive intake.

Sources: Sweet potatoes, kale, carrots, turnip greens, mustard greens, spinach, dried herbs, butter nut squash, lettuce, and collards.

Vitamin B Group

This group of B vitamins **has a vital role for the body to function at its peak level**. Who among us would desire less? They play an important role in many processes such as the breakdown and utilization of carbohydrates, fats, and proteins, as well as the synthesis of red blood cells, genetic material and the proper functioning of the nervous system.

Most vitamins in the B-group are involved in conversion of blood sugar to energy. Thus foods that are rich in B-vitamins are especially important for people who need more energy. I think it is safe to say seniors are in that category.

The government and scientific groups have focused a great deal of attention on B-vitamins. Many studies have been based on the vital role that this group has in reducing cardiovascular diseases, cancer, and mental disorders. Since January of 1999, the U.S. Food and Drug Administration has required food manufacturers of white bread and other refined grain products to supplement their product with folic acid, a B-vitamin. The FDA acted because folic acid helps prevent certain birth defects.

B-vitamins are essential for a healthy nervous system, normal digestion, energy, production of red blood cells, and muscle tone. It is also necessary for a healthy brain and heart.

Vitamin B-1 (Thiamine)

Heart abnormalities are also caused by the body's inability to burn sugar efficiently without B-1. Since the heart works all the time it must be continuously provided with energy. Digestive disturbance can also occur when B-I is deficient.

If a person does not get an adequate amount of this vitamin they can become tired and depressed. A severe deficiency can cause beriberi, but this is very rare in the United States. Malnourished people and alcoholics are a risk as are those receiving long-term dialysis or intravenous feeding. Symptoms may include visual disturbances, paralysis, staggering, loss of sensation in the legs and feet, psychosis, and congestive heart failure. No toxic effects have been reported for thiamin(B-1).

Sources: It is found naturally in brewer's yeast, sesame, sun flower seeds, dried herbs, spices, fish, corn, acorn squash, whole grain cereal, nuts, dry beans and lentils, breads and pastas. Cauliflower is a good source as well as lean beef.

Vitamin B-2 plays an **important role in the growth and production of the red blood cells**. It has a vital role in metabolism and contributes to the cells converting carbohydrates into energy. It may lower the risk of cataracts. The need for it seems to remain constant, but older adults may be especially deficient. This can lead to chapped lips, sores on the tongue, and vision problems.

The signs of multiple nutritional deficiencies are often a result of not obtaining enough of this vitamin. This is rare in the United States as vitamin B is easy to obtain. Studies at the University of California and elsewhere have indicated that a high dose of B-2 taken on a daily basis could help people suffering from migraine headaches. Seven hundred volunteers took 400 mg a day which is considerably higher than the recommended daily allowance. Almost four percent of the volunteers had fewer migraine problems. The researchers cautioned against taking such a high dose. [71]According to the researchers a smaller amount may work but only individuals having true migraine headaches should consider an increased amount of B-2 and it should definitely be under a doctor's supervision.

Sources: Liver and yeast, milk, yogurt and other dairy products, green and leafy vegetables (absorbed better after cooking), all foods made with whole wheat or enriched flour. Bread and cereals are often fortified with

---

[71] Neurology 50:46.1998.

B-2, another good reason to read the labels before you make your purchase.

Vitamin B-3 (Niacin)

Vitamin B-3, also known as nicotinic acid, helps to break down blood sugar for energy. Niacin **acts as a vasodilator widening blood vessels and increasing blood flow**. A deficiency of niacin causes pellagra. Symptoms can include eczema, intestinal and stomach distress, depression, thinning of the hair, and excess saliva production.

Anemia may occur, although this is probably due to an accompanying deficiency in folic acid.

Digestive problems may occur, including diarrhea and constipation, if the body does not get enough niacin. If the deficiency is severe mental problems such as depression and hostility may occur. Some doctors use high doses to lower the cholesterol level of their patients. In high dosage it acts as a drug and should be used only under a doctor's supervision.

Mega doses can be dangerous and cause severe reactions such as rashes, ulcers, gout, diabetes and damage to the liver. Mildly high doses can cause hot flushing of the face and shoulders, headaches, and stomach problems. Some who have increased the recommended amount have experienced heart disturbances and a decrease temporarily in their blood pressure.

Sources: Mackerel, salmon, swordfish, veal, chicken (reach for the white meat and remove the skin), lean meats, pork (lean chops), mushrooms, sun flower seed, nuts, dairy products, legumes, enriched breads and cereal.

Vitamin B-6 is **important for the normal functions of the brain**. It is essential before the unsaturated fatty acid linoleic and the many amino acids from protein can be utilized in the body. Without it tissues cannot be built, lecithin cannot be synthesized and blood cholesterol cannot be kept at a normal level.

B-6 can aid the functioning of the immune system and plays a role in white and red blood cell production. In one study when subjects were deficient of B-6 their memories deteriorated but the memories improved when B-6 was restored.

Low vitamin B-6 level is also associated with insulin resistance. Insulin resistance means that the insulin is less efficient at doing its job and delivering the goods and as a result sugar levels rise in the blood.

There is also evidence of increased carpal tunnel syndrome when the levels of this vitamin are low. Mega doses can cause sensory nerve disorders that can lead to pain and it numbness in the limb.

Sources: Oily fish, meats, fortified cereals and blood, poultry, whole grains, soybeans, rice, dried herbs, spices, raw garlic, avocados, baked potatoes with skin, watermelon, bananas, brewer's yeast, acorn squash and nuts.

Folate is a vitamin that is receiving a lot of recognition for its role in **reducing birth defects** such as spinal bifida. It is important for the normal metabolism of growing cells tissues and is used in the manufacture of neurotransmitters (chemical messengers in the brain), and also in preventing heart disease and for synthesizing DNA. It acts with B-12 to produce red blood cells.[72]

There are ongoing studies to determine if Folate and B-6 will lower the incidence of vascular and heart disease. Also being explored is if uncolored folate may protect against Correctol cancer. It may also lower the risk of cervical cancer and colon cancer. Folate may prevent the onset of cancer by preventing DNA damage. Other studies have demonstrated a link between deficiencies in the B-6 and B-12 vitamins, folic acid and elevated levels of amino acid.

A poor diet and alcoholism is the most common cause of folate deficiency. Conditions that disturb the small intestine can lead to a deficiency of folate. Smoking as well as high doses of aspirin can also contribute to this problem. High doses of folate can contribute to central nervous disorders and deficiencies of zinc. It can also delay the other B-12 deficiencies which can cause irreversible nerve damage. Symptoms include dementia and tingling or burning in the hands or feet. Always keep in mind there are virtually no nutrients

---

[72] New England Journal of Medicine, 337:230, 1997.

in animal based foods that are superior to that provided by plants.

While waiting reports of ongoing investigations and to be sure you do not take any excessive doses, enjoy the foods below.

Sources: Dark green leafy vegetables, spinach, citrus fruits, beans, bananas, lentils, wheat germ, fruits, green leafy vegetables, peas, yeast, cold cereals, foods that display on the label enriched whole grain flour. Eggs, milk and other dairy products, also liver, mushrooms, bananas, broccoli, tomatoes, whole grains, nuts, brewer's yeast and most of the other foods that supply B vitamins. Asparagus produces a healthy dose of folate. Biotin, as with all vitamins, is necessary for the metabolism of proteins and carbohydrates. It is also necessary with folic acid before pantothenic acid can be utilized. It is involved with the production of amino acid proteins and fatty acids. It is also produced by bacteria in the intestines.

Vitamin B-12 (cobalamin)

This is another vitamin in this important group that has a vital role in metabolism. It **helps in the formation of red blood cells and to maintain the central nervous system**.

According to a consumer report on health[73] B-12 prevents deficiency which can cause neurologic disorders. Even borderline-low levels have been tentatively linked with increased risk of cardiovascular disease, certain cancers, depression, and cognitive impairment.

Researchers in a study of 2,300 adults aged 72 or older indicated that roughly 7 percent had deficient levels of B-12.[74]

Most Americans get an adequate amount of B-12 in their food but 10 to 30 percent of older people lose their ability to absorb their naturally occurring B-12.

Mega doses can cause sensory nerve disorders that can lead to pain and numbness in the limb.

Sources: Oily fish, clams, crabs, meats, low fat milk, low fat yogurt, tofu, Swiss cheese, fortified cereals and blood poultry, whole grains, soy beans poultry, fortified foods as cereals.

---

[73] Consumers Report on Health Research, 1999.

[74] Am.Geriatr.Soc.60:1057,2012

Vitamin C (ascorbic acid)

When this vitamin is mentioned one will often picture a sailor munching on an orange or lemon to **prevent** the deficiency disease **scurvy**, a disease that played a major role in our history.

We can thank Columbus and other explorers from Europe. Scurvy is a rare health problem today because they brought oranges and seeds to our country.

Nobel Laurette Linus Pauling, PhD, who recommended **vitamin C for staving off the common cold**, is responsible for millions popping a pill to protect them from this ailment. Many researchers question his advice but I make sure to eat at least one orange a day because it tastes good and it is a healthy plant food that offers many benefits for the seniors.

Mark Moyad, M.D., of the University of Michigan reviewed, with fellow researchers, 100 studies of vitamin C. The results of the investigation pointed out how valuable it is in protecting our health.

Other studies say it can reduce danger of cancer and eye diseases.

Walter Eddy, PhD, at Columbia University said that if a senior citizen gets adequate amounts of ascorbic acid it will help them maintain their youthfulness.

Women's Health Advisor advises eating five to nine daily servings of fruit and vegetables an amount that supplies about 220-350mg of vitamin C rather than taking supplements. This is enough to almost completely saturate the blood and the food also provides many other disease-fighting nutrients and fiber. [75]

There are ongoing studies to verify the value of vitamin C. In the meantime it makes good sense to get it from the foods below.

Sources: The most popular source is citrus juices. They are high in this vitamin and a much better source of vitamin C than an apple, grape or pineapple. A group of substances known as bioflavonoid are in the pulp of the fruit (not the juice) and is also found in the rind.

Some feel that it is the bioflavonoid that reduces the need for Vitamin C and is the most effective. They taste almost the same as the fruit itself so it makes sense to eat it rather than discard it.

Oranges also provide a large amount of focalin as well as modest amounts of potassium, calcium, thiamin, niacin and magnesium.

Other good sources that will most likely surprise you are peppers, strawberries, broccoli, and peas. Also, according to the Department of Agriculture, papaya has as much as four times the amount of vitamin C as provided by one orange. Additional good sources are thyme, parsley, kiwi, fruits, strawberries, guava, cantaloupe, tomatoes, sweet and white potatoes, red cabbage, kale and acorn squash.

---

[75] Vitamin C supplements; Do You Need Them Women's Health Advisor ?December 1999

Vitamin D

Vitamin D is **important for the teeth, body tissue, and valuable to the nervous system, heart, blood, arteries, and bones**. If you live in the Sunbelt states and spend about 15 minutes outside at least three times a week you are most likely getting enough of this vitamin.

It could very well be called the sunshine vitamin for deficiencies are rare in sunny climates.

Do you remember the popular "Charles Atlas Advertisement" of the well-built man kicking sand in the faces of other men in the beach? It is fair to assume, because of his exposure to sun, that he had a substantial amount of vitamin D stored in his body.

For others who live in the north, there is concern that under exposure (especially for seniors) may put them at risk. Studies indicate that it may be a significant problem in the United States for seniors who live in the northern latitudes such as Chicago or Boston. A Massachusetts General Hospital study found that almost three in five did not have enough Vitamin D to keep optimum levels in their bones. By not getting enough of Vitamin D, they were 30-40% borderline deficient. The body is capable of absorbing only 10-15 percent of all calcium consumed thus endangering the patient to high blood calcium that may lead to kidney and heart disease. Deficiency can lead to bone loss and other disabilities such as osteoporosis and hip fracture and other disabilities troubling our senior population.

Bess Dawson Hughes, M.D., chief of The Calcium and Bone Metabolism Laboratory in the USDA Human Nutrition Research Center on Aging, states, "That aging unfavorably influences assimilation of vitamin D. First we know that women over 60 absorb vitamin D food less efficiently than woman under 30. As they age they lose bone at a higher percentage of loss due to menopause than their male counterpart."

A deficiency of Vitamin D can also cause a disease that weakens the bones and can make them break easier. As people grow older their ability to absorb **Vitamin D and, therefore, calcium** is diminished because of fewer intestinal vitamin D receptors, according to a status report on senior nutritional needs.[76]

Michael F. Holick, PhD, director of the Vitamin D Skin and Bone Research Laboratory at Boston University Medical Center, refers to vitamin D deficiency as a silent epidemic. As hypertension, it is also not fair. For adults over 50 it is usually silent and does not give warning until a lot of damage has been done.

Researchers[77] found that men with higher blood levels of vitamin D had a lower risk of lethal prostate cancer. However they found no link between vitamin D levels and overall prostate cancer or prostate cancers that were "aggressive" or advanced.

People with high levels of vitamin D in their blood have shown a lower risk of developing multiple sclerosis

---

[76] Status Report on Senior Nutritional Needs, Part 1 of a two-part series. Jan/Feb. 2000'

[77] Natl. Cancer Inst.104:1,2o12

an autoimmune disease that affects the brain and spinal cord that is believed to afflict more than 250,000 Americans, according to a Swedish study released in November 2012.

If you are vitamin D deficient, you will not be getting enough calcium. It is unlikely that you would receive too much of this vitamin from basking in the sun. Of course, you should use sun block to help prevent skin cancer and other problems. (Besides who needs more wrinkles?)

As with other supplements, mega doses can be dangerous. Prolonged uses of mega doses can have other serious effects such as calcification of soft tissue and life threatening kidney failure.

Another consideration is that certain medications can interfere with vitamin D absorption and retention.[78]

Sources: Oysters, cod liver oil, fatty fish, and dairy foods such as milk fortified with vitamin D. Breakfast cereals are usually fortified with this vitamin, fortified soy products, tofu, egg yolk, and mushrooms.

---

[78] American Journal of clinical nutrition 61: 1140, 1995.

Vitamin E

If there is one vitamin that is receiving a lot of publicity as a cure all for a variety of health problems, it has to be **vitamin E (also referred to as alpha-tocopherol)**; an oxidant that offers tantalizing hopes for the senior.

It **has been presented as a vitamin that plays a major role in slowing down the aging process,** by removing wrinkles from the face, and giving the skin a new vitality and youthful appearance. Vitamin E also is reputed to lower the risk of prostate cancer, cataracts, Alzheimer's, and heart disease. Is this "bailey-hoo", an exaggeration or for real?

Study after study came out with conflicting opinions. For example, researchers at Harvard University in 1993 studied this vitamin for eight years. Of 127,000 doctors and nurses that took supplements of Vitamin E all had about 40% less coronary disease compared to groups that did not. Needless to say, their report got the attention, of many seniors. It also stimulates drug companies to do more research.

Consumer's Report on Health made an encouraging statement in March 1999. The report states that Vitamin E protects against coronary disease and thrombotic (clot-related) stroke, may boost immunity, help prevent cancer, ease arthritic pain, slow arthritic pain, and slow progress of Alzheimer's disease[79].

---

[79] Health News February 2000

According to researchers from the University of Wisconsin, people with lower levels of vitamin E in their blood have a higher risk of cataracts. Earlier studies had shown that vitamin E inhibits the plaque in the arteries and that high amounts in the diet are associated with a declined rate of coronary artery disease.

Before you get too excited, the New England Journal of Medicine in January 2000 reported results of over 9,000 men and women who were at high risk of cardiovascular disease. There was an insignificant difference from those who took a placebo vitamin supplement.[80]

Researchers studied more than 69,000 men and women 55 or older. All had a poor health history and were a high risk group. After taking vitamin E daily for a period of four to six years no significant benefits were noted. A study in Europe also found a lack of significant benefits. Possibly it was because the people were at high risk. Perhaps it was too late to receive help.

Studies to see if vitamin E will slow the progression of Alzheimer's disease were conducted at Columbia University and elsewhere. High doses did slow the progression but Mary Sano, PhD, a member of the Cooperative Study, cautions healthy people against taking high doses of vitamin E. That may look safe but there are still a lot of unanswered question.[81] We don't

---

[80] New England Journal of Medicine. 342:154-160 January 20,2000 "The heart outcomes prevention evaluation study"

[81] 1 New England Journal of Medicine, 336:2167, 1997. 2 Study Finds a Lack of Evidence for claims of Vitamin E Wall Street Journal, 4-1100

know if the results can be generalized to people in the earlier or later stages of Alzheimer's or to people with other neurological disorders. "In earlier studies, vitamin E had no effects on Parkinson's or Huntington's diseases."

According to a report on dietary preference intakes from the Institute of Medicine of the National Academies, there is a danger in consuming large doses of vitamin E.[82] Investigations have shown that this can cause bleeding in people.

A Finnish study of 29,000 males who took both vitamin E (110 IU), beta carotene (33,000 IU) or a placebo for 5-8 years on a daily basis had no difference in the incidence of heart attacks.[83] In fact, in another investigation of the same group of men, those who had previous heart attacks and took the beta carotene were likely to die of heart disease.

"A direct connection between the intake of antioxidants and the prevention of chronic disease has yet to be adequately established," said Norman Krinsky, professor of biochemistry at Tufts University School of Medicine in Boston and chairman of the study committee.

Fortunately, for the health of the nation, there are many studies being conducted to help this dilemma pertaining not only to vitamin E, but of other vitamins and food supplements. While awaiting the results of the

---

[82] Journal of Internal Medicine, 1586 168, 1998.

[83] Lancet, 149, 1715, 1997.

various studies, it is wise and safe to obtain your requirements of the vitamin from the foods that you eat.

Do not expect a free face lift from a tube of vitamin E regardless of promises made by the advertisers. In regards to erasing wrinkles and making the skin more youthful in appearance, only time will tell. If it does rejuvenate the skin, it is likely due to the fact that it is an oil and will help keep the natural moisture from evaporating. Mineral oil will accomplish the same thing and it is considerably less expensive.

According to a 2011 study published in the Annals of Internal Medicine stated: that high doses of vitamins are dangerous and should be avoided. Most significant for the aging citizen is that you should not expect any pill or supplement to give you the benefits that can be provided by the foods you consume especially in the fruit and vegetable group.

Sources: Tofu, pumpkin, avocado, squash, wheat germ, nuts, seeds, fruits, green leafy vegetables such as spinach and broccoli. Vegetable oils are an excellent source and significant amounts are available in fortified cereals.

Vitamin K (alpha-tocopherol) natural

Vitamin K **has a vital role in the clotting of blood and prevention of bleeding**. It has also a significant role in maintaining healthy bones and healing fractures. The bacteria in our intestines manufacture most of this vitamin. The rest comes from the foods in our diet. Deficiencies are rare. However, patients who have problems absorbing fats such as seniors who have cirrhosis or are on long-term antibiotic therapy or taking medications could have a problem.

It interferes with Coumadin and other anti-clotting drugs. Easy bruising is symptoms of a deficiency of Vitamin K. Women who have a low dietary intake appear to increase their risk to hip fractures. It may cause insulin resistance. For people who have this problem the cells do not respond well and insulin builds up in the blood.

Sources: Bran, soybean oil, cabbage, Brussels sprouts, green leafy vegetables, spinach, kale, broccoli, cauliflower, collard-greens, Swiss chard, turnip greens, nuts, prunes, herbs dried and fresh, and cereals.

Choline

According to the National Academy, choline **is essential**

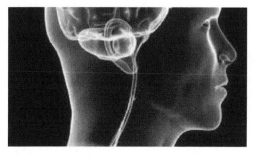

for fetal brain development and for learning and memory. For adults the level for choline was set at 3.5 grams per day; a higher intake could cause low blood pressure and a fishy body odor.

Sources: Richest source is brains, liver, yeast, kidneys and egg yolk. All are high in saturated fat. A better source of choline would be peanuts, wheat germ, vegetables, herbs, spices, broccoli, seafood, soy, and flaxseed.

Lutein is also getting a lot of recognition, and it is well deserved for it **has a number of potentially beneficial effects**.

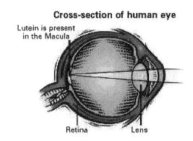

Cross-section of human eye

Lutein is present in the Macula

Retina   Lens

A study of over 77,000 nurses and more than 36,000 men in a follow up study indicated that those who ate lutein had about a 20 percent lower risk of cataract surgery than those who ate the least.[84] The National Academy of Science advises eating more carotenoid rich fruits and vegetables. Studies have shown the human body needs twice as many carotenoids as previously thought.

Sources: Oranges, egg yolk, fruits and vegetables (alpha and beta carotene), green leafy vegetables, sweet potatoes, and pumpkins. Seniors should add cooked kale and cooked spinach which are abundant in lutein which may lower the risk of cataracts and degeneration of the retina.

According to Steven G. Pratt M.D, an ophthalmologist at Scripps Memorial Hospital in La Jolla, California spinach may well be the better food to protect your vision.[85]

Zeaxanthin

[84] The ABC's of Vitamin A Veggie Revisited. U.S.News and World Report ,1-22 2001

[85] Amer. J. Clin Nutr. 70:432 509,517,1999

Zeaxanthin helps protect the eye from ultra-violet (UV) damage and prevents free damage to the retina and the lens of the eye that is associated with serious eye problems of the oldsters

Given the positive association between zeaxanthin and Lutein and age related diseases, it seems prudent for seniors to obtain higher amounts of these nutrients from their diet. However, the majority of people in the U.S. are not eating enough servings. Start and reach for the food below.

Sources: Cooked spinach, cooked kale, orange bell peppers, leafy green veggies, yellow and orange vegetables, fruit, egg yolks, orange juice, tangerine, collards cooked , turnip greens cooked.

> *Too Much or Too Little*

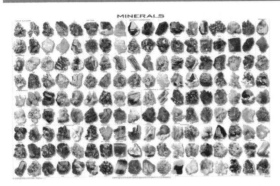

As with vitamins, **minerals are vital to the senior** to maintain a healthy lifetime. They are also readily available in the foods that are plentiful in our nation.

All of the unrefined foods grown on healthy soil contain minerals essential to normal life processes of animals, humans, and to the plants themselves. They are delivered to us by the soil, groundwater, and by the erosion of the sea, a continuous source to rely on to furnish our needs. There is considerable research regarding the minerals' role in chronic diseases that plague a high majority of seniors. Among them are coronary artery disease, high blood pressure, cancer, and osteoporosis.

Calcium

Calcium has an **important role in preventing osteoporosis** -- a loss of bone mass and sensitivity that increasingly makes bones fragile.

The levels of calcium in your body are very carefully regulated and kept at a low range so, if there is

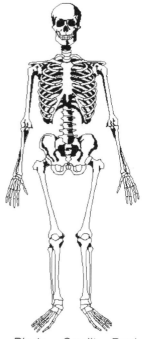

Photo Credit Paul Cooklin /Brand X Pictures/Getty

a deficiency, the body will absorb calcium out of the bones to maintain a constant level in the blood stream. If it does not, that means big trouble. Gradually your bones can suffer from this and develop osteoporosis. If the loss is serious, the bones will fracture more easily from even normal obstacles. This, unfortunately, is common occurrence. An estimated 25 million Americans suffer from it. Five million are men and 20 million are women. About 1.25 million skeletal fractures including 300,000 hip fractures occur annually in the U.S. as a result of osteoporosis.

It is not only the prevention of osteoporosis that should motivate seniors to get the proper amount of calcium. The cost of this problem to Americans was estimated in 1995 to be $13.8 billion. This includes the long-term care following a hip or other fracture.

Calcium is required for the blood to clot which could be a matter of life or death for the senior, especially after an accident. It helps to prevent hypertension. The proper amount decreases the risk of kidney stones. It is considered by some to be important in limiting the growth of cancer cells in the colon. Problems of insomnia can be ameliorated by getting enough of this valuable mineral.

Calcium deficiency is caused not only by too little in the diet, but by too much excretion of calcium in your urine. Even taking calcium supplements is not always the cure for this problem, and a problem it certainly is especially for seniors on a high animal protein diet. In fact, primary calcium excretion was 50 percent greater on an animal protein diet than on the vegetable protein diet. This is another good reason to limit the amount of meat in the senior's diet.

An interesting study of 6,500 Chinese found that although most consume no dairy products, osteoporosis is a rare problem in China. They get their calcium from the same vegetables they consume that helps them to prevent coronary artery disease. They may consume only one-half as much calcium as Americans, but the veggies help to make up the difference and to provide protection.

According to Chen J. Campbell, M.D., who was the author of the study, "Ironically, osteoporosis tends to occur in countries where calcium intake is highest and most of it comes from protein rich dairy products which cause the body to lose more calcium than consumed."[86]

It appears that caffeine in some older people may increase calcium loss. Therefore, Linda Massey Professor of Human Nutrition of Washington State University in Spokane states, "It's prudent to recommend that anyone over 65 get adequate calcium and no more than 300 milligrams of caffeine a day." That works out to two cups of brewed coffee, four cups of brewed tea, or six cans of cola or other caffeinated soft drinks.

According to Jean Mayer, PhD, U.S. Research Center on Aging at Tufts University in Boston, a three year study of 176 men and 213 women who were on average 71 years old concluded that people over 65 who

---

[86] C.J.Campbell TC,Li J, Peto R. Diet, Life style and Mortality in China." a Study of the Characteristics of 65 Chinese Counties". Oxford University Press 3-18-2000

do not consume three or four dairy products a day should consider taking a supplement to bring their total intake to 1,200 mg. of calcium and 600 IU of vitamin D each day. The recommendation is for both men and women.[87]

If you are taking 1,000 to 2,000 milligrams a day, according to Leon Ellenbogen, PhD, adjunct professor at Cornell University Medical College, the body may not be able to absorb larger doses all at once. He advises dividing the doses in half and takes one in the morning and one in the evening to get the best absorption. As with all supplements caution should be used.

Too much can lead to calcification in the kidneys and arteries. The danger of toxicity might be a larger problem than realized. For the senior, it is easy to furnish enough calcium to the body. You can get the recommended amount of 1,200 mg. by eating just three to four low fat dairy products. You can get the calcium you need from milk which is the foundation for all dairy products.

Yet, calcium and vitamin D are more deficient in the Western diet. Two cups of skim milk a day provides 27 percent of the RDA of protein for the average man, 33 percent for the average woman and it doesn't come with fat, unlike the protein in many meats.

Unfortunately, as previously mentioned, total milk consumption has been steadily going down. It has continued its slide during the past quarter of a century, giving way to cola's and other drinks.

---

[87] - N. Eng.J.Med, 337:670, 701, i1997.

At one point two main soft drink companies were contemplating an advertising campaign to encourage their consumption as a breakfast drink. Fortunately for the health of the nation, that idea was canceled.

Research indicates that diets that include plenty of calcium as well as fruits and vegetables may help lower blood pressure.

Sources: Cereals, soybeans, vegetables, turnip greens, orange juice, broccoli, beans, cheese, sardines, low fat dairy products. If you cannot tolerate milk try products with reduced lactose.

Chromium

Studies have shown that chromium **has a role in** 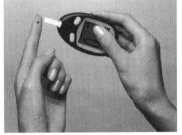 **stimulating insulin action in the body**.

It may lower the risk of diabetes and may help diabetics regulate blood sugar and insulin levels. Without it, the liver cannot function properly and excess fats cannot be removed from the blood.

Few serious side effects have been associated with an excess intake of chromium. As far as selected adverse effects there is inconclusive kidney or muscle damage. Since there is little information at the present time of adverse effects from chromium intake from supplements, no UL was set from the National Academy of Science.

Studies to determine the effect of reducing elevated cholesterol levels by using daily supplements of chromium were not encouraging. Chromium is widely distributed throughout the food supply.

Sources: Lean meat, poultry, seafood, sweet potatoes, vegetables, sweet potatoes, corn, white onions, brewer's yeast, fortified cereals, poultry, black pepper, mushrooms, fresh fruit juices, broccoli, whole grains and their products.

Chloride (chlorine)

 Chloride **regulates the balance of body fluids and acid base balance**. Chloride also activates enzyme in saliva, helps maintain proper blood volume, and blood pressure.

Sources: Vegetables, rye, tomatoes, lettuce, celery, olives, table salt and other natural occurring salts, fish, pickles, and smoked foods.

Copper

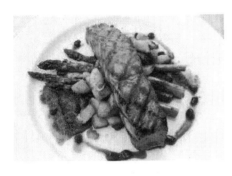

Copper is a nutrient that is **important for the liver and for the development of bones, nerves and connective tissue**. It is essential for the formation and synthesis of red blood cells. It also plays a part in the pigmentation of skin, eyes, and hair.

Sources: Seeds, nuts, sun dried tomatoes, spices, herbs, seafood, whole grain cereals, almonds, dates, beans, potatoes, and green leafy vegetables. Also available in chocolate, egg yolk, and liver. However, it would be better to obtain copper from the healthier foods mentioned at the beginning of this list. Beverages like coffee, black tea, coca, beer and wine have small amounts of copper.

Fluorine (fluoride)

Fluoride **has an important role in forming bones and teeth**. For that reason it is often added to water supplies. Many studies suggest that making fluoridated water available may reduce the incidence

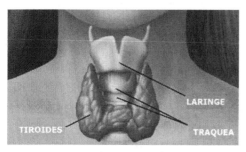

of not only tooth decay but the debilitating disease of osteoporosis.

Fluoride is part of thyroid hormones and is required for normal cell metabolism and reproduction. It can also lower resistance to infection. Deficiency, which is unlikely in the United States, can cause enlargement of the thyroid, mental retardation, goiter and dwarfism. You usually get enough from food. Larger doses can cause rotting of the teeth and bones. It is still a highly controversial issue in many communities that are concerned over potential health problem when fluoride is added to the water.

Sources: Sea food, pickles, grape juice, fluoridated water, tea, most animal foods and foods that are grown or cooked in fluoridated water, canned fish, gelatin, chicken, and cereal.

Iodine

Iodine is **an important mineral for thyroid heath**. It is

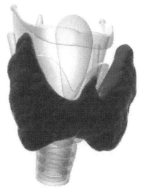

considered valuable in preventing iodine deficiencies including goiter. In an emergency caused by radiation exposure it is often used to prevent serious side effects.

The body needs iodine but cannot make it, so it must come from the diet. Most of the world finds it in the ocean where it is plentiful, especially in sea weed. An excess of Iodine can be harmful.

Sources: Sea weed, cranberries, cod, kelp, eggs, dairy foods especially yogurt, salt, turkey breast, potatoes with skins, navy beans, spices , herbs, fruits and vegetables.

Iron

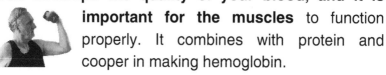Iron **develops the quality of your blood, and it is important for the muscles** to function properly. It combines with protein and cooper in making hemoglobin.

Hemoglobin transports oxygen in the blood from the lungs to the tissues which require oxygen to maintain the basic life functions. It is necessary for the formation of myoglobin which transports oxygen to the muscle cells for use in the chemical reaction that results in muscle contraction.

Iron is also present in enzymes that contribute to the protein metabolism and works with other nutrients to improve respiratory action. It is vital for the prevention of anemia.

An excess amount can cause gastrointestinal disease especially if taken on an empty stomach. Also there is a gene that raises the risk of too much iron.

<u>Sources</u>: Poultry, lean meat, seafood, liver, beans, lentils, dried fruits, eggs, leafy green vegetables, dates, wheat germ, and fortified cereals. In general the iron from animal foods is better absorbed than from vegetable foods.

Manganese

Manganese is **important in the formation of bones** 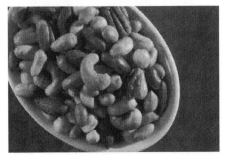 **and in the metabolism of fat, protein and carbohydrate.** It activates enzymes in the body. Animals deficient in this nutrient may show retarded growth, hyperactivity, abnormal bone structure, joint deformities, and uncoordinated movements.

Neurological side effects that were similar to Parkinson's disease were observed if a person consumed 15 milligrams a day. An excess amount may interfere with the absorption of iron.

Source: Whole grains, spices, herbs, green vegetables, nuts, beans, bran, wheat germ, and fruit. Mussels, oysters and clams, cocoa powder, and dark chocolate, seeds, chili powder, and roasted soybeans.

Magnesium

Magnesium **is important for bone formation and the** 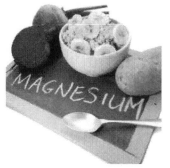 **function of nerves and muscles** including the regulation of the normal rhythm of the heart. It helps signal muscles to contract and relax. When the muscles, that line the major blood vessels, contract your blood pressure rises. It is also important for producing energy.

Studies have indicated that people who live in areas with hard water that contains magnesium as well as calcium and other minerals often have a lower incidence of heart attacks and stroke. It is suspected that too little magnesium could increase the risk of stroke, high blood pressure, osteoporosis, diabetes, and even migraines, but more study is needed to prove this theory.

Researchers have tried to give people magnesium to see if it lowers their blood sugar or makes their insulin work better.

A German study revealed that when 52 overweight people with insulin resistance,[88] were either given 365 mg of magnesium a day or a placebo, in six months, the magnesium takers had lower fasting blood sugar levels and less insulin resistance than the placebo takers.

---

[88] Diab. Obebs Metab.13:281,2011

If you are insulin resistant, your insulin doesn't work efficiently, and you have a higher risk of diabetes and heart disease.

Many Americans do not get enough magnesium to replace what they lose each day yet, it is plentiful in the foods so often mentioned.

Sources: Cereals, green leafy, beans, nuts and whole grain foods, vegetables, tea, bananas, apricots, milk, natural fruits and carrots, honey, blackstrap molasses.

Molybdenum

Molybdenum **is important for normal cell function**. It is essential for proper growth and development and plays a role in metabolism of fat, DNA, and the production of uric acid.

It is required to activate certain enzymes. Deficiency is rare in adults. According to the National Academy of Science impaired reproduction and growth in animals was present when there were high levels of chronic intake.[89] Toxicity symptoms cause diarrhea and anemia. A high intake may cause copper deficiency.

Source: Peas, leafy vegetables, cereal grains, organ meats, and nuts.

---

[89] National Academies Offices of News and Public Information, 1-30-2001.

Phosphorous

Phosphorous **works with calcium to develop and**
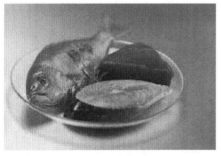 **maintain strong bones and teeth.** It is important for the growth and cell maintenance, to produce energy for muscle contraction and kidney function, and to transfer nerve impulses. It is also essential for DNA structure and cell membranes. High blood phosphorous levels may impact the body's use of calcium and iron. It may damage the kidney and the bones.

Source: Meat, fish, poultry, dairy foods (such as milk, nonfat yogurt, cheese), tofu, eggs, seeds, peas, beans, celery, whole grains, nuts, chard, pumpkin, string beans, and cucumbers.

Potassium

In previous chapters the importance of potassium intake

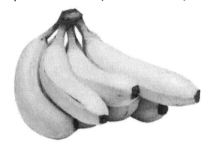 in **lowering blood pressure** has been discussed. But potassium does a lot more to keep us healthy. According to a study, **it helps to keep the arteries less stiff**. People with stiffer arteries have a higher risk of heart attacks, strokes, and memory loss.[90] Also in another study in the United States 1,000 healthy young adults without high blood pressure found that those who consumed more potassium and less sodium also had less thickening of the heart muscle.[91] Think of these studies when you peel that banana and thank it for its role in keeping you in good health.

Potassium and sodium help regulate water balance within the body. It is necessary for normal growth to stimulate nerve impulses for muscle contraction. It is vital for the proper functioning of heart and kidneys, and contributes to healthy skin. It unites with phosphorus to send vital oxygen to the brain. It also functions with calcium in the regulation of neuromuscular activity. Some evidence suggests that a diet high in potassium could reduce hypertension and stroke.

Source: Beans, spinach, dried apricots, fish, mushrooms, avocados, whole grains, seeds, nuts,

---

[90] Hypertension, 55:681, 2010.

[91] Hypertension 58:410, 2011.

oranges, bananas, dates, broccoli, potatoes, meats and yogurt. It is plentiful in many foods.

Selenium

Selenium **is essential for normal growth and development**, for proper functioning of heart muscle,

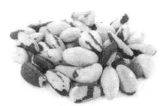

Selenium and iodine work together to keep thyroid function strong and consistent. Selenium is also important for proper immune response and is an antioxidant. It may lower the risk of certain types of cancer. Ongoing studies will help to determine its cancer fighting properties. Selenium intakes vary widely depending on the soil. There is not a specific area of the country where a person can be sure that fruits and vegetables have the proper nutrients and vitamins so eating a variety are recommended.

Researchers from Stanford University, the National Institute on Aging, and John Hopkins Medical School followed up on earlier studies liking selenium with the reduced risk of prostate cancer. They looked back at the blood levels of selenium that 52 prostate cancer patients and 96 healthy men had before any of the cancer appeared.

The men that had the lowest levels of this mineral were four to five times as likely to develop the disease as those that had higher levels. Since fish is rich in selenium it should be considered as a must for the senior's diet.

Sources: Seafood, poultry, pork, asparagus, mushrooms, whole grains, seeds, broccoli, onions, tomatoes, cereal and iron, brewer's yeast, garlic. Brazil nuts are loaded with selenium.

If you notice a loss of brittle hair or nails, you can be receiving too high amount of this mineral. Large doses, obtained with some supplements could be toxic. Other uncommon signs of too much selenium, can be gastrointestinal disturbances, fatigue, and nervous system abnormalities.

Zinc

Zinc is **an essential part of over 100 enzymes and is**

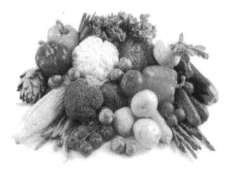 **vital for protein function and gene expression**. It is involved in digestion, metabolism, and wound healing. It is needed for proper taste and hearing.

Zinc is also a component of insulin required for blood sugar content. It contributes to a good working immune system. There are conflicting studies as to the effect of zinc on prostate and related disease. As with other treatments, the use of zinc supplements should be discussed with your doctor before using them. Too much zinc can cause nausea, impaired immunity, an increase in the LDL level (bad guys) and lower HDL level (good guys).

Sources: Sea food, squash, pumpkin, nuts, beef, lamb, pork, chicken, oysters, beans, yogurt, whole grains, fortified foods (such as cereals, milk), egg yolks, green leafy vegetables, peas, soybeans, brewer's yeast, and wheat germ.

Hopefully, after reading the chapters on vitamins and minerals the senior will appreciate the important role they play in helping the senior to "**Hijack the Aging Process**."

It is not complicated to furnish the body with an adequate supply of nutrients. Yet there is growing evidence that many seniors are not fulfilling their requirements. Aging may in itself make it more difficult for the senior to absorb and utilize certain nutrients. Many nutritionists are concerned that the vitamins and minerals that are insufficient in the diet for seniors are vitamins D, C, B-6, B-12, and folic acid as well as minerals such as zinc. There are many experts in this field that agree that supplementing the recommended daily allowance (RDA) of nutrients can help to reduce the risk of age or age related disease.

Yet, there are many studies that show a conflict of opinions as to the amount of supplement the senior should take and the possibility of a danger to their health from an excess amount.

If nutrients are to be used, the person may think I can keep increasing my intake. But according to George Blackburn M.D., Associate Editor, Health News, "It's tempting to think that more is better. But that's not always the case. A safe upper limit is especially important for healthy adults, who may have easy access to a plethora of vitamin and mineral supplements at any drugstore but no guidance as to how much to take."[92]

Since the needs of seniors vary and some supplements can interfere with your medications (hindering your wellness), you should not go on a program of your own. You may spend your hard earned dollars wastefully and dangerously. Registered dietitians, nutritionists, and your doctor can provide you with correct information for healthful living.

Do not be tempted to listen to individuals who are hawking their products without the adequate background to advise you about what supplements to take. Proper nutrition, exercise, and stress control (equally important and often overlooked) are all part of the equation to help you reach the numerical figure of 100 plus.

Select wisely from the food groups discussed in prior chapters for maximum health.

O.M.G.
- ➤ I'm Rich
- ➤ Silver in my hair
- ➤ Gold in the teeth
- ➤ Crystals in the blood
- ➤ Lead in the ass
- ➤ Iron in the arteries
- ➤ And an inexhaustible stable supply of natural gas.

---

[92] George Blackburn, M.D., The physician's perspective-safe amounts of vitamins. Health News, August 26, 1997.

> "The greatest discovery of our generation is that by changing the inner attitudes of their minds can change the outer aspects of their lives."
>
> **William James**

PUBLIC HEALTH ENEMY #1

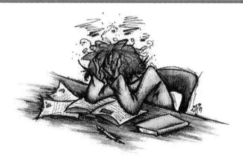

By now it may well appear the author has covered all bases so the senior citizen can march with a great deal of enthusiasm onto that 100+ mark. All you have to do is to **exercise on a regular basis, eat healthy meals, not smoke or consume too much alcohol. But** this is not the whole story. The risk factors such as genetics, cholesterol, blood pressure, obesity, age, gender, diabetes, and sedentary life explain only 50% of coronary heart disease.

What is that missing link preventing a full life for so many graying seniors? Dennis Burkett, M.D., a British physician in the 17th century may very well have answered that question when he stated, "Not everything that counts can be counted."

Shamefully, 400 years later, many physicians are just beginning to realize how stress can damage the body and, also, how easily the mind can heal the body. A doctor can measure one's cholesterol and blood pressure, and other lab tests can provide significant information about the patient's overall health. But it is difficult to measure the impact of emotional stress on the heart and other vital organs. As a result the importance of this association is commonly neglected, and a big part of the healing process is overlooked.

In 1985, the idea, "That psychological factors affect the course of disease was a dangerous myth," said Geoffrey Reed, PhD, a clinical and health psychologist, and a director of the American Psychological Association. More recently, studies that examine exactly those linkages have been published in major medical journals. Yet, very few articles on stress are presented compared to other medical subjects.

Many physicians tend to overlook the fact that the brain is connected to the heart and continuously sends messages that could damage the health of the coronary artery system. Medical technology mainly focuses on the treatment of heart disease rather than the cause.

You will meet in this chapter many of the doctors who are calling attention to the impact of stress on the health of seniors. Stress is finally becoming big news and is considered by many health experts to be the **"Number One Killer"**. Seniors are now dying at an - increasing rate resulting from life styles rather than infectious diseases. Stress-related diseases such as coronary artery disease, diabetes, alcohol abuse, depression and suicide are now considered to be epidemic.

Stress is usually defined as short-acute. Examples are: dodging a speeding car, being attacked by a dog, initial shock of a death in the family, or disasters such as a fire or flood. If it occurs suddenly the impact is much greater.

Chronic stress is more of a prolonged type, like being unhappy with one's work or family life, continuous poor health or financial problems. It can age you as much as any other single factor. This type of stress is manageable, and there are means to cope with it. Many seniors have developed remarkable coping techniques and thus be less susceptible to chronic disease.

New studies will be presented to show the relationships of stress, anger, and insecurity with heart disease and other serious problems. **Stress triggers a domino effect for the endocrine system**. The process starts in a part of the brain called the hypothalamus, which sends a message to the body's master gland, the pituitary. It signals the adrenal glands to release abnormally high amounts of stress hormone, Cortisol. This can result in abdominal fat storage and elevated insulin levels which have been linked to heart attacks, diabetes, stroke, high blood sugar, high blood pressure, a poor cholesterol profile, and other problems.

Yes, mental stress can either cause or aggravate the symptoms of most patients with ulcers, cancer, stroke, heart disease, migraine headaches, hypertension, and others. With care, however, stress can be brought under control and made to work for you, not against you.

Medical experts agree that over reacting to daily stress when combined with poor eating habits and lack of exercise can deal the final blow to the body's immune and other life-preserving systems.

According to one survey, during any six-month period approximately 29 million Americans or 18 percent of the population will have a stress-related drug abuse, or mental health disorder. Over 57 million Americans suffer from stress-related hypertension. Over the last several years 13 billion dollars has been spent per year on medical care for stress-related stroke. More than one in four Americans suffer from some form of stress-related cardiovascular disease. Men appear to be particularly susceptible to the effects of stress, which may explain the relatively lower life expectancy of males.

Stress, of course, is never listed as the official cause of a fatal heart attack or other chronic disease. Yet, stress can be brought under control and made to work for you, not against you. It is now rarely disputed that it is important for the senior to adopt methods (to be discussed) that will help you to do this. **Stress is inevitable**.

In a now-famous study, University of Washington psychiatrist Thomas Holmes, M.D., "Determined that the single common denominator for all types of stress is changing an individual's life pattern. This means that any change in your regular pattern of living, including taking a vacation, divorce, getting a raise, the death of a spouse, buying a house, and even Christmas creates stress, which may be positive or negative. Any out-of-the-ordinary event creates stress".[93]

According to a publication by the Office of Educational Research, U.S. Department of Education, stress is connected with life changes, personal and/or work-related. Too many changes at one time, either positive or negative, can overload an individual's capacity to adapt successfully and result in illness of one sort or another.

---

[93] Change in an individual's life pattern "Stress: Can We Cope? Time,6 June 1983

THE NEED FOR STRESS

We have come to **view all stress as harmful. The truth is; it isn't**. Hans Selye, M.D., director of the Institute of Experimental Medicine and Surgery at the University of Montreal, defined stress as: "The nonspecific response of our body to any demand made on it. It is immaterial whether the agent or situation we face is pleasant or unpleasant, all that counts is the intensity of the demand for readjustment or adaption."[94]

For instance, the mother who is told her son died in battle suffers a terrible mental shock. If years later, it turns out the news was false and the son unexpectedly walks into her room alive, she experiences extreme joy. The results of the two events sorrow and joy are opposite, but the stress they produce may well be the same.

The truth is that when someone says he or she is under stress, that person means excessive stress or distress. There is a great deal of evidence to indicate that every individual needs some stress for happiness. There are many individual differences, but stress is really the spice of life. As Dr. Selye said at a meeting of the Million Dollar Round Table of Life Insurance Executives; "Not only is stressing unavoidable, it is undesirable to avoid it. Any demand on the body causes stress, and is a great stimulus to achievement. You shouldn't try to avoid it; you should try to enjoy it."

---

[94] Understanding and Managing Stress in the Academic World. U.S. Dept. of education, Fall 1989

You could avoid stress by doing nothing but it would create a joyless world. Imagine living in the same room all your life. You wouldn't be bothered by stress, but you would wither away from boredom. Stress itself is not really harmful, since it helps us live life to the fullest. Without it life would be boring, boring, boring.

Always remember: Your life is not measured by the number of breaths you take, but by the moments that take your breath away.

Stress, of course, **can stem from simple or extremely complicated events**. You might, for instance, put yourself under stress by accidentally writing a check without funds to cover it. You handle it, however, by transferring funds from your savings account. It may cause a little bit of embarrassment, the need to make a phone call, and possibly the loss of a little interest of your funds but it is easily resolved.

Another example might be the theft of your wallet, containing cash and credit cards, while you are on vacation. This problem is more complicated than the first, but you eventually handle it by canceling the credit cards and duplicating the lost paper.

If you can control the situation including the many phone calls to an answering machine, the stress it produces is not harmful.

When individuals continually try to control an uncontrollable situation, they create problems for themselves. A good example is when a driver is stuck in traffic and becomes impatient and rants and raves over the problem, and continuously toots his horn. It will not ameliorate the situation but putting the radio on and listening to his favorite music station would be a more healthful reaction. It would certainly lower the potential for violence.

Richard S. Lazarus, PhD, points out that an essential factor in an individual's response to stress involves the person's appraisal of the situation and the manner in which the person copes with it. If complications of the situation don't outweigh the individual's ability to cope effectively, the effects of stress are minimized. But when the coping is ineffective and the stress prolonged, the individual who still struggles against it may well make himself or herself sick.

No-one knows if there is really more overall stress today than in the past, but many experts believe it has become more pervasive. It certainly is for our armed forces that are in harm's way and the families awaiting their home coming.

"A" May Be a Failing Grade!

How stress affects each individual, according to Meyer Friedman, M.D., a pioneer in the field of stress and its association with chronic health problems, depends on whether he/she is Type A or Type B.

The most dramatic proof that stress is a direct contributing cause of heart disease was provided by Drs. Friedman and Ray H. Rosenman,[95] who used behavior patterns to predict which subjects in a group of 3,500 would develop heart disease.

After eight years of follow-up, they found that the hard-driving subjects, whom they labeled Type A, had more than twice as much heart disease as the more laid-back subjects they labeled Type B, who go through life at a sensible and relaxed pace.

---

[95] R.H.Rosenman, et al.,"Coronary Heart Disease in Western Collaborative Group Study: Final Follow-Up Experience of 8-1/2 Years. "Journal of The American Medical Association 233 (August 1975):872.7.

Type A subjects had twice as much angina pain, twice as many fatal heart attacks, five times as many recurring heart attacks, and twice as many heart events.

Among subjects who died of other causes, the coronary arteries of the Type A subjects almost always showed far more disease than those of Type B subjects.

Among the subjects considered the most relaxed and whose cholesterol level was under 225, not one had a heart attack.[96] Dr. Meyer Friedman feels that the Type A factor is more important than exercise, diet, or heredity. Although he cautions against a diet rich in animal fats and cholesterol, especially for Type A men and women. He has found that Type A people have much higher cholesterol levels than Type B people. As we saw earlier, Dr. Friedman showed that tax accountants' blood cholesterol levels rose with the stress of tax deadlines and fell when -- the deadline had passed. Since the accountants were eating the same types of food during both periods and did not alter smoking or exercising habits, he felt the change in cholesterol levels could be due only to the added emotional stress. The researchers found also those individuals with extreme Type A behavior patterns exhibited every blood fat and hormonal abnormality associated with heart disease. Many cardiologists believe that these abnormalities may precede and possibly cause coronary heart disease. Doctors Friedman and Rosenman concluded that the Type A behavior pattern itself gave rise to the abnormalities.[97]

---

[96] M.Friedman and R.H.Rosenman, Type A Behavior and Your Heart (New York: Alfred a.Knopf, (1974}.

[97] Ratio of Type A's to type B's: "Altering Type A Behavior: UP for Debate." Medical World News, 14 April 1986.

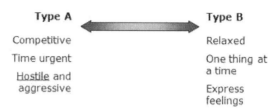

Type A	Type B
Competitive	Relaxed
Time urgent	One thing at a time
Hostile and aggressive	Express feelings

Are you Type A?

1. You feel a **sense of time urgency** -- that there is not enough time to do all the things you wish to do.

2. You are **impatient** with the rate at which most events take place. You frequently hurry others' speech and interrupt others to finish their sentences.

3. You often think or try to **do two things at the same time** (called polyphasic thought or performance). This happens when you talk to someone about one thing but at the same time are thinking about another. When you do this, you are neglecting to give the other person your undivided attention. A friend of mine brags that he can shave, read the newspaper, listen to the radio, and take care of his toilet needs all at the same time. You can often spot the Type A driver on the freeway using his electric razor, or talking into a cellular phone. A woman putting on makeup as she drives is exhibiting Type A personality, and if observed

doing so by an officer will be given an expensive ticket for negligence.

4. You have **difficulty just sitting and doing nothing**. Many Type A's feel guilty when relaxing Fortunately, I look forward to my quiet time each day when I can work in the garden or walk ,swim, or jog -- yes some Type A's can relax.

A Woman said to her husband "what are
   you doing."
He said, "Nothing."
She responded with anger, "That is what
   you told me you were doing yesterday."
He said, "I didn't finish"

---

5. You have **tense facial muscles** -- a facial expression of tension or anxiety.

6. You **jiggle your knees** or tap your fingers.

7. You frequently bring the **conversation around to your interests**. This can be a death-dealing characteristic. It has been shown in a study of over 12,000 adults that how often a person refers to himself or herself by using the words "1," "me," "my," and "mine" in an ordinary conversation actually -- predicted the recurrence of heart attacks.[98] A

---

[98] Scherwitz L,Graham L.E.2d,Grandits G,Billings J. "Speech Characteristics and Behavior-type assessment in the Multiple Risk Factor

good way to avert this problem is to ask others questions about themselves. It will also help you to maintain your social contacts.

8. You are **unobservant of life's details** and have little enjoyment of life.

9. You are **always short of time** and up against a deadline. Even in retirement you are always against a time factor and there's not enough time to do the things worth doing because of a preoccupation with the things worth having. Often a Type A Individual will say, "Sometimes I think that I never should have retired. At least then I had two days off."

10. You believe that success is the ability **to get things done faster than anyone else**. You fear not being able to do things faster and faster.

11. You feel **generalized hostility** and aggression--excessive competitive drive.

12. **Explosively** accentuating key words.

13. Playing all **games (to win** even with your grandchildren).

14. **Clenching fists,** pounding tables, forceful use of hands and fingers.

15. Facial expression of **aggression--clenching jaw**, grinding of teeth.

Intervention Mr.FIT structured interviews." J Behav Med. 1987; 10(2); 173-95.

16. **Irritation or rage** when asked about past events that previously caused anger.

Driving is especially hazardous to the health of the Type A driver. You can observe him or her as they speed down the highway honking his horn at slower drivers, tailgating and rolling through stop signs. They are undoubtedly responsible for a high incidence of the road rage episodes that are a growing problem. "They are driving themselves to death", says Malcolm Carruthers, M.D., a research pathologist, and Peter Toggert, M.D., a cardiologist. The doctors measured the heart rates of two groups of London commuters; one with a history of heart trouble and one supposedly fit.[99] The heart of a fit person beats about 70 times a minute at rest. After extreme prolonged exercise, the heart rate may rise as high as 210. The two doctors found that by the time the drivers had reached work the hearts of the fit person had sped up to 100-155, while those of the unfit had reached 180 -- the same level recorded for racing drivers after a Grand Prix. In both groups, the body produced extra adrenalin as it does during strong exercise. I often think of this when I feel tension mount while I am stuck in traffic. I know the healthy thing to do would be to get out and jog around my car to burn up the fatty acids, but I doubt if this act would be tolerated. I just sit back and listen to classical music. It works.

---

[99] P.Oglesby. "Myocardial Infarction and Sudden Death". Hospital Practice6(1971)

I am without question a Type A. My wife is a definite Type B. When she discusses events of the day with me, I constantly interrupt her and often finish her sentences which create tension for both of us. I get irritated when I have to stand in a long line in a bank to make a deposit, or at the post office, or wait to be seated at a restaurant. I hate paper work and I agree with the statement that, "A clean desk is a sign of a sick mind."

According to Dr. Friedman, I am a typical Type A personality. This does not make me a unique individual, for this behavior afflicts at least 75 percent of American men and 40 to 50 percent of American women. Dr. Friedman's recent studies show that the ratio of Type A's to Type B's may be as high as 8 to I or even 5 to 1. [100] I am learning to be patient, but it is not easy. The behavior modification techniques that were represented to me by Dr. Friedman have been a lifesaver and helped me to bring stress under control.

In terms of A's and B's, there are also overt A's. Overt A's have high drive, go at an accelerated pace, try to do too much in too little time, and are extremely competitive. When they start out to solve a problem they solve it. They, however, gradually give up on any situation which they cannot win and further struggle will only result in frustration.

I made an appointment with Dr. Friedman as I wanted to give him a copy of the Complete Prostate Book that I recently wrote, to thank him for all his support

---

[100] Adapted from M.Friedman and R.H.Rosenman, Treating Type Behavior and Your Heart(New York; Alfred A.Knopf,1984)

and inspiration. I arrived thirty minutes earlier as I wanted to beat the traffic. As I walked into his office he looked at his watch and expressed surprise, I said, "I know I am very early but I am type A. I have an urgency of time." We enjoyed a healthy laugh.

Dr. Friedman contributed so much to the wellbeing of our nation by his discovery of the relationship of Type A behavior to heart disease. His cardiac rehabilitation program which I observed has produced dramatic reduction against recurrent heart attacks.

Are you Type B?

If you are in this category and exercise daily and eat your vegetables you are on your way to becoming a centenarian.

1. You **do not feel time urgency** and its accompanying impatience. In my 64 years of marriage (to the same woman), this is one area where my wife and I had a great deal of conflict. My Type B wife is usually late. During our dating period, she could never understand my being 20 to 30 minute's early. Even currently, if we have a dinner date with friends at 6 p.m. I want to be in their driveway at 5:55. That is the time when she will start to put on her makeup and thus be late.

2. You have **no free-floating hostility**. You don't need to display or discuss achievements or accomplishments.

3. You **play for fun and relaxation**, not for superiority.

4. You **relax without guilt** and work without agitation.

Behavior modification techniques help the Type A make the transition to becoming a Type B. I work at it all the time. It is not easy, but it is worth the effort.

No longer do I wear two watches. I often don't even wear one. I take time each day to relax. My productivity, instead of diminishing, has actually increased.

Different personality types handle stress in different ways. A number of people have developed incredible coping abilities, self-control and personal strength. The results of this are not only increased mental and emotional strength and vigor, but also an enhanced ability to relax, stay calm, and be positive even under pressure.

When confronted with a stressful situation, the first reaction of the members of this group is one of calm reason and determination rather than resentment. These people recognize they can't afford to feel personally threatened by or even too concerned about the problem. Instead they take a lighthearted attitude, which seems to insulate them from the negative effects of stress.

One of the most notable examples of this quality is former president Ronald Reagan. Even with the stresses of running the country, Reagan always displayed the ability to let stress roll off his back while retaining a jovial attitude. In contrast the stress of the presidency aged Jimmy Carter considerably during his four years in office; Richard Nixon attributes the dangerous blood clots he experienced to the stress of Watergate.[101] Gerald Ford in contrast with his predecessor was most relaxed but did create stress for those who attended his golf tournaments and had to dodge his golf balls. George W. Bush has certainly

---

[101] **Richard Nixon:** "I Could See No Reason to Live" Time, 2 April 1990, 35.

displayed his coping powers. He was confronted with earth shaking problems yet he was able to guide the nation through the tense days that followed the September 11 catastrophe. He helped the nation to adjust to this calamity. Barrack Obama realized when the stress became overwhelming it was time for a brief vacation.

> *"I do not like political jokes. Too many get elected."*

The Type A personality is pretty well established as an aggressive and impatient, whereas the Type B personality as one who takes things more in stride and seems to enjoy life more without overexertion.

Dr. Friedman's researchers have found that **Type A victims have more of the so-called "struggle" hormone**, norepinephrine (noradrenaline), circulating in their bloodstream than non-Type A's.[102]

It is more difficult for Type A persons to rid their blood of the fat absorbed from their food. This is a characteristic of most coronary patients. Thus, decades before Type A's show any sign of coronary heart disease, they already possess one of the more notable biochemical attributes of the disease in its active state. A further discovery was the tendency of this abnormal accumulation of fat in the blood to cause red blood cells to adhere or clump together.

Reporting on his studies with animals, Baylor University psychologist Dr. James E. Skinner stated, "Having a blood clot in a coronary artery does not cause you to die. A psychological stress factor needs to be present." Dr. Skinner's laboratory blocked the coronary arteries of two groups of pigs, the animal whose cardiovascular systems are most like that of humans. One group was subjected to stress, the other was not. The animals under stress experienced a high death rate, while none of the other animals died, even though the major blood supply to their hearts was blocked. The psychological factor of stress was necessary for the blockage of the coronary artery to produce ventricular

---

[102] M. Friedman and R.H. Rosenman. Type A Personality and Your Heart. (New York: Alfred A.Knopf, 1974); Ernest and Roberts, Journal of Psychological Type 15(1988).

fibrillation, the death-causing rhythmical disorder of heart attacks.

Ventricular fibrillation is a kind of wild fluttering of the heart muscle in place of the regular contractions that normally enable it to pump blood to the brain and other parts of the body. Skinner reported, "It may be that brain activity alone is sufficient to cause the initiation of ventricular fibrillation without coronary blockage."

"Chronic stress," contends Robert Elliott, M.D., professor of medicine and director of the Cardiovascular Center at the University of Nebraska Medical Center, "can be a killer unless we learn to recognize it and effectively cope with it. "What can kill you", he tells his patients, "are hostility, impatience, and competitiveness."

He explains, "That although we don't yet know why, these behaviors increase the blood vessels' peripheral resistance to the heartbeat, acting as a clamp being forced down on a garden hose. The heart thus must pump against dramatically increased pressure, and there's a limit to what the heart can do."

He investigated the problem of aerospace engineers and technicians at the Kennedy Space Center in the mid-1960's. These highly specialized people who averaged only 31 years of age were dropping dead of heart attacks at an inordinately high rate. Their cardiac death rate was as much as 44.7 percent higher than that of an age and sex matched control group. Yet their cholesterol and blood sugar levels, blood pressure, smoking, and weight were well within normal limits. It was found that the main culprit was their fear of losing their jobs once their mission was completed -- a realistic fear since they had unique jobs in an unique profession and were not qualified to work in other areas.[103]

A good friend of Dr. Elliot developed a coronary problem which he attributed to stress that he couldn't handle. Although he had a master's degree in engineering, he left his field to seek a more relaxed career.

Occupations, Dr. Elliot discovered, such as air traffic controllers, are at risk. These controllers have five to six times more hypertension than a comparison group of aviation workers.

Dr. Elliot maintains that this distress is caused by a number of risk factors. Very specific events can increase the risk. For instance, he reports that of the 1,200 sudden cardiac deaths a week in the United States, almost half, 43 percent, occur on a Monday. According to Dr. Elliot's study, today's women are more stressed than men.

At the age of 44, Dr. Elliot had a heart attack while lecturing on how to prevent heart attacks. I think of this every time I give a talk on the subject. He was at the time a nonsmoker, not overweight, did not have high blood pressure, and had parents who lived to a ripe old age. He attributes his attack to a life that "had been a blur of over achievement to gain recognition." He now recommends to everyone to cope with modern pressures by relaxation, and suggests, "Rule number one is don't sweat the small stuff. Rule number two is,

---

[103] R.S. Eliot higher rate of sudden death. Stress and the major cardiovascular   disorders (New York: Future Publishing 1979 10

it's all small stuff. And if you can't fight and you can't flee, flow."[104]

---

[104] R.S. Elliot, Stress and the Major Cardiovascular Disorders (New York: Future Publishing 1979), 10.

Anger is only one letter short of danger. It is an emotion that is directly related to illness.

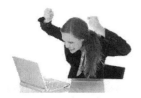

Everyone is burdened with some form of hidden anger and resentment but chronic anger or anger that is out of hand is dangerous to your health. Hidden anger tends to seep into our daily experience without our knowledge. Once the anger is lodged in the subconscious, it seems to take over with ill-fated results.

Studies by Redford B. Williams, Jr., M.D., of the Duke University Medical Center in Durham, North Carolina, suggest that high scores on a psychological test designed to measure hostility are associated with high risk of heart disease from all causes. These studies show that it is not the hard-driven workaholic who is at risk, but the hard-driving workaholic who is also angry, hostile, and distrustful.[105] You can spot them with their clenched fists pounding the table, a facial expression of anger correlation as rage. They have a lot of hostility toward many and are quick to point out all the negative things about friends, as well as enemies. They point out with irritation and rage about what is wrong with their workplace, country, and the world. Higher cholesterol levels as well as blood pressure are certainly not unusual in their health profile.

---

[105] Bottom Line-Health-Anger Trap, 4 1999, p.14.

Dr. Williams believes hostility is the critical component of the Type A personality and a potent predictor of heart trouble. Hostile people are more likely to meet daily challenges with large increases in blood pressure. The Type A might get extremely angry for example, if a customer ahead of him in the supermarket express line has 15 items in his basket instead of the permitted 10. He might even complain about it out loud to the checkout clerk or manager. Such situations just annoy the average person. The hostile Type A person may produce not only sharp increases in blood pressure but also a surge of adrenaline that is equivalent to the amount produced during heavy exercise. The extra adrenaline, however, is not burned up but instead releases fatty acids that clog arteries.

His research also found that a study of a group of doctors with high scores on a hostility test given during medical school were more likely to die during the 25-year-follow-up period than were their more relaxed peers. Only 2 percent of physicians with low or average hostility scores died, while 14 percent of physicians with above average hostility died during the same period.

In a related study, researchers followed a group of 118 lawyers who were given the Minnesota Multiphasic Personality Inventory test. Twenty years later those with the higher hostility scores died at a rate of 4-12 times higher than those with low scores.

According to Murray Mittleman, M.D., having a hostile disposition is also likely to set you up for a heart attack. The doctor, who is a cardiovascular epidemiologist at the Beth Israel Deaconess Medical

Center in Boston, interviewed 1623 men and women who had experienced a stressful incident, on average, four days prior to their heart attack. The risk of having an attack was more than twice as great as expected if they had been very angry in the two hours before the attack.

Suggests Mittleman: If stress mounts so high that you begin snapping at people, ask yourself, "Is it worth having a heart attack over this?"

A study by epidemiologist Janice Williams indicated that people who are highly anger-prone are nearly three times more likely to have a heart attack.

The connection between anger and heart attacks held true even after researchers took into account other major risk factors such as high blood pressure, high cholesterol, smoking, and obesity.

"Anger could potentially lead to heart attacks, especially among middle-aged men and women with normal blood pressure," said Williams.

Previous studies have shown stress hormones constrict blood vessels and may trigger a blockage in the arteries.

An eight year study of 2110 men was presented at a meeting of the American Heart Association by Susan A. Everson, PhD, MPH, department of Epidemiology, University of Michigan School of Public Health at Ann Arbor. The study disclosed that men who, when angered, lost their temper in explosive outbursts were twice as likely to suffer a stroke as men better able to control their feelings. The exact connection between anger and stroke is unclear, but being careful to avoid anger-provoking situations may help.

So seniors, keep in mind what Horace Greely stated in 65 B.C.: "Anger is short-lived madness."

If you identify with the angry type person no need to blush or fret. You can modify your behavior. The next section will direct you so you can join your more relaxed type of senior on the pathway to longevity.

Before we discuss how to let go of stress, this test will help you know how vulnerable you are. This test was developed by psychologists Lyle H. Miller and Alma Dell Smith at Boston University Medical Center. Score each time from one (almost always) to five (never), according to how much of the time each statement applies to you.

1. I eat at least one hot, balanced meal a day.

2. I get seven to eight hours sleep at least four nights a week.

3. I give and receive affection regularly.

4. I have at least one relative within 50 miles on whom I can rely.

5. I exercise to the point of perspiration at least twice a week.

6. I smoke less than half a pack of cigarettes a day.

7. I take fewer than five alcoholic drinks a week.

8. I am the appropriate weight for my height.

9. I have an income adequate to meet basic expenses.

10. I get strength from my religious beliefs.

11. I regularly attend club or social activities.

12. I have a network of friends and acquaintances.

13. I have one or more friends to confide in about personal matters.

14. I am in good health (including eyesight, hearing, and teeth).

15. I am able to speak openly about my feelings when angry or worried.

16. I have regular conversations with the people I live with concerning domestic problems; such as chores, money, and daily living issues.

17. I do something for fun at least once a week.

18. I am able to organize my time effectively.

19. I drink fewer than three cups of coffee (or tea or cola drinks) a day.

20. I take quiet time for myself during the day.

To get your score, add **up the figures and subtract 20**.

Any number **over 30** indicates a vulnerability to stress.

You are seriously vulnerable if your score is between **50 and 75**, and extremely vulnerable if it is over 75.

Type C Personality

Now medical researchers are talking about the Type C personality. They love details. They are not assertive and most often suppress their own desires even if it relates to something they dislike which often causes tremendous stress and sometimes depression. They are very vulnerable to depression compared to Type A and Type B.

Lydia Temoshok, PhD, psychologist at the University of California, San Francisco, says that Type C's are completely opposite to the hard-driving, get-out-of-my-way Type A's.[106]   For example, the patients afflicted with melanoma were super cooperative, nice to a fault, and without a visible trace of hostility. Their feelings are so far beneath the surface that they have lost awareness of how they really do feel. The energy required to prevent feelings from bubbling to the surface. Dr. Temoshok says, may weaken the system and open the door to cancer. When asked about the difficulties of coping, these individuals passed off the idea as being related to other people and not themselves.

Cancer patients who talked about past emotional experiences, discussed their feelings openly, and actively sought to overcome their disease had a far greater survival rate than patients with a stoic attitude.

Canadian physician Gabor Mate, M.D., studied Type C personality for many years. He found that they are susceptible to illness because they are unable to

---

[106] Gary Kamiya, the Cancer Personality," Hippocrates, November/December 1989:92-93.

express anger or recognize the primacy of their own needs. They are always doing things for others.

Many researchers also now believe that cancer, arthritis, ulcerated colitis, asthma, migraine headaches, and numerous psychosomatic disorders are associated with very distinct personality types and specific clusters of personality traits.

It used to be thought that the mind and the immune system existed independently of each other, but extensive research shows that they may very well act as a single unit. For example, if you feel stressed, you can be more susceptible to whatever virus is going around. But if you are feeling in good spirits, your immune system will be more resistant and better able to protect you. Expectation plays an important role. If you expect to be healthy you will increase your chances of enjoying good health.

A good example of stress is:

You pick up a hitchhiker, a beautiful girl. Suddenly she faints inside your car and you take her to a hospital. Now that's stressful. But at the hospital they say she is pregnant and congratulate you on becoming a father. You say that you are not the father, but the girl says you are. This is getting very stressful!

So, you request a DNA test to prove that you are not the father. After the tests are completed, the doctor says that you are infertile and probably have been since birth. You are extremely stressed but relieved.

On your way back home, you think about your 3 kids at home.

Now that's Stress!

HANDLING STRESS

Fill your bowl to the brim and it will spill.

Keep sharpening your knife and it will blunt.

Chase after money and security and your heart will never unclench.

Care about people's approval and you will be their prisoner.

Do your work, then step back the only path to serenity.

Tao Ching

(four thousand years ago.)

LETTING GO OF STRESS

You have heard the expression, '**think positive**'. This is 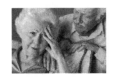 a significant recommendation for letting go of stress. According to a study a positive emotional state may help older adults live longer and more independently.

"Positive affect, defined as a state of emotional well-being, appears to protect against the physical declines of older age" reported Glenn V. Oster, PhD, and colleagues of the University of Texas Medical Branch, Galveston. The study included a group of over 2000 Mexican-Americans aged 65-99 who all had good daily functions.

Emotional well-being was assessed by four simple questions:

1. They felt they were as good as other people.
2. They felt hopeful about the future.
3. They felt happy.
4. They enjoyed life.

The result suggests that seniors, who have a positive attitude, are health conscious, exercise regularly, and have a good circle of friends and family to provide social support, have a greater chance of aging with youthful vigor.

Sliding down a spiral of declining energy and health is largely a matter of personal choice not fate, according to Richard Vulliet, professor of pharmacology at the University of California at Davis. He further states, "It's dismal to think that there is nothing that you can do but sit and waste away."

Negative attitudes and not being able to prevent stress from converting to distress are self-destructive and are depleting to your physical and mental wellbeing. Often, it is not possible to change your environment, or your current situation as a means of eliminating stress. If you do eliminate stress, the same stresses may crop up again in other situations. Fortunately, research has shown that it is only necessary to change yourself and the way you relate to stress to really make a difference.

Harry Truman used to say, **"If you can't stand the heat, get out of the kitchen."** During the last days of World War II, President Truman was asked how he managed to bear up so calmly under the stresses of the presidency. "I have a foxhole in my mind," he replied. The same way a soldier retreats into his foxhole for protection and respite. He periodically retreated into his mental foxhole where he allowed nothing to bother him. In doing so, he was following the wisdom of Marcus Aurelius, who wrote, "Nowhere either with more quiet or more freedom from trouble does a man retire more than into his own soul."

Stress often leads to a state of depression. More than two million of the 34 million Americans age 65 and older suffer from some form of depression, according to the National Institute of Mental Health.[107] It has become more commonly recognized and diagnosed among the senior population. More frightening is the fact that major depression, the order most associated with suicide in elderly Americans, is a widely unrecognized and under treated medical illness. Yet, depression is not a normal part of aging. The techniques, that can be used to

---

[107] Depression- Department of Health and Human Services. National Institute of Health, NH Publication No.00561, 2000.

prevent and treat chronic stress as well as depression, are workable and worth the effort to engage. According to the National Institute of Health, the cost in human suffering cannot be under estimated.

Following is a list of the most common signs of depression. If any of these last more than 2 weeks you should seek help.

1. An empty and sad feeling of being alone with anxiety.

2. Lack of energy and always feeling tired and irritable.

3. Loss of interest in activities that generated a lot of pleasure including sex.

4. Having problems with sleeping and awakening much earlier than usual.

5. Problems with eating and sudden gain or loss of weight.

6. Crying often when negative thoughts surface in your mind.

7. Aches and pains that pop up in areas that were not present before.

8. Finding it difficult and unsettling to make decisions.

9. Worried about the future and your lack of ability to improve it.

10. Seriously contemplating suicide.

Sadly, although this illness is devastating to the individual and to the family, most people do not seek help -- and help is available. As a result of years of productive research, even the most severely depressed individual can be helped. If stress or depression is a severe problem to you -- help has arrived.

Guidelines will now be presented to further your ability to get rid of the listlessness, hopelessness, and the events that are diminishing the quality of your life.

There are nine ways to help you let go of stress:

1. **Start the day** with this brief prayer.

> "God grant me the serenity to accept the things that I cannot change, the courage to change the things that I can And the Wisdom to know the difference".

2. **Minimize the source** of your concerns.

3. **Participate in activities** that will hold your attention. Going outside to garden, even watching television, diverts the mind away from negative thoughts (depending on the program). This can relieve the hopelessness you feel and contribute to the attitude that there may be a way you can ameliorate your predicament.

4. If you are **Type A, try to avoid others** with a similar personality. I do not enjoy playing tennis with other type A's especially the angry type where winning is the only thing that matters.

5. **Eat healthy**. There is a definite link between diet and mental and emotional well-being. If a senior eats right it will promote more of a youthful feeling and certainly affect their appearance. Improper eating habits contribute to obesity, poor complexion, and loss of energy which adds a lot of unwanted and unnecessary stress to the elder person. Looking in the mirror can start you off with a positive or negative

feeling. The statement that "you are what you eat" is an old but truthful one.

6. **Get a pet**. No doubt about it! You can talk to them all day or night and they will listen and only give you positive feedback. Erika Friedman, PhD, associate professor, Brooklyn College, finds in her research that pets have a tranquilizing effect that markedly lowers the heart rates of Type A participants. Regular contact with pets, she reports, can provide direct health benefits by reducing stress. Pets provide companionship and love and help calm the individual down. It also gives you another good reason to walk each day.[108]

U.C.L.A. has developed a People Animal Connections program, an innovative plan that brings dogs into the hospital to spend quality and happy time with patients.

"The hospital environment is very high-tech, very sterile, and a person can feel so deprived," says Katherine Brown-Saltzman a clinical nurse specialist. "When suddenly into that environment you place an animal, you're bringing back some of the normalization of nature."[109] The concept is so popular that there is an ever-increasing need for volunteers to share their pets -- not only with older

---

[108] A.H.Katcher, E., Friedman, A.M.Beck, et al. "Looking, Talking, and Blood Pressure L the Physiological Consequences of Interaction with the Living Environment, in A. H" "Katcher and A.M.Beck (eds). New Perspectives in Our Lives with Companion Animals (Philadelphia; University of Pennsylvania Press, i983) 351-59.

[109] Julie E.Bowles Good Medicine. U.C.L.A. Magazine, Spring 2001, p42.

patients in hospitals but in rest homes. The volunteers say that it is so gratifying to see their faces light up and the big smile as they enter the room. The pets also look forward to the visits and the wagging of the tails increase as they make contact.

Mary Oliver, 80, of Encina, spent several weeks at UCLA while preparing for bypass surgery and received several visits from four-legged friends "they are just adorable when they snuggle up on the bed with you," she says. "They brighten up your day. I say they're more human than humans."[110] There is no question in medical centers that animals do play a significant role in reducing anxiety and depression as well as loneliness. Yet, it is not a new realization. As far back as 1792, animals were used in the healing process in York, England. Currently volunteers are observed at the Beth Israel Hospital in New York City roaming through rooms to comfort patients in pediatrics, rehabilitative medicine, neurosurgery, and to the delight of seniors -- geriatrics.

Cuddle a dog, or pet a cat, and the patients will most likely forget for the moment the fear of their illness. Hopes for recovery brighten up.

7. **Laughter**. As discussed earlier and worth repeating, a laugh is a total body experience. It not only helps to relieve stress; it is good medicine. Laugh, laugh again and you will grow old later, much later.

---

[110] Ibid.

8. **Be friendly** -- be sociable. They are great stress busters. Loneliness increases the level of distress for the elderly. Scientists are convinced that if the senior is socially isolated the less healthy they will be both psychologically and physically, and the more likely they will be to die. But inversely, if they have good social and family relationships, they have a greater chance to live to make it to 100+. The physical and psychological benefits of support from friends and family can be dramatic.

Studies conducted over a nine-year period in Alameda County, California, for example, have indicated that people who have extensive networks of social support may live longer than those who do not. Social support can reduce stress symptoms following the loss of a loved one. It helps speed recovery from surgery and heart attacks, and alleviates the symptoms of asthma and other disorders. Good friends are essential for good health. Former President Lyndon Johnson said, "Make friends before you need them."

While surveying unemployed workers in the Detroit area, University Researcher Louis Ferman found one hard-luck victim who had been successively laid off by the Studebaker Corporation in 1962. Then in the 1970s, he was working for a truck manufacture that went under. Later, he was released during cutbacks at a Chrysler plant. By all accounts, "he should have been a basket case, yet he was one of the best adjusted fellows I've run into" says Ferman.

Asked his secret, the man replied, "I've got a loving wife and go to church every Sunday."

A close-knit family and a social structure that provides a lot of tender loving care may be the best guarantee the graying senior will live a long and healthy life.

A study of 3,809 Japanese men aged 30-79 years, who maintained the traditional life style of close family and social contacts revealed a reduced risk of coronary heart disease. In fact, the investigators found the Japanese-American men with the greatest social isolation and most traumatic life events had twice the risk of dying of coronary heart disease.

S. Leonard Syme, PhD, of the University of California, Berkeley, School of Public Health, who reported on the study also said, "The lowest rate of coronary heart disease in the United States is among Seventh Day Adventists who also have more extensive social relationships than most Americans. It seems that people need people." Perhaps this factor is as important as the low fat diet of the Japanese and Seventh Day Adventists. Some researchers say that T.L.C. (Tender Loving Care) may be one of the best protections against the build-up of cholesterol deposits in the arteries. While studying the effects of various diets on rabbits, researchers at Ohio State University accidentally discovered that the animals that were cuddled, fed individually, and talked to showed only half the number of lesions (considered the forerunner of heart disease) of the others. Amazed, the researchers tried the experiment again several times with identical results -- "dramatically reduced arteriosclerosis."

According to Fred Cornhill, M.D., of O.S.U.'s College of Medicine: "Although they have no explanation for these results, they speculate that T.L.C. may affect the growth of the endothelial cells that line arterial walls and that provide a barrier between the wall and unwanted materials like cholesterol." Or, said Dr. Cornhill, "It may be a myriad of other factors, we just don't know about yet." A study published in the February 1997 Lancet (which is considered a most reliable publication in Great Britain) identified withheld and denied emotions, social inhibition, and lack of social support as risk factors for heart disease. Many consider it as great a mortality risk as smoking. Anything that contributes to making a person feel "alone out there" can build up to chronic stress.

Being with others can help the senior live longer and more independently. It will help the adult develop a positive emotional state that will contribute to a healthier immune system.

9. **Spend time with your grandchildren.** If you do not have any, borrow someone's. Your friends would be delighted. They are great stress busters. Take them to the zoo or park. You can go on the same rides, play on the swings or games such as "Hide-and-Seek." You can be silly, forget about the stock market or what's happening to Medicare. You can even take them to a good old fashioned western and not worry

about being seen at a movie for youngsters. Needless to say they are a lot of fun. As one senior remarked, "If I knew they were so much of a joy, I would have had them before my children."

Seniors love jokes about their grandchildren.

A grandson visiting his grandparents asked his grandmother: "Grandma where did I come from?" She answered, "God made Adam and Eve and they had children and then all mankind was made."

He was a little confused at this answer and went out to the garden where his grandfather was working and asked him the same question.

It was hot and his grandfather was tired from picking weeds for the past hour and in a grouchy mood.

He responded with a crusty voice, "We all came from monkeys. The human race evolved from monkeys."

Now the boy was even more confused and returned to his grandmother and said, "Grandma, how is it possible that you told me the human race was created by God and Grandpa said we developed from monkeys."

His Grandmother answered, "Well dear, it's very simple to explain. My side of the family came from God and his side came from monkeys."

An 8 year old girl went to her grandfather who was working on his car and asked him "Grandpa what is couple sex?"

He was amazed that she would ask this question at such an early age, but decided that if she was old enough to know to ask this question, he should give a straight and honest answer. Steeling himself not to leave anything out, he proceeded with telling her all about human reproduction and the joys and responsibilities of intercourse.

When he finished explaining, the little girl was looking at him with her mouth hanging open, eyes wide open in amazement. Seeing the look on her face, the grandfather asked "Why did you ask this question, honey?"

The little girl replied, "Grandma says that dinner will be ready in just a couple 'secs'."

A grandpa walked in to his daughters home to babysit his grandchildren. As soon as they saw him, they shouted together "Grandpa please imitate a frog". He responded "No, I don't want to." They persisted in asking and he inquired "Why"? They answered "Grandma said when you croak we will all go to Disneyland."

A 5 year old boy was visiting his grandmother one day. He was playing with his toys while she was dusting. After a while he looked up and asked "Grandma, how come you don't have a boyfriend now that Grandpa is in heaven?"

She replied: "Sweetheart my TV is my boyfriend. I can sit in my bedroom all daylong and if I am sad, I can listen to religious programs, or if I need a good laugh, I can tune in and watch comedians".

In fact you reminded me my favorite program is on now. She tried to turn on the set but nothing happened. She tapped it again, but still no picture. She got mad and started to bang it but still no response. She banged it again but still no picture.

The doorbell rang and with an angry voice told her grandson to open the door. It was their priest who said, "Hello son is your grandma home? I came to visit her and offer my support for the loss of your grandfather."

He replied, "Wait I will get her she's in the bedroom banging her boyfriend."

A little girl watched fascinated as his grandmother gently rubbed cold cream on her face. "Why are you rubbing that on your face grandma? The little girl asked. "To *make myself beautiful," the grandmother answered.*

The next morning she saw her removing it and asked "Are you giving up Grandma?"

Up to 30 million Americans live alone. As the population grows older it will increase. Living by yourself doesn't necessarily mean you will feel isolated but, for most, it takes some time to get used to this feeling. Attending a church or synagogue or mosque may be a good way to make a connection.

One key to overcoming loneliness is reaching out to other people. An investigation by scientists at the University of Michigan studied 2,754 people over a ten year period and found that "men who did no volunteer work were 2-1/2 times more apt to die during the study than men who volunteered at least once a week."[111] Give of yourself. Doctors and researchers are now finding that people with an altruistic spirit tend to stay healthier and live longer. The converse also seems to be true: According to research done at the Medical Research Institute of San Francisco by Larry Scherwitz, PhD, self-centered people are much more likely to die of a heart attack than less self-centered people.[112]

---

[111] House, J. S. Robbins, C., Metzner, and H. L. "The Association of Social Relationships and Activities with Mortality   Prospective Evidence from the Tecumseh Community Health Study." Am J Epidemiol 1982:116)1): 123; 40.

[112] Emotional Well-Being Linked to Improved Functioning and Survival of Older Adults. Journal of the American Geriatrics Society.3=1'00.

I am surprised that the Red Cross, United Welfare agencies and others that are always in need of volunteers have not been active in publicizing this study.

Today more than ever you can receive support by mail, phone, e-mail, and Facebook. The Internet provides for the first time a method to cultivate a new range of contacts. The exchange of humorous stories, political and international news, and sharing personnel times can be a safe and comfortable means of support.

A positive emotional state may help adults live longer and more independently. A "**positive effect**" (defined as, "a state of emotional well-being) appears to protect individuals against the physical deadlines of older age," reports Glen V. Oster, PhD, colleagues of the University of Texas Medical Branch, Galveston. A positive emotional state might protect health in many ways. "The senior will be more inclined to exercise, be more health conscious and socially active. Think sick, be sick."

Being down in "the dumps" over a period of time is not a normal part of growing old. However, it is a common problem, which may require help. Friends to "talk-to", and share a good joke may be all that is needed. If there is pain and serious depression, medical help should be sought. There is so much that a senior can do for themselves -- without drugs and without medical intervention.

You have the internal power to relieve yourself of depression, loneliness, anger, and other factors that foster the angry process. Just as with physical activity, it is possible to lower high blood pressure without the use of hypertensive drugs. There are many techniques that have proven effective to lower the pressure on your mind. In looking for that Fountain of Youth, one may look not outside the body but within.

By now the reader should be far ahead of other graying citizens by realizing that lifestyle is the one main thing, above everything, that determines how successfully you age. Hopefully, you are developing the health practices that will prevent, slow, or modify the chronic diseases that afflict the older person.

To add to our list of anti-aging activities and to relieve and control stress here are techniques that Eastern cultures and religions have long recognized.

Skills to **"Ease the Mind and Heal the Body"** that have
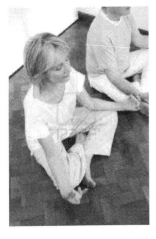
only recently been addressed by physicians in the United States. A good choice could very well be meditation. Its techniques have helped many people to adjust to stress. If you read an ad that promised to shave ten years off your biological age, or help you keep your vision and hearing, to normalize your blood pressure, to keep your libido intact, and do it on your own time schedule with no cost, would you be interested?

Meditators were tested for their vision, hearing, and systolic blood pressure, and found they actually scored on the average seven years younger than their chronological age. In addition, the longer a person meditated the more age resistant they were. Later investigations of the same persons showed even more favorable results. Abilities that usually decline with age (like motor speed, reaction time, visual memory and creativity) did so at a much slower pace.

Many others, worldwide, say that meditation does work. The president of Mozambique in 1996 said that meditation had cured his headaches and brought peace to his war-torn country. In fact, it was part of basic training of his military. He meditates twice a day, every day. He sits quietly with his eyes closed, and focuses on his mantra -- a word used to charm the mind away from thoughts and distractions and into a different level of consciousness. The type of meditation he uses is called Transcendental Meditation more commonly referred to as TM.

At one time this was very popular and was used by many corporations that encouraged their employees, especially their executives, to use TM. Over six million in the late 1960's and 70's used it including the Beatles.

This classic Hindu practice was mass marketed by the Maharishi Mahesh Yogi.

According to the mass marketers, as the mind "transcends", the body will relax. The blood pressure drops and the breathing slows down. It relaxes the person and combats stress.

A prominent supporter of meditation is Dean Ornish, M.D., who uses it in his health retreats and recommends it in his books. He has been meditating since 1972. According to Dr. Ornish, meditation simply helps to quiet your mind.

Many do not accept the fact that doing meditation for 20 minutes once or twice a day can affect the way they will function for the rest of the day, but after they try it, not only do they become believers but encourage others.

It works for me. If I have an especially stressful day and have trouble relaxing, I will close my eyes, picturing myself at the ocean (the waves reaching for the sand) and often the problems flow away.

A major proponent of meditation is Herbert Benson, M.D., who demonstrated this is a simple and effective mind/body approach to relieving stress. Benson has theorized that the relaxation response is the body's protective mechanism against over-stress. TM is a built-in buffer against the negative effects of norepinephrine (noradrenaline). He points out that the physiology of stress is the exact opposite of that of the relaxation response. Stress increases heart rate, respiration, and blood pressure, while meditation slows them down.

When one compares it with the cost of antidepressant drugs which often have adverse side effects, meditation sounds like a winner. When you consider the fact that it is estimated that stress contributes to around 75 percent of all visits to physicians. It should motivate you to give it a try.

You can do it anywhere, anytime, in anyplace that provides a quiet environment. According to Dr. Benson,[113] "Begin by breathing deeply, allowing your mind to focus on one object or sound. It could be the word 'one,' a candle, a flower or some other object or sound. For example, if you select the word 'one', then think the word 'one' each time you breathe out. Breathe slowly in, and as you breathe out, think 'one.' If other thoughts come into your mind, notice them objectively, then go back to noticing your breathing and think 'one' as you breathe out. Continue this for 10 to 15 minutes as desired."

Very simply, meditation is the ability to focus on one's awareness of an external or internal point of concentration, such as the breathing process or an

---

[113] H Benson." Your Innate Asset for Combatting Stress." Harvard Business Review, July-August.1974.

external object. It is the ability to concentrate without interruption that allows you to relax. It is most beneficial when it is done twenty minutes each morning and evening. The meditation exercise included in the TM training involves concentration on the breathing process.

As with most forms of mediation, TM has its roots in religion. All the major religions include some form of continuous chant that puts one into a deeper level of consciousness. In every religion the instructions of how to meditate are basically the same. Whether you say "Hail Mary, full of grace" or use the word one, the techniques are the same. Focus on the word or phrase selected and other thoughts are pushed away when they appear in your mind. A telephone call or ringing of the doorbell is very disruptive and should be avoided.

Prayer is a form of meditation, and some people believe that regular churchgoers have fewer heart attacks than non-churchgoers. An Israeli study showed that among people who went to synagogues, 24 per 1,000 suffered heart attacks as compared to 56 per 1,000 for people who rarely went.

Praying with others offers a form of social support. The music and solemn setting is also relaxing and often leaves the person with a feeling of optimism and exhilaration.

Most of us have often turned to prayer when confronted by an illness or an illness of a close relative or friend. Today, an increasing body of experimental evidence suggests that prayer may also help the healing process. Prayer has shown to have positive effects on

Yoga system goes back somewhere between 5000 BC

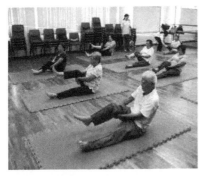

and 300 AD. You may immediately picture a swami standing on his head. Quite the contrary, it is **an established way to strengthen the body and to also relax the mind** through breathing, meditation, and a variety of positions that will tone and strengthen the muscles.

"Yoga" comes from the Sanskrit word meaning to bring together "yoke." It focuses on making one aware of what is happening to them not only physically but emotionally and spiritually.

Doctors in the United States have been slow to recognize and suggest the therapeutic effects of yoga. This should not come as a surprise for most look at the body as something that can be helped mainly through surgery or drugs. But with the increasing popularity of holistic medicine yoga is gaining recognition.

Stretching, exercising, breathing and visualization are all part of yoga and an important way to complement the typical approach to medical care. There are many schools, health clubs, and other organizations that offer classes in yoga for the senior.

These techniques are well worth the time of the senior citizen and will most likely slow the aging process as well as providing physical strength and emotional vitality.

Choose a class wisely. Remember, it's your body that has gotten you here and you do not want an inexperienced teacher in yoga to stress your body past its limit.

The techniques in this chapter have been successful for many older Americans.

They have helped the senior who has lost a companion. They have helped others who are recovering from the many chronic diseases that afflict the older person.

The author believes that all seniors have a great deal of power to prevent and ameliorate mental and physical problems. At the same time when problems are long lasting, and will not go away, and interfere with your ability to function, seek help.

In addition to your family doctor there are mental health specialists, geriatricians, psychiatrists, psychologists, social workers, mental health counselors, and organizations to help the seniors.

> "Do not let sadness come over you, for all your white hairs you can still be a lover"
>
> Debeal Voit
>
> The Coming of Age 1993

Yes, there is sexuality in the later years. Contrary to the misbelief of too many graying adults impotency is not inevitable. Many seniors look forward to an active and satisfactory sexual life with good reason. They are still physically attractive and capable of enjoying and achieving sex. Snow on the roof doesn't mean there's no fire in the furnace.

Yes, your body has changed as you age. Of course, you look and feel different. If you can accept these changes and can be open with your partner, you will share many romantic years. Honesty is a strong emotion to foster trust and relax your partner. There is no time schedule that assures that as one ages their desires for sex will shut down. There may be a gradual slowing of activity but it doesn't have to come to a complete stop. There are too many false stereotypes about the seniors. The assumption that as we reach the 60's we start to lose interest is far from the truth.

Abe, an 80 year old man, told his physician during his exam that he wanted to lower his sex drive. The doctor responded "Now come on Abe. At your age it's all in your head." He said, "I know it. I want you to lower it."

The older woman in good health does not commonly lose her desire or capability for an orgasm. A man does not necessarily lose his desire or ability to develop an erection and ejaculation. The sex may not be as intense and it may take a little longer to attain an erection than in earlier years. It may not be as firm or as large but the enjoyment is still there.

Thinking positive about your ability to continue your sexual relationship will help you to overcome the false concept that seniors are unlikely to enjoy sex as they age.

In our society, the male is indoctrinated to achieve at everything, and sex is no exception. Many boys and men are brainwashed with many false myths and pulp literature into believing that they should always be ready to have sex, and that all intimate contacts should result in sexual relations.

Numerous amounts of money are wasted on products that will up lift (no pun intended) the senior's sexual activities.

During adolescence when the penis always seemed to be in one position, firm and ready for action all was well. But now as men become older the hormones no longer charge through our body as they did when younger.

We should not find this embarrassing or discouraging. After all we cannot walk or run as fast or stay up as late as we used too. We shouldn't expect to be an active sex machine. But still active: yes! Sexual activity is a means of renewing the passion and affection that existed through the years of marriage. It will provide not only pleasure, but a feeling of self-confidence.

Unfortunately, there are no shortages of negative attitudes about the sexual behavior of the elderly which does have its effect on the senior.[114] Kinsey et al. reported that there was a reduced frequency of intercourse among adults to one in every ten weeks by age 80.[115] Many following investigations implied you should not expect too much sex in the golden years which most likely had a negative impact on the attitude of the aging. Let us also not forget the most satisfying reaction derived from a firm hug, a light kiss of welcome or good bye. Kinsey [116] et al. reported, according to S. H. Spence[117] and other specialists in this area, the negative attitudes within society and the media do influence the

---

[114] Hall A., Sell J. and Vanclay, F.M. (1982} Sexual Ageism. Australian on Aging, p'29-34

[115] Kinsey.A.C, Pomeroy, W.B.Martiin, C.E.: Sexual Behavior in the Human Male. Philadelphia   W.B.Saunders, 1943

[116] Morley, J.E.Kaiser, F.E.Aging and Sexuality.   In Albard J.I., Campbell, A.J. Grimely-Evans J.et al (eds: Facts and Research in Gerontology. New York Springer,1992

[117] Spence.S.H. Psychosexual Dysfunction in the Elder Behavior Change,1992 p.55-64

senior's expectations and attitudes toward sex in the later years. The stereotype that older people are generally disinterested and not capable of achieving satisfactory sexual activity is still out there.[118] For those seniors who have been inhibited by these studies or other factors that are interfering with a healthy sexual relationship, read on. You have many amorous years ahead.

---

[118] Vasil.,& Wass H. Portrayal   of the Elderly in the Media : A Literature Review and implications for Educational Gerontologists Educational Gerontology, 1993 p.71-85

Emotional and Physical Problems

There are however emotional and physical problems that do effect the sexuality of the senior.

Diabetes: A disease affecting many seniors that can put an end to a satisfying sexual relationship. However, it can be treated with good results by your physician and potency be restored.

Arthritis: A disease that is no stranger to many seniors and can limit sexual activity. However, exercise and planning sex during hours when pain is usually not intense can keep the couple experimenting with different positions that reduce pain and also assist sexual activity.

Alcohol: Excessive downing of alcoholic drinks will certainly put a damper on your sexual drive.

- Yes, a glass of wine, soft music and exotic lingerie can set the stage for pleasant sexual experiences but alcohol if used excessively can put a damper on the plans. Seniors especially are affected for alcohol tolerance decreases with age.

- Moderate use can be helpful in relaxing one and stimulating desire but too much will discourage sexual activity.

Drugs: Some prescription drugs can cause impotency. Antidepressants, common high blood pressure drugs, tranquilizers, and others may seriously affect your libido.

- Some drugs claim that they stimulate sex activity but there is always the danger of adverse side effects and should be discussed with your physician. This is another good time to remind you to read the labels of all products.

Heart Problems: Angina (a type of chest pain which is a result of a reduced flow of blood to the heart muscle). This will inhibit sexual activity.

- Nitroglycerin is often used but this may prevent using drugs to treat erectile problems.

- Arrhythmia -- in some cases, but not often, this condition can occur after any form of exercise and can be inhibiting.

Stroke: It may prevent the ability of a person to maintain sexual activities. The danger of sexual activity causing another stroke is not as great as with a person who has had coronary artery problems.

Fear: Most patients are fearful of sexual activity after a heart attack. But contrary to common belief, sexual activity is the norm and not dangerous.

As expected after a heart attack, the patient may lose interest in sex for a while and also be reluctant to express his or her fears. Sometimes, the partners are reluctant to make love because they fear a heart attack during sex. Surprisingly, the fear of having intercourse can be as much of a risk factor for a coronary artery attack as sex itself. For most people, it is safe to partake of sex in two weeks following a heart attack. You should, as with all physical activities, progress gradually. Your confidence will increase and you should be back to normal.

In the early 1970s, researchers in Cleveland[119] were able to document that sex with someone you have had a long and stable relationship with is entirely safe. The energy expended while having sex is simply equivalent to the energy it takes to climb one flight of stairs, walking at a brisk pace, or scrubbing a floor. In another study, conducted by the Japanese, the investigators analyzed the autopsy records of 5,000 people who had died suddenly. Of this group, 34 had died during intercourse; of the 34, 30 were with someone other than their spouse, and the partner was on average 18 years younger. Moreover, all had blood alcohol levels close to or within the range of intoxication. The results are not conclusive but suggest that extramarital affairs, especially those involving a younger partner, produce more and potentially lethal stress.

Performance anxiety is certainly not a new event and has been referred to since ancient times. This fear

[119] The Medical Form, Cleveland and Japanese Studies, HMC Health Letter. March 1986, 5-6 Medical Forum.

concerns not only the middle-aged man but, as doctors now realize, the eighty to ninety-year-old male as well. Problems in performing, as sexual investigators, Masters and Johnson, and Dr. Ruth are quick to point out, are often due to the emotions of the individual.

Erectile dysfunction is certainly not a unique problem. By the way, erectile dysfunction is a more acceptable term than impotence. The term impotency creates a mental picture of a male being sterile or weak with little vigor or power. In 1992, the National Institutes of Health defined erectile dysfunction as the inability to sustain or achieve an erection. According to the American Foundation for Urologic Disease, it affects ten million to thirty million men in the United States ages forty to seventy.

Stress again pops up. This time it is as a contributing factor to inhibiting sexual activity. There is no doubt about it: stress will put a hold on your sex life. Most men realize that their stomachs can become upset when they are under stress. However, as says Richard E. Berger, M.D., a urology professor at University of Washington Medical School in Seattle, "They don't realize that erections can be affected by the same thing stress."

According to a study by K. LaMott, M.D,[120] when stress is present there is a reduction in the level of sex hormones of the husband and wife which

---

[120] K La.Mott, Escape From Stress. (New York: Berkely Nedallion, 1975).

in turn reduces their sex drive. This problem does not affect only graying citizens.

Robert Rose, M.D., at the School of Medicine at Boston University, studied soldiers during the Vietnam War. He analyzed the urine samples of men who were waiting to carry out combat missions and found abnormally low levels of testosterone.

This same phenomenon was observed in soldiers at officer candidate schools. During the first few weeks of the training program when they were most worried about being washed out, the testosterone level went way down. Later, as they felt more secure, the level rose as well as their interest in the opposite sex.

Unfortunately, seniors are less inclined to discuss their problems related to sex. Sex education is not just for the young. There are many books, articles, and websites that can provide information to assist the senior to overcome any problems that may develop. Avoid the junk material and consider the qualifications of the author.

Radical Prostatectomy - This is a procedure where the entire prostate is removed including the surrounding tissue and structures to eliminate cancer.

There are nerve spanning techniques to allow the patient to continue sex activities. If the patient however becomes impotent the urologist may suggest devices to alleviate this problem.

There appears to be a strong correlation between a healthy life style and good sex. This is another good reason for seniors to follow the advice provided in the earlier chapters and to hit the gym.

A Harvard study showed that men who exercise three to five hours each week have a 30% lower risk of erectile dysfunction than those who are sedentary.

A study done at the University of Texas at Austin showed that women are more sexually responsive after just 20 minutes of vigorous exercise. Researchers believe that in both men and women, improved blood flow and circulation play a key role.

Kegel Exercises

A survey from the Chicago's National Social Life, Health and Aging Project, showed that senior sexual activity was closely tied to overall health.

The Kegel exercise **used to treat incontinence (loss of bladder control) is also used to improve sexual activity**. This involves alternatively tightening and relaxing the muscles on the floor of the pelvis to improve their tone and strength. The exercise is done throughout the day. You probably do this often without realizing it, for example, when you are urinating and suddenly stop before you are through.

This exercise was developed by gynecologist Arnold Kegel, M.D., for women who had trouble holding their urine after childbirth. Thousands of women and men have also increased their sexual responsiveness by doing this exercise. It is recommended by many therapists. Many males report stronger and more pleasurable orgasms as a result. It's also been helpful to men with erection problems and those who do not experience much feeling in their pelvic area. To do the exercise your contractions can be brief. Hold 3-5 seconds, start with 10 a day and work up to 50-100.

If the senior's sexual desire still goes limping along and the pattern of activity slows up, masturbation may help to maintain sexual interest and abilities to perform. As with other health problems do not look for a quick fix.

There is a multimillion dollar industry claiming that their pills, powders, and potions will stimulate your sexual drive. Magazines, brochures, and books are published daily with impressive endorsements that will definitely intensify your sex drive. Some of their recommendations are almost humorous but can be dangerous. Plus the parts from tigers, elephants, bears, and other animals that are supposedly valuable as aphrodisiacs are depleting many protected species.

Once again exercise may be of great help. It may not convert you into a passionate lover but give you more energy. Rather than make you tired, according to several studies, it will give you vigor and a more active sex life.

According to Cedric Bryant, PhD, Chief Exercise Physiologist for the American Council on Exercise, "Regular exercise may enhance sexuality through a variety of mechanisms that affect the mind and body." He also cautions to be careful not to over strain. "Too much exercise can actually decrease the testosterone level leading to a less robust sexual appetite."

So, the next time your husband or wife complains of a headache you may want to suggest that they jog around the block.

Working with your doctor or a registered sex therapist is the logical place to look for assistance. It helps to talk to someone about your concerns and worries.

Perhaps discussing it with your spouse, a close friend or family member can help you to see your problem in a different light. If you feel your problem is serious you might seek professional help from a psychologist, psychiatrist or a qualified licensed therapist. You want to be careful to seek help in the right place. Knowing when to ask for help may avoid more serious problems later.

In the meantime, to provide great sexual satisfaction, a cuddle, a snuggle, a whispered "I love you" is a powerful way of expressing love for your spouse or partner and for many is just as satisfying. A hug or warm embrace can help to compensate for the slowing down of the earlier torrid sessions, not to say that they are history. Far from it, you should be able to look forward to many more romantic years.

Hugging is healthy

✓ It helps the body's immune system.

✓ It keeps you healthier.

✓ It cures depression.

✓ It reduces stress, it induces sleep.

✓ It's invigorating, it's rejuvenating.

✓ It has no unpleasant side effects and hugging is nothing less than a miracle drug.

✓ It is organic, naturally sweet and contains no pesticides, no preservatives, and no artificial ingredients and is 100% wholesome.

✓ Hugging is practically perfect.

✓ There are no movable parts or batteries to wear out, no periodic checkups, no monthly payments, and no insurance requirements. Hugging offers low energy consumption and high energy yield while being inflation proof, nonfattening, theft proof, nontaxable, nonpolluting and of course **FULLY RETURNABLE**.

You should be able to look forward to many more romantic years.

A man brought a dish with two aspirins and a glass of water to his wife who was lying in bed reading. She jumped up and asked, "What are you doing? I do not have a headache." He answered, "Good I got you."

Frank, age 90, asks his physician for a prescription for Viagra. "Don't be foolish it would be like putting a flagpole on a condemned building," was his reply.

Jim, age 86, and Lillian, age 78, were getting married but only if he would consent to a pre-nuptial agreement. He says, "Fine." She said, "If the marriage doesn't work out, I want to keep the BMW."
He responds "Fine." She adds, "I also want the house." Same response: "Fine."
And the condo in Sun Valley. "Agreed."
  "One more thing I want to have sex 7 nights a week."
He replies, "Fine put me down for Fridays."

Jacob, 90, and Sarah, 85, are all excited about their decision to get married.
They go for a stroll to discuss the wedding and on the way go past a drug store. Jacob suggests they go in.

He addresses the man behind the counter. "Are you the owner?

The pharmacist answers, "Yes"

Jacob: "Do you sell heart medication?"

Pharmacist: "Of course we do"

Jacob: "How about medicine for circulation?"

Pharmacist: "All Kinds"

Jacob: "Medicine for rheumatism?"

Pharmacist: "Definitely"

Jacob: "How about Viagra?"

Pharmacist: "Of course"

Jacob: "Medicine for memory?"

Pharmacist: "Yes, a large variety"

Jacob: "What about vitamins and sleeping pills?"

Pharmacist: "Absolutely"

Jacob turns to Rebecca, "Sweetheart, we might as well register our wedding gift list with them."

A senior was in a terrible accident and his manhood was terminated. However, his doctor told him that it could be restored but his insurance wouldn't cover the surgery.

Since the cost was $10,000, he suggested that he discuss it with his wife.

The man called her and asked what to do. She responded "I would rather remodel the kitchen."

One night an 87 year old woman came home from Bingo to find her 95 year old husband in bed with another woman.

She became violent and ended up by pushing him off the balcony of the 20th floor of their assisted living apartment. He was killed instantly, and she was brought before the court on a charge of murder.

The judge asked her if she had anything to say in her defense. She said rather coolly, "Yes your honor, I figured at age 95, if the old geezer could have sex he could fly."

CONCLUSIONS

> **"Age is a lusty winter frosty but kindly."**
>
> **Shakespeare**

As I conclude this book, I assure you that the author did his homework and diligently tried to cover all bases to show you how to **"Hi Jack the Aging Process."** Well, I sincerely hope that I have motivated you to use this knowledge so that you will enjoy a healthy and pleasant passage into your Golden Years.

At the danger of being repetitious, it is worth reviewing the book and reminding you that aging can be a blast and how to make it last.

The reader may think that life is indeed too short but it is much longer than it used to be. In theory, even the centenarian might very well have another quarter to a half of a century to enjoy healthy living. Your real age (the actual age of your body) depends on how well you live and how positive your mental outlook is: A combination which is a pre-supposition for healthy living.

The bottom line is the time schedule is up to you. Good health is not a matter of luck or inheritance. You can reset the aging clock to run slower. It is not up to your doctor. He is not the possessor of your health or facilitator. You should realize that you must take charge of your own life. You are the biggest factor in determining your health. Don't take your own body to the doctor as if he was a repair shop.

Aging cannot be reversed but it can be enhanced. How often you exercise is important. Seniors who say that exercise definitely keeps them young are probably more correct than skeptics think.

The author found that there was irrefutable evidence that consistent exercise lowers the risk of the most serious diseases that attack the seniors. There is no magic elixir for a long and healthy life but exercise is the closest -- so get moving.

Many investigators as reported in this book also reveal that much of the decline once expected from seniors, as they age, is in reality due to being physically inactive. The common expression, "Use it or lose it" applies not only to the importance of your muscles but the brain as well.

Research from Mankato nuns and supported by researchers such as Arnold Scheibel, M.D., at UCLA have found evidence that throughout life the brain continues to grow dendrites (connections) between nerve cells that allow them to communicate with each other.

Continually challenging the intellect seems to promote this growth. Research has shown that animals kept in stimulating environments have more dendritic growth than un-stimulated animals. And recent studies suggest that older people who are mentally active face a reduced risk of Alzheimer's disease.

Scientific evidence also established the realization that good nutrition is essential for the health and self-sufficiency of the high quality life. "With the right food choices, physical activity, and not smoking, we could prevent about 80 percent of heart disease, about 90 percent of diabetes, and about 70 percent of stroke," says Walter C. Willett, M.D., chairman of the nutrition department at the Harvard School of Public Health in Boston. "Those are the three pillars. They really do make a difference."

Choose wisely. Watch your weight, do not smoke or consume too much alcohol, and control stress. This will put you on track to enjoy the golden years rather than derail you into the blue years.

The encouraging news for seniors is that it is never too late to start on a healthy program. Stress is too often overlooked and it can impair your health as much as any other single factor. A positive emotional state will help you to live longer and more independently. A happy marriage, family and support from a circle of friends will have a lot to do with your real age.

Maintaining a positive stereotype about yourself as you age is important. A Yale study revealed that the older person's beliefs about aging can have a direct impact on their health. According to Becca Levy, PhD, assistant professor in the Department of Epidemiology and Public Health at Yale School, "We were able to reduce this cardiovascular stress by introducing positive stereotypes of aging."

You see yourself as others see you. Unfortunately, too many of the younger generation still picture us as old geezers shuffling along or spending our days in a rocking chair or glued to the television set. Not so in China where older people are beloved and respected. Do not accept the negative stereotypes that many senior encounter. It is a major contributing factor to our longevity.

Thanks to major breakthroughs in the area of heart disease, many of you who already have had a heart attack or stroke and were fortunate enough to survive can look forward to a long and healthy life. One day you even may look back at your illness as a blessing in disguise. Most likely, Mother Nature's warning caused you to sit up and notice that you were not taking good care of your circulatory system, not eating properly, not exercising or relaxing enough, not listening to that cigarette cough.

If you have problems related to cancer or other chronic disease, your chances of living a full and healthful life are better than ever and improving all the time. You have a lot of fun-filled years ahead of you. It is not the end but could be a new beginning.

The outlook for older Americans has never been better. On the average they are living longer and healthier. If you have reached the 50's, 60's, 70's or more the opportunity to stay healthy into the 100's is definite.

A happy marriage, family, and support from a circle of friends will have a lot do with your real age.

There are also many support groups to help you. They will share their personal experiences and how they are adjusting to their problems and overcoming its difficulties.

Social interaction is a good way to reduce tension and develop a positive attitude. Be open about your feelings with your family and friends as well as others; to not do so is an unwise decision and will contribute to a feeling of hopelessness and helplessness.

Ask your doctor or hospital where support groups meet. You can also obtain information by contacting your local Cancer Society or American Heart Association Chapter or other groups related to your disability.

And to quote Charles Chaplin (he lived to be 88) "A day without laughter is a day wasted." He probably was responsible for making more people laugh throughout the world and proved without a doubt that everybody laughs the same because laughter is a universal language.

I sincerely hope that the information provided in this book will help you to stay healthy and enjoy the golden years.

To quote the sixteenth century poet John Donne: "Any man's death diminishes me because I am involved with mankind."

ABOUT THE AUTHOR

Lee Belshin M.S. was born on a farm in Lexington, Massachusetts. After serving in the Navy during WWII, he graduated from the University of California at Los Angeles (UCLA) with a Master of 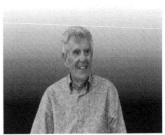 Science degree in Health Education. He worked as a Public Health Educator for the Los Angeles County Health Department. In this position he was one of the first to organize and teach classes in gerontology. He is Past President of the Golden Empire Northern California Chapter of the American Heart Association, and a recipient of its Distinguished Service Award.

He is the author of the book "Love Your Heart" and a second book on preventing a fatal heart attack entitled "The Love Your Heart Guide for the 90's." A third book, "The Complete Prostate Book" discusses one of the main killers of mankind. (A more accurate title would be "To Pee or not to Pee".) The book has been translated into several languages and is on sale in several countries including Russia and Spanish speaking nations.

He has always been interested in the relationship between humor and health. At an age when most comedians retire, Lee has fulfilled his lifetime ambition and became a Stand-Up-Comic.

Made in the USA
San Bernardino, CA
12 March 2018

Foreword by Rosemary Radford Ruether

THE INSIDE STORIES

13 Valiant Women
Challenging the Church

Edited by Annie Lally Milhaven

TWENTY-THIRD PUBLICATIONS
Mystic, Connecticut

To honor the memory of
my father, Thomas (Bob) Lally, who set a match to
my fire,
and
my mother, Delia (Murphy) Lally, who coaxed the
kindlings along.

Twenty-Third Publications
P.O. Box 180
Mystic, CT 06355
(203) 536-2611

ISBN 0-89622-350-7
Library of Congress Catalog Card Number 87-50841

Edited by Hilary Cunningham
Designed by William Baker

Photo credit: P. 101: Mary Gordon photo by Fay
Godwin

FOREWORD

Women have always either existed in equal numbers within, or comprised the majority of, the Roman Catholic church. They have played prominent roles as saints, as heretics, and as the ordinary church members who have been more likely to be faithful churchgoers than have adult males. But it is only in the last ten or fifteen years that Roman Catholic church leaders have been aware of Catholic women as a "dissenting" group in the church. For the first time, theologically well-educated Catholic women, with some access to public media of communication, have been able, as a consciously feminist group, to mount a public critique of Catholic ethical and theological teaching. This dissent comes from both nuns and laywomen. This collection of interviews with critical Catholic feminists includes five nuns and eight laywomen, some of whom are married, and others who are single or divorced. Despite these differences in experience, these women express criticisms of Roman Catholicism that are remarkably consistent.

One major reason why Roman Catholicism now consciously has a "women's problem" is that Catholic women today experience a sharp gap between women's possibilities in secular society and their treatment within the church. A medieval abbess, such as Hildegard of Bingen, might have been less privileged than her brothers in the ecclesiastical hierarchy, but, relative to other women, she had more power, status, and access to education than did the laywomen of the period. Even aristocratic women, who might occasionally have the leisure to cultivate learning, would be restricted by their relationships to their husbands. Moreover, there was a cultural unity of religion and society concerning a woman's place within an overall church and class hierarchy. There was little space or cultural support for a feminist dissent against the church.

Although secular society has hardly overcome patriarchy, it nevertheless today offers women considerably more space than does Roman Catholicism. Women can attain the highest advanced degrees in secular universities, while many Catholic seminaries still will not admit them for theological study. Women can run for political office and, at least in theory, be elected to the highest levels of leadership. They have independent control over property and money. In the Catholic church, however, they are still treated as permanent dependents, the lowest class in a hierarchy of clergy over laity, men over women. As church workers they are expected to accept low pay or to work as volunteers, to receive orders, to refrain from shaping their own ideas and programs, and to be grateful that they are allowed to "serve" at all. They are expected to have their minds, their bodies, and particularly their sexuality directed by celibate males who "know better."

This gap between church and society has been compounded in the last two decades by reform movements. In society, civil rights, peace and feminist movements have challenged in new ways the continuing racist, sexist, militarist and colonialist patterns of national communities. In the Catholic church, the Second Vatican Council marked a monumental departure from the church's entrenched resistance to modern liberal social and theological ideas. This unleashed reform movements in liturgy and expectations of more democratic participation in both religious orders and local parishes.

Many American religious orders both upgraded the educational level of their members and revised their constitutions to allow for a more consensus style of government. For Catholics involved in liberation movements in society and reform of the church, these changes became an integral part of their understanding of authentic Christianity. They felt themselves part of a new trajectory in the church's self-understanding, and they thought their sense of the church was shared by the church leaders who had apparently unleashed these movements for change.

LEADERS OF REFORM

The Catholic women in this volume have not only been deeply affected by these changes in the church and in society, but have for the most part been important leaders in those changes. These are the nuns who have been shaping their orders to allow for a more consensual process, and redefining the vocation of the nun to include ministries of social advocacy. These are the laywomen who have been reshaping theology and biblical studies to integrate feminist and liberation issues into the Christian understanding of redemption. These are the women who have founded new social advocacy organizations. A feminist liberation perspective is not simply a set of some new ideational symbols. Rather, it defines both a vision and a way of being and relating to others that is integral to women's personal integrity and their identities as Christians and as women—thus their outrage when church leaders show neither understanding nor respect for these basic premises.

A number of themes run through the accounts of these women's lives, as revealed in the interviews. First of all, there is a profound critique of patriarchal, hierarchical, institutional functioning within the Christian church. Such patterns of authority, for them, have been rendered ethically and theologically illegitimate. It is not only that such patterns conflict with more democratic processes presumed to be in effect in civil society, for these women indeed know how oppressive much of secular society is. Rather, such patterns of power are seen as sinful, as based on psychic and physical violence between domination and subject people. They are fundamentally in contradiction to the redemptive mission of the church. These women expect the church in particular to be a paradigm of mutual, respectful relationships.

They know very well, however, that a different norm has prevailed for most of Christian history. For Bernadette Brooten and Elisabeth Schüssler Fiorenza, this is an issue of New Testament hermeneutics. They are involved in showing how patriarchal domination, and even violence to women, children, and slaves, is contained in Scripture. And yet another norm, one of mutuality and equality, is the authentically Christian one, for many women. Their exegetical task, as I perceive it, is to vindicate this view in the face of contrary scriptural evidence. For other women in this collection, patriarchal violence is much more immediately a matter of personal experience with the church as an institution. They have experienced themselves violated and betrayed by the Vatican, by bishops, and by superiors of their religious orders who have failed to defend their own best insights against such authoritarianism. They have experienced violence at the hands of parish priests and even other members of the laity.

STRENGTH IN COMMUNITY

These experiences of violence and betrayal have not shaken these women's faith in mutual respect, which many hold to be as the authentic Christian ethic of community. But they have thrown them back upon themselves, and upon small, supportive communities, as their primary base of religious nurture. Several of the women speak of needing to find their own spiritual power, rather than being dependent on validation from the outside. This suggests a shift from what Paul Tillich would call "heteronymous" to an "autonomous/theonomous" understanding of spirituality. No matter how those who claim to represent God may negate these women's experience, their experiences can no longer shake either their own integrity, or their sense of being rooted in divine being, or their confidence that their own values well up within themselves from the authentic God of love and justice. This is the ultimate base of their ability to withstand ecclesiastical contempt.

For a number of the women in this volume, this autonomous spirituality has found expression in an alternative feminist liturgical community. "Women-church" among such Catholic women is both new a vision and a new practice of worshipping community. It allows feminist women to claim Christian community as a community of liberation from patriarchy. It provides some beginning of a new experience of this possibility in practice, in communities of experimental liturgy and mutual support. Here, in a feminist, base-community movement that has been pioneered by American Catholic women (but is rapidly finding echoes in other countries and other branches of Christianity) a new religious culture is being developed. For the first time in Christian memory, and perhaps for the first time in history, women have become the active subjects of liturgical celebration, not only as actors, but as the shapers of the symbols and texts of worship in a way that speaks to their own experience of oppression and liberation as women.

If claiming one's own spiritual power is one important theme, claiming the rights of women to their own bodies, to the control of their own sexuality, is a parallel theme that runs through these writings. This is not necessarily because these women, particularly the nuns, have chosen this battlefield. Rather, it is because the patriarchal, ecclesiastical authorities have forced this battle upon them. The Catholic hierarchy seems literally obsessed with a battle to reassert control over female sexuality. Virtually all the major conflicts with church authority that these women have experienced have, in one way or another, been based on this effort to reassert control over female sexuality, or sexuality in general. Birth control, abortion, homosexuality, divorce, married priests: all these issues, in one way or another, show the anxiety to subordinate the sexual to a clerically controlled realm of the sacred.

HIERARCHICAL POWER
AND SEXUAL DOMINATION

In some profound sense, these women have come to realize that clerical hierarchical power is integrally related to sexual domination. Any kind of autonomous existence of women, particularly women's right to make decisions about their sexuality and fertility, threatens this psycho-social celibate clerical power system. Whether it be a nun, who is forced out of her order because one of the marginal aspects of her job with a state social service agency is provision of medicaid payments for abortion, such as Agnes Mary Mansour, or a woman integrally involved in providing birth control and abortion services, such as Mary Ann Sorrentino, or defending women's rights to such services, such as Frances Kissling, this power struggle over sexuality is at the heart of the explosive conflict between Catholic women and the Catholic hierarchy.

Not all these women have experienced these conflicts in quite the same way. But one figure in this collection stands out as a person who reflects on this historical moment in Catholicism in a distinctively different way. This person is novelist Mary Gordon. While the tone of most of the writers is one of resistance, but, nevertheless, confidence and hope for the future, Gordon has much more a sense of the tragic. She is deeply divided between an old religious aesthetic which she loves—but which today is only an expression of reactionary politics and theology—and new movements in theology and politics that she supports, but that seem to lack totally the aesthetic that can nurture her soul. She also has much deeper doubts about the instinctive rightness of women's ethical insights. For her, female power in antiquity has more to do with the cruelty of an impersonal nature that sacrifices the individual to the species, while it is patriarchy that has risen above this cruel, impersonal nature and formulated the ideals of justice. Whether or not the other women would agree with this evaluation of cultural history, her reflections nonetheless form an important counterpoint and corrective to the tendency of the others to unquestioning confidence in the particular *zeitgeist* that has emerged in Catholic feminist liberation circles in recent years.

MARJORIE TUITE

There is also a ghost who stalks these pages, a woman who might have been one of the prime candidates to be an interviewee, if it had not been for her sudden death in June 1986. This ghost is that of Marge Tuite, a personal mentor to at least half of the women represented. A Dominican nun, Marge Tuite represented that extraordinary transformation of American Catholic nuns from docile agents of a male, clerical church to vigorous counter-cultural activists on behalf of the poor and the oppressed in North American society and in the Third World. She was empowerer of the women of this church to organize, to fight oppressive power in the church and in society.

Caught in the middle of the conflict between hierarchical power and control over sexuality, Tuite found her very existence in the Catholic church threatened over an issue which is the last issue she would have chose to "go to the wall" over, namely, the right of dissent on abortion. For most of the women who knew her, this conflict with its ruthless demands for submission from the hierarchy killed her, or, at the very least, hastened her death. This death makes Marge Tuite close to a new Christ figure for Catholic feminists. They renew their own commitment to struggle now "in her name." She is present in the continued breaking of bread, sharing of wine, in women-church.

"WHY DO THEY STAY?"
Given the profound and destructive character of this conflict between Catholic feminists and the Catholic hierarchy, one can well ask, "Why do they stay?" While I cannot speak for all these women, it seems to me that, in one way or another, each of them affirm that they "shall not be moved" from their membership in the Catholic church, as they define and understand it. Why? There seems to me to be three reasons.

First, they have made an appropriation of Christian identity which is integral to their own being. They refuse to let the hierarchy define them outside of the church, but rather insist on disputing the territory of the true meaning of church with the hierarchy, challenging their right to define its meaning and boundaries.

A second reason why they refuse to be defined outside this particular historical church is their own ethnic, historical roots in this community. For most of them this is their family, their roots. No one can falsify who they are and sever kinship ties that have been forged by blood and not simply by baptismal water or creedal statements.

A final reason for staying in this church is not spelled out, but I think it may be the most powerful reason of all: these women, on the whole, sense that they have clout precisely by remaining as dissidents within this particular church. This might surprise some of them, because, from an institutional, legal point of view, they would seem to be quite powerless. But institutional power does not lie only in possession of control over property and juridical authority. It lies, in the church particularly, in a cultural hegemony to define the meaning of the community and its mission.

The Catholic church is today one of the most powerful constructs for the legitimization of patricarchal values in Western culture, and perhaps in the whole world. But cultural hegemony is fragile when it fails to connect with most people's real experiences. These women, although few in number, have enormous power because they articulate alternative experiences shared by most lay women and men, and, indeed by many priests as well. Thus, they pose a serious threat to the credibility of Catholic authority. When that authority loses its credibility, its hegemony will quickly crumble. The hierarchy senses the full magnitude of this threat, and this, I think, is why they respond to these women with such repressive fury.

The ability of these women to persevere as spokespersons recognized by their fellow Catholics as part of the Catholic family spells the handwriting on the wall for Catholic patriarchy. Out of its death throes, a new church must emerge. This is the significance of these female voices within Catholicism in the last decades of the twentieth century.

Rosemary Radford Ruether

PREFACE

Once upon a time I loved saintly men and women who suffered ignominy in silence. Their going to their graves without vindication appealed mightly to my sense of sainthood. But now, I love courage. I admire those women—there seems to be more of them—and men who take rightful risks in spite of their fears. Such valor seeps under my nerve endings, stretches the ecclesial horizon, and provides hope for the future. The most engaging women I know are those Catholics who stand up to hierarchical oppression, who name the evil done them and others, and who refuse either to be victimized further or to leave their church.

They are the kind of women I engaged in conversation for this volume. These thirteen Catholic women of vision, courage, and scholarship are dedicated to the creation of a new *ecclesia*—a church of justice and love. The reader must not expect to meet Mother Theresas or Little Flowers of Jesus. Rather, these women speak with a sense of freedom, responsibility, and independence beyond that of a Catherine of Siena or a Teresa of Avila. They, as Gerda Lerner suggested, challenge the script written eons ago by men for men; they insist on changing the direction of their church, and demand an equal point of action.

Viewing the Catholic church today, one sees a drive to diminish the gains, the few steps toward liberation that women fought for since the time of Pope John XXIII and Vatican II. It is like the drive by the government to stamp out the hopes and expectations of Ameria's underprivileged in the 1960s. But the women in this book refuse to be passive or victimized in a church gone arwy. Nor will they wait for the grave and a heaven beyond in hopes of eventual justice and love. They believe as the Hebrews did that Yahweh is behind the Exodus, that God is always on the side of the oppressed. With Ghanian theologian Mercy Amba Oduyoye, these women know that if American Catholic women "make it," women everywhere will be emboldened in their struggles.

Speaking of courage: I want to thank Twenty-Third Publications and my editor Stephen B. Scharper for his unfailing civility. I am vastly in the debt of the women who so effortlessly and spontaneously described a church few know to exist, and to Rosemary Radford Ruether for so ably leading them forth. My thanks also to John Giles Milhaven for his enthusiastic support and to Shelly our daughter for her skill with the word processor as this manuscript took shape.

CONTENTS

"Nothing can exist unless it is properly described."
Virginia Woolf

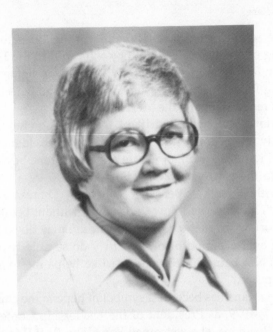

THERESA KANE

". . .I call it the new consciousness. It is the historical evolution which [demands that] women be acknowledged in the twentieth century as human beings in their own right. . . .[To say that] some ministries can only be performed by one group, and the group happens to be men, is to say somehow they're in a higher and better ministry. It raises the whole question of hierarchy of ministries, and we must start looking at questions of idolatry."

Born in the Bronx, New York City, of Irish immigrant parents, Theresa Kane is one of eight children—she has six sisters and one brother. Educated in Catholic schools, she was eager to learn about economics at the time she entered the Sisters of Mercy in 1955. The order fostered this interest; after graduating from Manhattanville College in Purchase, N.Y., she was appointed finance minister in a health agency.

Because Theresa Kane was at one time caught between two worlds, she offers a striking model of emergence from the old monastic semi-cloistered religious life of the 1950s to the full flowering of renewal called forth by Vatican II in the 1960s and 1970s. In fact, because she held high offices for eighteen years, including President of the Sisters of Mercy, she herself helped lead this renewal among the Mercy nuns.

She views the current drift of the Catholic church philosophically. One Mercy nun, Mary Riley of Providence, states, "Theresa Kane is a woman whose anger has gone beyond frustration to the clarity of truth. She apears to be a woman at peace with herself." Speaking of herself, Theresa Kane observes, "I have learned how to be angry without being hostile. It is important for me to correct injustice. I may do so immediately, or over a period of time. I may do so quietly or not so quietly. Not being hostile and warlike helps me to a deeper sense of peace."

Theresa Kane has become a symbol of hope in the church. On October 7, 1979, as President of the Leadership Conference of Women Religious, she welcomed Pope John Paul II to the United States. During her brief remarks she challenged him to give women access to all ministries in the Catholic church.

Energy to advocacy for a new historical moment for women. She describes the price she continues to pay for this celebrated but difficult role she adopted because of her four-minute greeting to Pope John Paul II.

THE 1979 PAPAL VISIT
It seems that the name Theresa Kane burst suddenly on the Catholic scene causing quite a stir. How did this happen?
Kane: It was October 7, 1979. "Bursting upon the scene" was occasioned by the papal visit to the United States. I'll give you my recollection of what it was about and why that date was important. I was serving at the time as the President of the Sisters of Mercy of the Union. The Union is an amalgamation of several independent orders which came together in 1929. We have nine provincial headquarters, with our national headquarters in Washington, D.C. We number close to five thousand nuns.

Serving as president of the order, I was also active in the

Leadership Conference of Women Religious (LCWR). I was elected vice president in 1978 and automatically became president in 1979. In that capacity I was asked to greet the pope when he participated in the prayer service at the Shrine of the Immaculate Conception in Washington, D.C. His schedule had been planned for the week: he arrived in Boston, traveled to Chicago [and] Des Moines, returned to Philadelphia, New York, and [went] finally to Washington, D.C. Washington was actually the last stop of the eight-day papal visit. At that time, I was living and working in Washington, D.C. One of the sisters on the Leadership Council said that the pope would be at the Shrine on Sunday morning for a prayer service. He would also address the sisters. Somebody would be invited to greet him. In the conversation, I recall saying it would probably be a local nun.

About two weeks before the event, I received a phone call from the director of National Shrine of the Immaculate Conception, saying that as president of LCWR, I was asked to greet the pope in the name of the sisters of the United States. There wasn't a lot of preparation [time] for it. I looked on it as part of my job. There was little advance publicity; it just seemed like an event that would happen.

It was part of a normal day's work, except that every day the pope isn't here.

Kane: Yes, that's true. In many ways it seemed right for a sister to greet the pope since many sisters were expected in the Shrine. The only other woman I knew who had done anything publicly was Rosalind Carter. President Carter asked his wife to be the official greeter of the pope to the United States. In the New York event, sisters did readings in St. Patrick's Cathedral, but no other woman was asked to address the pope in a public way. I was conscious of very few women actually doing any kind of public function while he was here. The only instruction I had was that the greeting be brief, not more than three or four minutes. The entire service would last maybe 45 minutes.

I put together thoughts which I considered important for the greeting. I planned to warmly welcome him among the sisters. I thought it very important to acknowledge what the sisters have done in the United States. My perception was that sisters were functioning beings here in the church. They did a great deal to build it up. But, in a sense, their work was behind the scenes, quite private, and not given enough public credit. I remembered thinking very clearly how important it was to acknowledge the work of the sisters throughout the century, and their contribution to the development of the Catholic church in the United States. The third point I wanted to make was to acknowledge that in the one year he had been pontiff, he was very strong about our responsibilities to and with the poor. He had focused attention on the plight of the poor. I felt it was important to express solidarity with him there. We, too, were struggling with that question, and particularly in the American context where so many times our poor seem to be more invisible than in other countries. The fourth point I wanted to make was the question of women, thinking it was important, appropriate, and right for a woman to speak of women in the church. . . women in ministry in the church. Basically those were my four points and I spent most of my time trying to reduce the greeting from twelve to three or four minutes. That was my big struggle.

A couple of days after the phone call, one of the sisters working with me in administration asked, "Are you going to say something about women?" And I said, "Yes, I am." I guess her question raised a question in my mind. I said, "Do you think I should?" And she said, "Oh yes, yes, I think it would be wonderful. I just didn't know if you were going to do it." It was probably the first inkling I got—a question raised in my mind, you know—should I, or shouldn't I say something that might be controversial? For myself, it seemed a very natural thing to do. I had no doubts, no reservations, and no deep questions. I felt what I wanted to say was certainly not shared by everybody. I didn't expect it to be. What I asked actually was, "Will women be provided the possibility of being in all ministries of the church?" The fact is that women are called, and they should be [accorded] the possibility of being in all ministries of the church—that was what became controversial.

What went through your mind as you formulated the words for your greeting? And what did you say?
Kane: I reflected and reviewed my words several times. I wanted to speak in a manner that expressed what was in my heart and mind. But I did not want it to be done in a way that

was harsh or judgmental, like, "This is your fault," or "This is your problem." I see it now (as I did then) as a structural, systemic problem, something that we really need to struggle with, grapple with. It's a new consciousness. A totally new moment has come to pass in [the] church and in society on the question of women. I struggled most [with] how to say it in a way that shared my convictions, my beliefs, all of which I wanted to communicate.

But without being confrontational. . .
Kane: On behalf of women; well, I knew it was going to be confrontational.

CONFRONTATION VITAL FOR A NEW CHURCH
You see confrontation as a positive thing then?
Kane: To me confrontation is not a negative thing. It is important to confront each other in a respectful way. But I knew it would be controversial. I have a feel for confronting if it isn't done in a militaristic way.

In other words you feel confrontation is a necessary tool?
Kane: Absolutely. And I think one of the reasons why we're having such real struggles in our church now is that we never developed that tool: how to confront each other. We've never developed ourselves as church-people to sit down, be diverse, and disagree with each other.

Nuns, however, have grown through that experience, and our church has to do the same thing. We must reverence diversity, not be afraid of it. If I don't know how to do anything but agree and conform, then I've never been taught that it's okay to disagree and to dissent, and to be quite different one from another. As it is, we don't really handle each other well when we are different. When we see people who dress or think differently, we want to shy away rather than sit down and have a conversation with them.

Essentially what you were doing was quite consciously looking at and using that tool of confrontation, which is part of the American political dynamic.
Kane: I did not tie it in with the American political dynamic. I learned it in the renewal efforts in the religious order. It is one of many tremendous things we learned through our renewal ef-

forts. It was based on the integrity and dignity of the individual, each of whom is graced differently. Our struggle had been to come out of uniformity of dress and procedures, and having the honorarium similiar in every convent. We diversified and realized that it is all right to look and dress differently. It is that experience that helped me to bring up a controversial point. In fact, it was only appropriate that I do so.

Even if it jarred the pope?

Kane: Yes. I didn't know if it would jar him or not. I knew it would jar people other than the pope. The point I make here is that in writing and giving my greeting, I knew it would be controversial.

Now what were the words you used?

Kane: In the first two sentences, I spoke on behalf of the sisters of the United States, but I did not speak for *every* sister. But when I came to my fourth point, then I knew I was switching from just speaking on behalf of sisters to speaking on behalf of Catholic women. It was a conscious shift, and it became significant, and important for me to say that I don't see the woman's issue in the church as in any way exclusively a nun's issue. I wanted to speak on behalf of *women*. As women we have listened to the call of Vatican Council II, we have dwelt upon the many insights that have come from Vatican II, and our ponderings lead us to raise the question of women being provided the opportunity to serve in all ministries of our church. That's really the substance of it. Here are my exact words:

"As I share this privileged moment with you, Your Holiness, I urge you to be mindful of the intense suffering and pain which is part of the life of many women in these United States. I call upon you to listen with compassion and to hear the call of women who comprise half of humankind. As women, we have heard the powerful messages of our church addressing the dignity and reverence for all persons. As women, we have pondered these words. Our contemplation leads us to state that the church in its struggle to be faithful to its call for reverence and dignity for all persons must respond by providing the possibility of women as persons being included in all ministries of our church. I urge you, Your Holiness, to be open to and respond to the voices coming from the women of this country who are desirous of serving in and through the church as fully participating members."

You did not mention women being ordained?
Kane: No, I didn't use the word ordination. I deliberately omitted it. It is a much bigger question than ordination, although I certainly have become aware that ordination becomes the focus, the linchpin of the question. Ordination is, in many ways, the access to those other ministries. It is a very important consideration which I would not leave out. I said women in all ministries, and I continue to say so. To take any one ministry in the church and say it is exclusively for men is not really to look at ministry as service. I feel wherever people are to be served, women and men are equal beings ready to serve.

So when you say churchmen are not looking at service, what then are they looking at?
Kane: To take some ministries and say they can only be performed by one group, and the group happens to be men, is to say that somehow they're in a higher and better ministry. It raises the whole question of hierarchy of ministries, and we must start looking at questions of idolatry. That is how I interpret it.

What do you mean by idolatry?
Kane: Take the priesthood. To say you have to be a male is somehow to idolatrize that sacrament, [to set it] apart from the others. All the others can be received by women and men and can be administered in certain circumstances by women and men. But this one can only be held by men, and that really, I think, puts it in the idolatry category. It becomes a godly thing; it doesn't belong to all humans.

DEFINING WOMEN AS FULL HUMAN BEINGS
Implied in our discussion, therefore, is the fact that women are essentially not viewed as fully human by the church.
Kane: Yes, that is the belief. That is a strong belief in the church. It's been there for centuries. [Beginning with] Thomas Aquinas and. . .[continuing through] the fifteenth century, it was questioned if women had souls? Were women fully human? Do women have rational abilities? It's [a] very strong [trend], and even goes right into the twentieth century. It is an underlying emotional belief still strongly with us: as long as I consider a woman my mother, my wife, or my grandmother, she isn't up

on those pedestals. The men are a bit above her. What I've done is put her down below me. I look on this view as evil. We can see a whole pattern where men do not see women as equals. Obviously, if we talk about the [early] twentieth century, women did not have political equality, [and] do not now have economic equality. Yet, ours is in the most "advanced industrialized country" in the world, and we know from the U.S. that equality is not happening in many other countries, either. It is a question of women being incorporated into the mainstream of not just of private but political life. Women, it is obvious, are very much the cornerstone of private life. In no way are they seen as the cornerstone [of], or central to, public life. Hence, we have questions about a woman being capable of the vice presidency [of the United States].

As if the office itself were a great thing. . . ?
Kane: Well, of course, it is a great thing. The whole ethos through the centuries is that women were property, men's property. They still are. A woman marries and immediately she assumes his name. She becomes not only his last name but Mrs. John Thomas, or whatever the man's first name happens to be. Recently, *The New York Times* has an advertisement by Sarah Brady, wife of [former Reagan Administration press secretary] Jim Brady. She strongly favors handgun control. But she's listed as Mrs. James Brady. You see?

You take exception to this?
Kane: Oh yes. My exception is that the woman is not woman in her own right. She's only there as the appendage: the wife of, some relation to a man, known only by his name.

CHURCH OPPRESSION OF WOMEN
The Catholic church has its roots in Christ's call to free the prisoners, feed the poor, and take on oppressive establishments. Yet it seems that women have somehow been ignored as part of this call. How, over two thousand years, has the church maintained an oppression of women?
Kane: It was not a question in the Catholic church before the present age. If it is not a question, then you are not maintaining oppression. . .in the same sense as being blind to the fact that there is a problem. That is why I call it the *new consciousness*.

It is the historical evolution which [demands that] women be acknowledged in the twentieth century as human beings in their own right.

Previously, women could not be lawyers, or doctors, Now, nuns cannot be politicians. We talk in our circles about political ministry. Can sisters be in political ministry? Well, it's still considered a great, great exception, and I compare it to the fact that nuns who wanted to be doctors in the 1920s had to get special permission. Becoming a doctor was something nuns then did not do. Now nuns are not considered fit for political office, and we will see that anomaly die out in another twenty or thirty years.

Well, not only is it an exception, but are not nuns like Arlene Violet and Liz Morancy forbidden to hold political office?

Kane: They are not forbidden; the possibility is there as an exception. Approval is to be given by the local bishop, because it is seen as an exceptional ministry. Sisters wanting to be doctors were considered to be an exceptional ministry in the 1920s. The women who became medical missionaries [did so] five or seven years before Rome gave them approval to be doctors.

Meaning only a man could be a doctor?

Kane: It meant certainly that doctoring was not something for women; it was probably far too public to think about cloistered nuns performing such a service. But teaching was considered appropriate, and so was nursing, yet medicine was not considered appropriate for women.

As a nurse, I know that physicians were seen as gods.

Kane: It is very true that when we have a group of experts we raise them up, consider them somehow godly. We appropriate too much authority to them, without assuming enough authority for our own life. I found it very helpful myself, in relating with a physician, to realize the physician is not the one who truly knows me, or knows my body. Nobody knows it as well as I do. He or she can provide some good technical information. I'm the one to make the decisions. It is important to obtain professional advice and consultation, and to think about recommendations we receive. But I am responsible for my own direction, and for authoring my own life.

We're really talking about a caste system, then. In the upper strata we find men, those who are god-like; then one top man in the church who is very god-like. And then we have women. Do you agree with that?

Kane: I do, and that's why I spoke to your question, which was very important: how did we maintain this oppression for twenty centuries? Vatican Council II provided a development of spirituality of church as community. I have heard a number of expert church people confirm that what we're doing now in the Catholic church is similar to what Christians did in the early centuries. They developed a church community; structural questions were minimal.

Over twenty centuries, though, we also developed an empire. The hierarchical system of the Catholic church acts in the same way as government in the civil arena. In developing those systems we keep a certain amount of oppression. We insist that all have to think alike, believe alike. It leads to lack of diversity. We lack this richness, this branching out to many creative developments through the centuries. I believe strongly in the Holy Spirit who moves in our midst. Periodically, we get a total change, a new and creative approach to church life. Certainly, the religious orders are an example of it. Certain spontaneous and creative flowerings develop which do not get legitimized for some time.

So is that what is going on with the nuns?

Kane: It certainly is going on with the nuns, but also with the women. It is very, very obvious in the women's movement in the Catholic church: the development of feminist liturgies, feminist theology and spirituality, a whole array of things. Mary Hunt and Diann Neu [co-directors of Women's Alliance for Theology, Ethics, and Ritual (Water)] are examples of the kind of things happening. In Massachusetts, [you have] Plainville Women's Center, and a number of other women centers are developing around the country. They are Catholic, sponsored by Catholic women, but open to women of all faiths. A lot of exciting and creative things are happening.

THE PAPAL GREETING

Let's get back to the papal greeting. You delivered it, and what did you do then? Did you kiss the pope's hand?

Kane: There was quite a bit of tension in the Shrine; sisters inside knew that women were demonstrating outside, handing out leaflets, and going to stand in protest at the service. The directors of the Shrine were also aware of it. They tried to strategize to prevent it. When they realized that was not possible, they asked the women not to stand in one block but to distribute themselves throughout the Shrine. And they did so.

What do you think of that?

Kane: Well, I wasn't at their meetings. I think they weighed carefully all the factors. They were concerned in their dialogue about safety. Secret Service people were around the Shrine, but it was almost all sisters who organized the protest. They did not feel they wanted to stand in one block and have any kind of safety incidents. It was hard for them, because they would have felt easier standing in a group rather than trying to stand alone.

If they all stood together it would have been more powerful. Interspersed, it could be viewed as women who were unorganized, divided.

Kane: But they had the blue armbands on which is the symbol of the Women's Ordination Movement.

Did you face the pope as you spoke?

Kane: I faced the audience. He was behind me. I actually wanted to go over and say hello to him, greet him. I even asked if I could shake hands with him. A priest, directing all of the activities, said to me: "When it's time for you to greet the pope, I will come over to your seat and escort you to the podium." I said: "Well, I'd like to go up and greet the pope." And he said: "No, that would not be appropriate. Just get up and bow and then go to the poduim and when you're finished, bow again and go back to your seat." I was not comfortable with that; I felt the person to person approach was what I wanted. I thought it was only decent, really.

Were you able to overrule the priest?

Kane: I did follow the instruction to bow. I then went to the podium. There was extensive applause three or four different times during my talk. When it was finished, I was very conscious that there was a lot of tension in the air. I turned to the priest and said: "Father, I would really like to go and greet the

Holy Father." So I just walked away from him and went over to the pope.

Good for you! So what did you do?

Kane: Well I got over to him, and I was conscious that I did not know Polish, and I did not know how well he knew English. I did shake his hand and the two of us tried to say a couple of words. It just didn't seem to work right, either. Then I said: "May I have your blessing?" I knelt down very spontaneously. I knelt for his blessing. Then I got up and walked back to my seat.

As you described the scene, and the four points that you had to boil down to four minutes, there's nothing earth-shaking about it. Yet it was a watershed event in this country. Why?

Kane: I don't really know! One thing, it was the pope's first visit to the United States. Pope Paul VI came once and went to the United Nations. He returned to Rome the same day. This pope stayed for eight days. Bear in mind he had only been on the job a year. He was very charismatic, very appealing to people. He skis, and to many he is a man of inspiration. People were eager to hear about his visit. It was like having royalty in the country; witness how we reacted to [Princess] Diana and [Prince] Charles more recently. So, too, the pope was kind of a curiosity.

He spoke in different places: the Midwest; the farm country; then in Philadelphia and New York. In Philadelphia, he spoke to the priests saying very strongly to the applauding clerics that only men could be ordained. Then on Sunday morning, he prepared to speak to all the sisters. He had seen the activity, the blue armbands, and the demonstration outside the Shrine. I spoke, and my short greeting was clear about women being in all ministries of the church. It was immediately interpreted as ordination and speaking for ordination exclusively. Several people felt that since it was a Sunday morning many people were at home. They had more leisure. This larger audience knew that the pope had two or three more events before leaving the country. With people watching, there was more tension because of the sisters' protesting.

Ordination of women is an issue in the U.S. Catholic church, and my speaking as I did symbolized its importance. All these factors led it to being the event it became. People, I believe, were expressing their feelings. One man in the media told me that he felt during the visit that things seemed to be repressed, not expressed. Everybody was trying to make a smooth visit, that there be no problem, and that the pope have no final hurdles. In a sense, he would have had it made, because if there was to be any kind of controversy, it would have happened in the United States. Until Sunday morning, it did not happen. Or it was not allowed to happen, I guess.

That event was catalytic; perhaps its importance went beyond even your own expectations.

Kane: For some reason, it was a moment which became important to many people. Important to women, as I said earlier. Catholic women, and women who are not Catholic, saw it as something very symbolic. The same excitement happened in this country with Geraldine Ferraro. It was a exciting moment when she was chosen candidate for vice president. I was in South America at a conference of sisters when someone called from the United States. When it was announced in the dining room all eighty-five nuns, mostly South Americans, cheered. These nuns were women who never imagined having a woman politically prominent in their countries.

When did you get a sense that your statement was causing some trouble?

Kane: I had heard on Friday that the prayer service at the Shrine would be televised in Washington, D.C. It would be a local audience. On Saturday someone called me from New York and said that it would be televised in New York City. I remember feeling anxious, knowing that sisters sitting in the Shrine would not be where I was on the questions of women and the church. I was very sensitive to that fact. Yet, I felt it was important for me to speak. I was reflecting a growing number of Catholic women in the United States and I made the judgment to speak out. Hearing it was televised regionally, I felt it was a bigger audience than I had anticipated. The more people, the more possibility of controversy. I got back to the motherhouse early afternoon of that Sunday. The nuns told me of phone calls and telegrams from different parts of the country: Washington, North Dakota, California. These messages began almost immediately after 11:30 a.m. Only then I realized that there was national coverage. Only then I anticipated that there would be more controversy.

REACTIONS OF THE MERCY NUNS

Was there controversy within your order about your stand?

Kane: Yes, there was. Within the order, the sisters are very much a microcosm of people in general. I had written ahead to all the sisters telling them I was to give this papal greeting. I wanted them to be aware, thinking they would not see it. Many of them were surprised that I said anything about women. Many of them were very, very pleased, but a number of the sisters were very upset. A few were shocked. These said it did not reflect them and they did not want the head of their order speaking like that. So I got a mixed response.

As president of their order, how did you respond?

Kane: I made a very deliberate effort to visit sisters in all parts of the country. I ordinarily visited sisters anyway, but I made a deliberate effort to engage them in conversation. Coming into an area, I asked the provincials to set up meetings and invite the sisters to attend. I did not mandate it, but said simply that I would welcome their presence. I made an effort to explain to them what I had said, why I had said it, and how it came about. I opened it up for conversation. I encouraged them to speak up, particularly to tell me if they disagreed with me, and to share their feelings. They were very vocal about it. Initially shy, they did not want to speak publicly against me. I continued to encourage them because I felt it was important. After a while, they became more comfortable in saying: "I just disagreed with you; " "[I am] sorry you did it"; or "I wish you hadn't." That was very healthy, I think, for our community.

I'd like to see something like that going on in Rome.

Kane: Yes, I would, too.

ROME'S RESPONSE

Speaking of Rome, you went later to Rome in your capacity as president. How did those visits go?

Kane: Before I gave the greeting, we, the executive committee of LCWR, asked to meet with the pope when he was in the United States. We had listened to his messages, heard his talks to sisters, and we felt what he was saying about religious life and what we were living were not in harmony. He was talking about the nun's habit quite a bit at that time. . .wearing the religious habit. He was talking also about what we thought was a highly cloistered, secluded form of religious life from which we had moved after Vatican Council II. What we heard him saying and what we were living were not connected.

And did you feel this had something to do with the models in Poland?

Kane: I cannot tell. His view of religious life was more of an enclosed, cloistered model than ours. The sisters in Poland are very much into the religious habit and religious dress. They may do these things for a sign to the government, a sign of the presence of the church. That may be part of his model.

So what you nuns were trying to do was to meet with him and get some kind of a synthesis, because you were on one wavelength and he was on another?

Kane: That is right. The bishop who arranged meetings while the pope was in the U.S. said too many groups asked to meet with the pope. We decided that since we were going to Rome in November, we would arrange a meeting with him in Rome. But his secretary in Rome replied that it was not possible for him to meet with us. The pope was involved in special sessions dealing with financial and bank problems of the Catholic church. The secretary said to write again and ask for another meeting. We wrote again; we asked for a meeting. In March 1980, we got a letter saying that the pope was willing to dialogue with us; however, the appropriate forum for any meeting with us was the Congregation for Religious, CRIS. He encouraged us to meet with them. Indirectly it was a no, but we made a judgment after we read that letter that CRIS is our appropriate, normal channel in Rome. We, in this instance, however, thought it was important to meet directly with the pope so we wrote a second letter. We felt it was important to see him personally. We welcomed the presence of CRIS with us also. We never got an answer to that second request.

Did you feel you were locked out of Rome? Were you being punished?

Kane: No, I didn't feel locked out. What I said at the Shrine was controversial. When I went to Rome in November 1979, I asked several of the officials there whether they thought the pope agreed, appreciated, or liked my statement. They said he really had not expressed any opinion on it.

Do you believe that?

Kane: Well, my sense is, not from him personally, but from a number of the other Vatican officials, that they don't have a problem with speaking your mind on an issue, but do not do it publicly. My sense of him is that he would prefer I had not done it publicly. If we sat down and talked about it over a cup of coffee, it would have been acceptable. But not in a public forum though.

The Vatican therefore was very much aware of what you call "this moment in history"?

Kane: When I went to Rome, right after the event, I had a letter from the head of CRIS requesting that I clarify my greeting at the Shrine. We went through our meeting agenda first. Then they asked me if I would clarify my greeting. "I certainly will," I told them, "but what is it that you want clarified." They replied: "Anything you'd like to say about it." So I thought the best way to handle it was to tell them everything that I've just told you. At that point, in late November 1979, we had probably three to four thousand letters from people. I brought positive and negative letters, and I told these CRIS officials that I understood they were getting many more negative letters in Rome. They, I felt, should hear from both sides. I went through the entire experience, and when I finished, we got into the question of all ministries in the church. They said they [CRIS] had been directed to ask me about this question of ordination. The ordination document had come out in 1977 and therefore in light of it, how could I make such a statement?

I replied that the ordination document did not in anyway close the question off forever. It was an important question and it needed to be raised. In fact, the document itself invited us to dialogue on the the mystery of priesthood, and to come to a better understanding of priesthood. I told them basically the document invites us to do so, and that's what I was doing. I was following the spirit of the letter, raising the issue. It was an issue then, and it is an issue *now*. Their point was: "Well, when does dialogue end and when does obedience begin?" And I said: "On this particular question, the dialogue has just begun."

Really, the document itself in 1977 opened up the whole question.

The tone of the document appears to invite dialogue, but, in essence, it sounds like dialogue is finished.
Kane: Once a document comes out, that is right.

But you, as an American, look at dialogue as discussion.
Kane: From the time of Vatican Council II we nuns were asked to critique and study everything, and raise questions. We opened up our chapters to every member of the community. Any sister could come up to the microphone. We urged her opinion on any issue. We were trained to do that. Dialogue also comes out of John Courtney Murray's spirit in the Vatican II document on *Religious Freedom*. Actually, there is a connection between what we did in Vatican Council II renewal, and what's been the traditional kind of atmosphere in U.S. politics. They are very close.

As president of an order of nuns, how does it happen that you are caught in a position which sounds pre-Vatican II?
Kane: Yes, I think that is a very important question. It comes out so often, this monolithic approach. What is even more interesting is [that] many of the officials in CRIS are Americans.

AMERICAN CLERICS IN ROME
How many American clerics are there in Rome?
Kane: I don't have the numbers, but of the men and women we met in high positions, many of them are Americans. Hence, it is not simply European versus American. It really comes down to how closely and how long you work in the bureaucracy. There one gets into a whole mind-set. The same thing happens in all levels of government in the United States. Those in staff positions get inculcated into a particular system and mind-set. But then there are employees who raise questions and who want to change the bureaucracy. It happens in even the smallest organizations: people on staff raise questions. The administrator says: "How dare you raise a question? This is the way we do it here."

I am surprised to learn that many of these officials of CRIS are American. John Tracy Ellis wrote in the past

that these types became more Roman than the Romans themselves. Can you comment on that?

Kane: Yes, I've heard that a number of times. I also hear that when the some American bishops go over, they act more like *servants* of the Roman staff people. They seem inhibited by them. They are afraid of them. There is a certain awe which intimidates. I myself experience it in Rome. Roman procedures seem out of the last century; things are much less organized, and that has many advantages. Facing the seat of power of the Catholic church, one gets intimidated. When these men go from the United States, they are in awe of all these systems, all these congregations, and of their own staffs. The question of power is pervasive.

These men don't want to rock the boat.

Kane: Correct. None of us likes to rock the boat. It's an odd place to be, especially when you start rocking. The American nuns also are a phenomenon in Rome. We are not like [some other] nuns from around the world, [who are] very protected, very much under their bishops, and certainly not seeing themselves in any way equal with these bishops. Not being formally educated, yet, certainly very smart women, they are not always very articulate. They see themselves more as children with their father rather than as adult women working with adult men.

Adult women working with peers. . . ?

Kane: With peers. When we go to Rome we are professional, confident, assured of who we are, and what we are. We appear as educated and seasoned women. Some of us have gray hair, and even with all of that, we still feel a sense of intimidation. It is somehow overwhelming. I've met people on the street who say, "Oh! the American nuns." It's like we are a real curiosity around Rome. I remember being there after I greeted the pope. I met a priest on the street who was very hostile and he said, "You're Sister Theresa Kane." And I said, "Yes I am." He asked, "What are you doing over here? We don't want the likes of you here!"

Did you ask for clarification?

Kane: I did not. He was in a hurry, and I was so taken aback. When someone attacks, you need a few minutes to recover, to analyze what is happening. In addition to American nuns being a threat to these men, people began to be nervous seeing us around Rome. This priest was apparently one who was unsure.

THE LIBERATION OF WOMEN
Professor Mercy Amba Oduyoye, a scholar born in Ghana, and a teacher at the University of Ibadan in Nigeria who also taught at Harvard in 1986, has argued that African women look to American women. She suggests they feel that if American women achieve liberation, African women will also. Would you respond to that?

Kane: That is very much the spirit women from many other countries have expressed. A few days after I greeted the pope at the Shrine, I traveled on a plane with a woman who recognized me. She thanked me for what I had done. She was a professional Islamic woman from Iran; she noted that women in Iran had just had their uprising about the veiling in 1979. She said the women in the United States are giving courage to women all over the world, and certainly giving courage to women in Iran.

I went to the United Nations *Conference on Women* in 1985, in Nairobi, Kenya. Women attending from all over the world are becoming more and more conscious of their abilities, their gifts, and they want to articulate and promote them. Men in all parts of the world are becoming more and more nervous, not only about the woman's role, but about their own roles. It's as much an adjustment for the men as it is for the women.

Isn't it criminal, though, to deny the gifts of women to the universe?

Kane: Well, part of my mission for myself and other women is to infuse the world with our gifts. I admit that it is criminal to deny women's gifts. People who disagree with this philosophy feel that we are causing deterioration in traditional values. Consequently, we are in a very conflictual time. We must acknowledge the conflict, and yet not be overcome by it. Our greatest challenge is to be convinced about our mission, our vision, what we want to do, and how we want to do it. We must be realistic, knowing that many obstacles will be placed in our way. Yet, if we believe, we will continue.

U.S. blacks in their demand for civil rights in the 1960s went through a similiar experience. Some of the sever-

est opposition at that time came from other blacks.
Kane: That's right. Political leaders in the black community asked Martin Luther King, Jr., how to get across to white people what he was trying to promote. He said he spent all his time trying to get it across to black people. It was black people whom he had to somehow inculcate, encourage, and energize with their own sense of dignity. It is the same for us women. We must not be afraid to promote ourselves. Frequently men do not know how to act when they meet women of equality, and, similiarly, we're not always comfortable being equal with the men. We have the sense that a woman is to be protected. Recently an older woman who visits her husband in the hospital said, "I don't like to go out at night, and if I do, I have a man drive. Now Sister, I know you're not going to like that." I said, "I'm a very competent driver. I am a woman, and as competent as any man to drive day or night." This is kind of thinking we live with. Some of us believe and behave that way. We've been inculcated and [socialized into the belief] that there are certain things women can do, and certain things only men can do. Some women may be uncomfortable fixing a car; but many, many men are uncomfortable fixing dinner in the kitchen. Yet, women and men are capable of both.

MERCY NUNS IN POLITICAL MINISTRY
The Mercy order has blazed a trail in political ministry. Yet, you have gone through three political turmoils.
Kane: Very early in the 1970s, we held strong general chapters which gave social justice a special thrust. The move coincided with the bishops' synod, *Justice in the Church.* Justice was taken very seriously by large numbers of Sisters of Mercy, because we have been in the works of mercy. Sisters felt a human need to move in with the poor, to open up soup kitchens and things of that nature. We set aside monies for sisters who were not funded either by government or by church. They opened up soup kitchens, like the one in Providence, Rhode Island. It became a very natural thing, then, for Liz Morancy, working at McCauley House, to move into the advocacy role. She became an advocate for the poor, ran for office and was elected. The last pope didn't have a problem with it. I think it was so new he did not give it that much attention. A Vatican document issued in the

late 1970s seemed to imply that if a nun was to run for office, all she need do was to call her bishop. But things changed radically in Agnes Mary Mansour's case. For the first time, political ministry became controversial for the [Sisters of Mercy]. There were a lot of local dynamics in Michigan politics. The whole CUFF group was working in the church at that time. . . . Catholics United For the Faith is one of the rightest groups in the Catholic church.

These people are extremists?
Kane: Yes. They became aware of Agnes Mary's position on the governor's cabinet. She was very careful on her position on abortion. Nevertheless, political ministry and the abortion issue got intertwined there. We still see political ministry as something special—a position of advocacy. Changes in structures and systems cannot occur without political involvement. Hence, we sponsor political ministry. This past summer our general chapter affirmed it as appropriate for Sisters of Mercy. I anticipate continued conflict with the church officials. What we must do is acknowledge the conflict, try to negotiate, and work something out. You cannot say it is never allowed because that is not the position of the church. Right now it *is* allowed, but with the approval of the bishop.

Do you have any thoughts on why you have experienced three political conflicts?
Kane: A number of people have asked. It is difficult to document. People tend to put my views and the position of these three Mercy nuns together, giving reasons for the conflict. My intuition indicates a connection, but I have no documentation to prove it.

EXTREMISTS SETTING THE AGENDA?
Please comment, Theresa, on why you think the extremists are setting the agenda for the Catholic church?
Kane: Well, I'm not sure that they are. This particular pope is very orthodox on questions of sexuality and reproduction. The question of birth control was a very conflictual one with the last pope. It is more so with this pope. He considers abortion unjustifiable in any circumstances. He has not said what should be the civil and legal resolution of the issue. In the United States this state-church question is important, and since he is

opposed, certain people take advantage of his position.

Somewhat like Ronald Reagan...

Kane: Yes, that's right. Nationalism, rather than a sense of faith, is becoming the religion of the day. It is something of an idolatry. . .if you're not an American, then somehow you're not connected with God. It is a critical time, because the more we move toward national security, the more we find countries beginning to tighten up. It tends to hold back creativity, the energy of individuals, and the spontaneous, free spirit of people. We seem to have more faith, yet that is unhealthy, because we are not living in a faithful time.

Was there any incident that changed your life?

Kane: What happened to me when I gave the greeting at the Shrine: it was so public, and the response never ceased. Even this interview is a response. In a sense, it helped me to become very conscious of the importance of the question of women. That changed my life, in a kind of quiet, long-range way more than just overnight. It led me along another path: women's groups, speaking with women, and listening to many, many women. Now I'm interested in women's studies and women's history. These I've chosen over a more spiritual approach, and I want to connect them with what has happened to women in the Catholic church. It is a very creative and exciting time for us women.

Essentially you are at peace?

Kane: I try very hard to keep myself in peace. I have my normal anxiety and nervousness. I'm someone who does not often get angry but when I do, I try to work through the anger in a way that is direct. I have learned how to be angry without being hostile. I have just anger where something really isn't right, and I want it corrected. It is important for me to correct it. I may do so immediately, or over a period of time. I may do it quietly or not so quietly. Not being hostile and warlike helps me to a deeper sense of peace. All injustices are not going to be righted, but at least if I'm aware of them, I like to work towards righting them.

You keep connecting how we are and how we live based on our American ideals, and political orientation. I only repeat that a lot of who I am and where I came from has to do with my upbringing in the Sisters of Mercy and the fact that I entered the order in 1955, just eight years before Vatican Council II. After a few years, I heard sisters raising questions during our general chapters. I was led into adulthood asking questions. I listened a great deal, learned a great deal, and saw the need for change. All of it produced who and what I am. Add to that my experience in the Leadership Council of Women Religious (I went to their national conventions every year). The question of women in the church was consistently addressed. The words I used in the greeting in 1979 were similiar to a resolution we passed six years earlier. We resolved and affirmed that women, as well as men, must be in all ministries of the church.

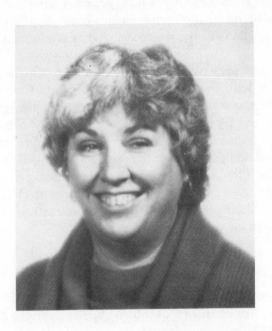

RUTH McDONOUGH FITZPATRICK

"When Margie Tuite died recently, I went to her wake and funeral. . . .I stood up and gave her talk, to remind all present of her words. And over in the corner was her casket, covered with a peace quilt. I quoted her . . . . 'I still have a dream. . .Just do it. Take it. . . .' The next day I realized that moment was the beginning of our taking church to ourselves, saying to women, 'We are church. We are coming out as church.'"

Ruth McDonough Fitzpatrick coordinates Women's Ordination Conference (WOC) from her Fairfax, Virginia, home. Associated with the movement from its inception, she is a walking warehouse of information on Catholic women's struggle to be ordained. Born into a military family, Ruth has, since childhood, yearned to become a Roman Catholic priest. Only once had she a desire to be a nun. She told her mother she felt she had a vocation. Her mother replied, "Hold on; it will go away."

Married and the mother of three grown children and growing grandchildren, she has seen women's ordination goals change from ordination at any price to demanding a reformed and new church.

The desire to be ordained has not vanished. On the contrary, beginning with the first Women's Ordination Conference in 1976, Ruth's vision of women-church became gradually clarified. She is one of many Catholic women who, in desiring ordination, wish to create their own ministry. Providing provocative inside pericopes of the pope's visit in 1981, she shows fascinating glimpses of the "collaboration" between press and pope. She describes a vision of powerful men in church circles and their disconcerting, behind-the-scenes methods of intimidating Catholic women.

COMING OF THE SPIRIT

You await the day when women will be made priests, bishops, popes in the Catholic church. Where did your interest in this come from?

Fitzpatrick: In 1976, I was convinced that I would never be a priest. I decided that the only way to deal with that loss was to live the priesthood without ordination. This is one reason why my home is also the office of the Women's Ordination Conference. I cannot merely live in a middle class home, being a middle class woman. Once I became active in church, I then began to give my total life to social justice issues. These issues put me sometimes with, sometimes against, the hierarchy. One day I may organize a prayer vigil for the bishops in Lafayette Park; earlier that day I may demonstrate outside the Hilton Hotel against the bishops . . . .

At one time I was a non-entity Catholic. After I married, I bundled up the kids, went to church every Sunday, sat through and endured. My son attended CCD classes. He came home one day and asked me if I knew that there was a bad angel on one shoulder and a good angel on the other, both urging us on. I said to myself, "That is not right." So I moved out of that conservative parish into a more progressive one run by Belgian priests. There I learned about Vatican II, studied CCD methods of teaching, and fell in love with the Scriptures.

Then the time came for [my children] Kelly and Michael to be confirmed together. A friend and I went to the confirmation, which was performed by the Bishop of Pusoli, Italy, where we were then stationed. It is important to know that the Catholic chaplain in the military is evaluated and ranked for promotion. Our particular chaplain was an extremely ambitious Italian priest. He said the only reason he had gone into the seminary was, being the youngest of thirteen children, he would, for the first time, have a bedroom of his own. He bragged, "I have never read a theology book since I graduated." Of course I had read a lot of theology. The night our children were confirmed in the Pusoli church (where St. Paul is supposed to have landed on one of his three missionary journeys), we went there early. Marines in full-dress uniforms and white gloves met us at the door. Since they were ushering us as if it were a wedding, these men asked, "Are you invited guests?" We said, "Invited guests? We are parents of the confirmands." And they said, "You stand in the back here and if there are any seats left over you can have them." What that chaplain of the base had done was to invite what is called the "protocol list"—all the marine VIPs. We, the parents, could not even sit down.

Afterward, with our families, we went to the Officer's Club for dinner. We walked by this private room and saw the Bishop of Pusoli, the chaplain, the VIPs. . .who didn't even know what was happening, all celebrating. Some of them said to us, "We got an invitation to this confirmation. What's a confirmation?" We parents were quite outraged. We made an appointment with the chaplain, but he said, "If you want to get involved in anything, join the women's group. That's where everything is done." This event radicalized me. I then realized that the chaplaincy, which is supposed to be ministering to people, became caught up in a military promotion system, and that this priest was not pastoral. His ambition was preventing him from serving the people as he was paid to do.

What was the effect of this incident?

Fitzpatrick: It filled me with rage. That was to me the coming of the Holy Spirit. I was confirmed at the age of seven by Cardinal [Richard] Cushing before the war broke out. It meant nothing. Neither did my first communion. But this outrage—I felt like I had just been confirmed—filled me with the Spirit.

From Vatican II, I knew this was not what church should be about. That was the beginning of my becoming actively involved: experiencing the suffering, seeing the injustices, and trying to do something about them.

What did this transformation drive you to do? What have you done?

Fitzpatrick: On my return to the U.S. I went to Georgetown University [Washington, D.C.]. Georgetown people looked at a person like me as if my mind had been asleep for eighteen years. There's no way, they seemed to say, that you can get in here. But I was determined to be accepted just so I could tell them to "forget it." McDonough Gymnasium at that university is named after my great uncle; my father and all my uncles are alumni. They, of course, were all very much caught up in the male hierarchy and its patriarchy. I wanted to be the first woman in the family to break this tradition. And so I did!

Monika Hellwig became my advisor in theology, and I became updated in what Vatican II meant. I had some outstanding courses with Jesuit Jim Walsh. The Hebrew Scriptures gave me an indescribably new understanding of the God of love and the God of justice.

After graduation, I went to work for Georgetown's School of Education. I developed programs in church ministry, religious education, social justice, and one for the divorced and separated. This last program, though I could never prove it, got me out of Georgetown. The bishop wrote to the Jesuit president [of Georgetown] (who was leaving, and wanted to go out in a burst of glory). The president "freaked" out when he received the letter, insisting that these courses could not go on under his watch. I was told I must leave in six months. Subsequently, they had one or two religious programs, but nothing on social justice or the divorced.

I then went to work for the Women's Ordination Conference (WOC) and later moved the office to Washington, D.C. On June 6, 1977, we celebrated its official opening in a storefront. Drug dealers were plying their trade in the back, and [they were] derelicts in the front of our offices. I tried to make the statement that women's ordination is being with the poor, the oppressed and the forgotten . . . .

While working for WOC, I got involved with a local community called Tabor House. It was a "dialogue center" where people lived a simplified community lifestyle. It was founded by former missionaries from Latin America. I went there for lunch each day. Gradually I became closer and closer to the group and to another experience of alternative lived church—not something we're *philosophizing* about, but something we were *living*. It was a mixed community of lay people, nuns, priests, married priests, kids. People came there who had been tortured or had other terrible experiences in Latin America. Tabor House helped them to talk to this Congress person, or to that official, and to go to the U.S. Catholic Conference and tell their story. That's when I became aware of the importance of telling one's story. After dinner, in Tabor House, we sat around the dining room table, and said, "Now tell us your story."

WOMEN'S STORIES

Current women writers, such as Rosemary Radford Ruether, place great emphasis on women telling their stories. Why do you also see it as important?

Fitzpatrick: It's the only way to change the world of women. Much of what we did in the past was an intellectualizating and a philosophizing that is somewhat separated from our lived experience. Only by telling the story can an Argentine person show me what her (or his) experiences are. As a North American, I can then somehow have some empathy, establish some bonding, and in that way enter into and become worthy of the body of Christ. We are brothers and sisters even though we are very different. I found through hearing and sharing our stories we became friends, and we experienced something even deeper than friendship.

Do you think this is the insight women contribute to ministry?

Fitzpatrick: Well, the women certainly have picked it up. At Tabor House, Peter Hinde, a Carmelite priest, encouraged the form. He and Betty Campbell, the Mercy nun who founded the house, taught us the importance of one's story. Coming from their missionary experiences in Peru, they had learned the value of letting go the hospitals, parishes and property. Hinde turned his parish over to the Peruvians; Betty released the Mercy hospital to the Peruvians. She went to the mountains and lived with the Indian women as a midwife. She helped deliver babies, but mostly she was just there, you see.

What you seem to be saying, Ruth, is that in the past, the church supplied an answer for everything. And you're saying that such an approach is too intellectual. Womens' stories add a new element to the way we now envision church. This new element allows other facets of the human person—feelings, sufferings, and a vision of new church—to emerge.

Fitzpatrick: There has always been a split, a dualism, between the spiritual and the secular, the flesh and the spirit, the body and the soul. It is one of the problems of Christian theology. I have to thank my Latin American friends for helping me deal with Greek iconography. "Away with that," they taught me. Instead, the sharing of the story is the sharing of the totality of life and the reality of personal experience. Now I too try to incorporate this approach into the WOC newspaper. *New Women, New Church* tells stories and from those stories we get a true picture of a human being.

You were involved in the Latin American Bishops' meeting in Puebla, Mexico, in 1979. How did it influence you?

Fitzpatrick: Two conferences of Catholic bishops in Latin America changed the face of the church there. One was in Medellin [Colombia] in 1968 and the other in Puebla [Mexico] in 1979. It was at Medellin especially that the Latin American bishops took Vatican II and began to deal with it. They affirmed what they called an "option for the poor" and oppressed. Although lay people were present, few women participated. But, in 1979, a follow-up meeting was held in Puebla. I went and met Betzie Hollants there.

Betzie had been to Vatican II as a journalist. She was a marvelous, wonderful woman who worked with Ivan Illich in Cuernavaca. Active in grass-roots organizing [and] women's issues, she called women together to make sure that they would not be forgotten in the findings and recommendations of the Puebla meeting. At Medellin, women, it so happened, were not even mentioned. Consequently, the group of us who went to Puebla held seminars and workshops. We met women from all over the world, and the bonding from that experience is still alive.

Outside the walls where we women were, workshops, press conferences, and meetings were held every night. The bishops were locked in meetings inside the walls. One bishop said, "We are dead men in here. The living are outside those walls." And some of them came out and shared our meetings. People like [Archbishop] Oscar Romero [of El Salvador] came late (he had to bury people just killed in his diocese). The relatives of the disappeared from Argentina were present. These women and men asked the bishops, "Where are our disappeared relatives in Argentina?" Every issue, every conceivable subject, was discussed by the women at Puebla. We educated the press from all over the world. It was a wonderful experience of how the institutional church is just really walled in, and life is outside those walls. And if they wanted to come out, they were welcome to do so.

And some of the bishops acknowledged this?

Fitzpatrick: Yes they did. And it was a very important moment in my development. It was also the first time I was ever called a communist. The women meeting there had been offered hospitality by a number of fine Catholic families in Puebla. Somebody phoned these homeowners and said, "Why are you housing these women? They are communists. They are against the pope. If you don't stop the hospitality to them, you will be excommunicated." These families were so terrified that they disinvited us women. Only one family gave us a brunch at the end and said we were welcome any time, *"Mi casa es su casa"* (my house is your house). We wondered, then doubted, that a priest made the calls. Who would ever believe one would be excommunicated for housing a group of women? And who would ever believe I would go down to Mexico to be called a communist?

WOMEN'S ORDINATION

Where do you see women's ordination at the moment?

Fitzpatrick: I keep saying we will not see it in this pope's lifetime. Certainly one day we will have women ordained in the Roman Catholic church. But when I look at WOC newsletters and the recorded pictures of all the different episodes along the way since 1976, I find much of its past has been protest. Demonstrations, organizing, trying to hammer through that wall, so the hierarchy will acknowledge that women exist, and throw us the bone of ordination. Yet we all know from the Episcopal women's experience that ordination is not the answer. It marks the beginning of another big struggle. I now see that we're not asking any longer simply for ordination. We still have to work for the ordination of women. But my book of photographs of WOC's activities in the last year shows that we women now have our own prayer meetings, our own liturgical celebrations, and our own workshops. Women are now ministering in a renewed Christian ministry. In some ways we are living out that ministry. We would be reined in if we were ordained.

Are you therefore less fervent in agitating for ordination, because now you feel that the women are really doing ordained ministry anyhow?

Fitzpatrick: I think we're coming into our own. I learned this especially at one workshop-dialogue session with the bishops. When these men saw two thousand women meeting simultaneously with their annual meeting, the bishops panicked. They declared they must do a pastoral on women. "We must pay attention to these women," they claimed, "because they're leaving the church and taking their children with them." That is why I say now we're not asking any more; we're beginning to realize an alternative reality and that's a gift. If they had given us ordination ten years ago, they would now have us. But we would not be free. Now we are free.

So you feel denial of ordination is a blessing?

Fitzpatrick: I feel it's a blessing in many, many ways. Part of the blessing is that WOC existed for ten years and has grown a great deal during that time. We are not saying, "Just hand us that cup, give us those vestments, and put us up there on the altar." We realize, now, when we talk about *renewed priestly ministry*, that it is not an abstraction; it has to be something that's lived out of our experience. That lived experience will change the church. It is the only way the church will change. The church has always changed by people acting. New practices. . .bring along the institutional church. It finally catches up, and validates what had already changed.

You think that women are going their own way, emptying the pews and bringing their children with them?

Fitzpatrick: I know it has happened to a large extent. There are many who stay, no doubt about that. But every time we have an incident like the current Charlie Curran affair, more and more people, like my nephew, say, "I don't want my child to go to Catholic school after all this. I don't think I even want my child baptized." Yet, when he was married ten years ago, he and his wife were going to have their children baptized and attend Catholic school.

How has it come about that the conservatives and the extremists are setting the agenda of the Catholic church?
Fitzpatrick: Because they have the power. The Knights of Malta are a good example. Some are members of the Reagan Administration, powerful people in his administration: [the late] William Casey, head of the Central Intelligence Agency, and James Buckley, who once headed US propaganda against Eastern Europe at Radio Free Europe and Radio Liberty. Current members who are knights (after the feudal fashion) include Lee Iacocca, John McComb, William Buckley, Alexander Haig, Otto Von Hapsberg, and various leaders of the fascist Masonic Lodge in Italy, who are closely tied to the Vatican and the Vatican Bank affair. There are many very key people: J. Peter Grace, president of W.R. Grace Company, belongs and he was the key figure in Operation Paperclip [the Reagan Administration's project to cut government spending]. The Knights had also been funding the Contra war [against the Nicaraguan government] before it was made legal. Now, sadly, the Congress voted that it was legal to fund this disgraceful war.

These men also have the ear of the pope; women do not. Theresa Kane was able to welcome the pope in Washington only because she was in the leadership position at Leadership Conference of Women Religious. She welcomed him and said, "Please listen to the sufferings of the women and open up the church to ministry at all levels." And he said he didn't hear her: the acoustics were such that he didn't hear her. Now, she has never been able to get an appointment with the pope even to explain what she said. But [I presume] any Knight of Malta can pick up the phone and talk to the pope.

THE PAPAL VISIT TO WASHINGTON, D.C.
You were in the Washington Basilica when the pope visited? Can you tell us about it, and your vigil which

preceded the visit?

Fitzpatrick: Well, it was an exciting time. The Quixote Center and other groups formed a coalition of people concerned for rights in the church. This coalition met and strategized about what should be done. I remember saying we should dog his footsteps from the minute he lands at the airport until he gets back on his plane. Luckily, the Pope came to Washington, D.C. last. Every place he went there were demonstrations not against the pope personally, but against sexism in the church. We didn't know him well enough to evaluate whether or not we liked him.

In Philadelphia he spoke to a big audience of seminarians and said there would be no women priests. And the seminarians stood up and cheered and clapped! Every place he went he said something that got more and more people angry so that by the time he came to Washington, we were ready. We decided to use blue armbands (blue for Our Lady) in protest. My interest in the Nicaraguan base communities made me appreciate Mary's Magnificat: he will cast down the mighty and raise up the lowly. We used that prayer. We reclaimed Mary, printed posters and banners, and put out press releases.

Priests for Equality issued another call from the Washington area. Around the country lay people had become accustomed to distributing communion. Yet, for the pope's masses, no lay person was allowed to give communion. The excuse was there were plenty of priests. Priests for Equality asked all priests to pull back from giving communion, to withdraw themselves so that lay people would have to do it. We also encouraged people not to go to communion.

Bill Callahan was one of those priests calling for the pull back. He is a Jesuit who started the Quixote Center and had been at the Center of Concern [a Jesuit-sponsored reseach project in Washington, D.C.]. He works with the "no-no" issues in the church: the "new waves" ministry, and ministry to homosexuals. The thing that basically got Callahan in trouble was the issue of women's ordination. The pope silenced him.

Why? What did this Jesuit say?

Fitzpatrick: He came out for women's ordination in the 1970s. He also said the pope doesn't understand [the U.S. situation] because he's Polish. Eventually, his superiors got orders from

Rome through the Jesuits (as you know, they too work on the hierarchical system) that he should be silenced on the subject of calling for women's ordination. . . .Because he was the first to be silenced on the issue of women's ordination, he knew how to use the press. The press loved him because he's extremely articulate. At the pope's visit he wore his collar, and he spoke to the journalists, something the church cannot stand.

Why not?

Fitzpatrick: Because it's the only alternative that the voiceless people have. And Rome can't control the secular press, much as they would like to. During the pope's visit we went to the apostolic delegate's home where both were spending the night. We decided to hold a liturgy across the street, a women's liturgy with men, women, and everybody. It was a candlelight event; we sang songs like "We Shall Overcome" and "We Shall Equal Be" across from the house where the pope was. Our press releases had gone out; even the press van was there with guys sitting in it as we held our liturgy. They didn't move out of their seats, didn't even take a picture, and, of course, did not print anything. We stayed all night.

Next morning, standing several yards from us was a big group newly arrived from St. Mary's of the Lake Seminary in Michigan where the pope had once visited. Word spread that he wanted to see these people from St. Mary's. Suddenly, the big French doors opened over the balcony, and the pope appeared waving. [People were] cheering, singing, and yelling. We too ran up; we all mingled right in with the group. We couldn't hear a spoken word because of all the traffic on Massachusetts Avenue. We women sang at the top of our lungs,"We Shall Overcome," "We Shall Equal Be." The Michigan people were saying, "Oh, Holy Father." He came down the steps suddenly, before we knew what was happening. The Secret Service stopped all the traffic. The pope walked right out to the curb. We of Women's Ordination Conference called to him, even louder.

Did he recognize the women?

Fitzpatrick: I don't know if he even saw us in all the excitement. I did know that he was not there for the women, but for his friends from St. Mary's. The important thing was that the television cameras never turned on for our all-night vigil. Also, we realized that all across the country there had been demonstrations, but there had been no report of them in the major press.

After our demonstration, Dolly Pomerlau of WOC went to a bar with someone for drinks. The mainstream press people told her at that bar that they had an agreement: *self-censorship*. If they reported something the hierarchy did not like, subsequently they would be excluded from the press pool. Hence the press self-censored. The major story was the pope; the minor story was the fringe activities and the protests of sexism. The protests were massive around the country, yet the press simply did not report them.

THE PRESS AND THE VATICAN
So you feel there was collusion?
Fitzpatrick: We figured that there was collusion. It was verified by another story from these press people. They told us of the secret arrangements. When the pope waved to beckon the multitudes, they could take pictures. However, when he put his fingers together in a certain way they were supposed to focus in on his face, and that meant not on the women or the men demonstrating on the sidewalk.

This is similar to when President Reagan went to Ireland. . . .Independent sources told me that there was sustained opposition to his visit. The Irish had very strong feelings against Reagan because many Irish missionary priests in Nicaragua and Central America know first hand of the brutality that goes on there with American support. But reading the press reports in the United States, other than The New York Times, **this opposition was not covered. . . .**
Fitzpatrick: The thing that's really frightening is that the press leader in the stories is *The New York Times*. If it carries something "that's fit to print," then *The Washington Post* and *The Los Angeles Times* and all the others will pick it up. But in our protest, *The New York Times* did see it as news, and the others did not pick it up. You have to look at who owns the newspapers and realize how deeply, deeply mired it all becomes.

Now before we leave this issue of women's ordination,

let me ask what is the missing element in women that prevents them from being ordained? I believe the pope called it the "ineluctable" maleness, or whatever it is that makes the male ordainable. What is that missing thing?

Fitzpatrick: It's anatomy! The missing part in women is the penis. It really gets down to that; people don't want to hear it. This is the first argument used in the Vatican declaration against the ordination of women. Women do not "image" Jesus in the male form and Jesus came as a male. He could never have come as a female in those times and circulate as freely as he did. Had he not come as a man he could never have related to people as he did. If he came today, he probably would be a black woman or a Third World woman. That is history. This pope has changed the argument a bit, saying that not only are we women not ordainable, but they don't have the anatomy. It goes back to Freud's "anatomy is destiny." The pope [essentially] said in Belgium that it's very simple why women cannot be priests: there were no women at the Last Supper.

But if one adopted this kind of logic, one would have to admit there were not Poles there either. . .

Fitzpatrick: Of course there were no Poles. There were no Romans, there were no Italians, there were no Gentiles. That we know of. But we know that there were women there. The women—Jewish women prepare the Passover meal—were everywhere. They never left him as the men did. Who did the dishes? Who cooked the meals? It was the Seder supper, the Passover supper, which is a family affair. Women are always included.

VATICAN REPRESENTATIVES
AND WOMEN'S ORDINATION

During your involvement with WOC, have you had any encounters with the Vatican representatives in this country?

Fitzpatrick: I want to talk about two instances. One dates back ten years, and one dates to 1986. Ten years ago, right after the Vatican Declaration on Ordination, we had a very wonderful apostolic delegate here. Jean Jardot was a Vatican II-type bishop who appointed a number of very, very good bishops in the United States. As the co-ordinator of the Women's Ordination Conference, I was invited to a meeting of Christian feminists. Jean Jardot agreed to attend, just to listen. He was not going to dialogue, nor get into any discussion. He decided to listen to what the women had to say about ordination. We had a very interesting evening.

I was not told that the event was off the record. In an interview with David Anderson for an UPI article, I said we had met with the Apostolic delegate. Well, I got a call from Jean Jardot, saying I should not have said he attended a WOC evening. I wrote him and said I thought he was a man who would stand behind what he said. If he said something to a group of women, I didn't see any harm in mentioning it. We were exchanging letters back and forth, each holding our own. Gradually, I realized that Jardot needed to write those letters, more or less to cover his situation. He had to cover his situation because UPI went all over the world and I'm sure the Vatican asked him what he was up to. I had another view of how the hierarchy has to cover itself simply because it is the hierarchy.

Before we move on to the second incident, could you comment on what seems to be a lack of solidarity among the male clergy—for example, where are all the "progressive clerics" now that Charlie Curran is in trouble?

Fitzpatrick: I really don't know. Many of them have chosen their issues. Walter Sullivan is Jardot's bishop and he defended Curran. His issue is social justice and he has been very involved in peace issues, in the peace pastoral letter, and in Central America. Bishops may have to choose which road to go down. I don't know who is choosing Charlie Curran as his issue. The United States does not have prophetic bishops like Archbishop [Oscar] Romero. There's no cardinal here who would go to Rome with Charlie Curran like the three Brazilian cardinals who went with Father [Leonardo] Boff.

You said there was a second incident with Vatican officials?

Fitzpatrick: The second incident occured in October 1985, when the Women's Ordination Conference held a convocation— "Ordination Reconsidered"—in St. Louis. It was a meeting for

Catholic women who were trying to discern their call to the priesthood. We wrote to the Leadership Conference of Women Religious, asking them to co-sponsor the event. Our brochure listed twenty-five or so sponsors who had responded in time for the printing. We also had lay sponsors like Mary Gordon, the novelist, and Marianne Kelly of our office.

Months later, I received phone calls from religious orders asking for a copy of the brochure. I asked these callers, "What's happening?" Someone finally told me that they had gotten letters from the new apostolic delegate.

Who is he?

Fitzpatrick: Archbishop Pio Laghi. He had taken it upon himself to search out the list from A to Z, beginning with the Adorers of the Precious Blood nuns. He searched out the names and the addresses of the women in leadership positions in these orders. He wrote each of them a letter asking, "What does co-sponsorship mean to you? How did you decide whether to co-sponsor this meeting which was called by the 'Women's Ordination Conference?'" He put Women's Ordination Conference in quotes. He inquired if the entire community made the decision. Or was the decision made by the superiors alone?

I saw this as a very manipulative form of harassment to intimidate the women whom the archbishop figured were major funders of the Women's Ordination Movement. Not only to intimidate them about giving money, but to divide lay women from nuns. Rome would love to do this, because they are very fearful of that bonding. The harassment was designed further to divide the community members from their leaders by asking them "Did *you* decide, or did all your nuns decide?"

The women were not intimidated. Unlike abortion, which is a more emotional issue, women's ordination is clear. We have done the theology; we have done the research; we are very clear. One nun wrote, "We'll have no trouble answering Pio Laghi. I'm on the funding committee for my order and I'm going to make sure that you get a large amount of money." Two months later her order sent a "lovely" sum.

Did you communicate with Archbishop Pio Laghi?

Fitzpatrick: Yes. I realized that he was never going to write to Women's Ordination Conference. I wrote him a letter which mirrored back his questions. I asked him in ten different ways why he was doing this and who asked him to do it? Did the Knights of Malta set him up? Are Catholics United for Faith the ones? Who's sending him the brochure and saying, "Look at this horrible thing?" Or did Rome ask him to do it? Did he notify the American Catholic bishops he was harassing these nuns?

I asked for a meeting with him and with lay women. I wanted to get the heat off the nuns. I wanted to take advantage of his office to arrange a meeting with the pope to talk on this issue. His letter to me did not, of course, answer any of those questions. He ignored my request for dialogue, [and] insisted that ordination of women was a matter of doctrine and discipline.

I noticed also how he addressed your letter: Ruth McDonough-Fitzpatrick, P.O. Box 2693, Fairfax, VA.
Fitzpatrick: He did not even acknowledge our letterhead—the heading of our letter and its envelope. He ignored my involvment in any way with WOC. I thought that as history views this incident, somebody going through these files will see a letter from Pio Laghi to some woman, some housewife with a post office box in Fairfax, Virginia. He could not even acknowledge that the conference exists. If he acknowledged that it existed, he would in some ways, in his eyes, legitimize it.

I reviewed my canon law commentary, talked to canon lawyers, and it's very clear to me that he was either shooting across the bow or harassing us. It is clear that we see the tip of the iceberg now; there's going to be a lot more—a lot more repression.

MARJORIE TUITE: WOMAN MARTYR
You wanted to mention Marge Tuite. . . ?
Fitzpatrick: I'd like to talk about Margie Tuite. Margie was one of the founders of our conference and served on the first board of directors. I've known her since 1976 and worked closely with her in National Assembly of Religious Women. I also worked with her on Central American issues. We asked her to give the keynote talk at the 1985 WOC Awards dinner. She had grave doubts because she had moved so far from wanting ordination to the point where she cried, "They don't want you women, they've never wanted you, they're never going to want you." Prophetically she added, "My friends know that some-

day I will sit up in my coffin and I will say: "Wait a minute. I still have that dream and it's a collective dream of renewed priestly ministry. They never will give it to you. *You must take it.*"

When Margie died recently, I went to her wake and funeral, and we sang, "Oh Margie, don't you weep, don't you moan." We came to the part where it said, ". . .makes no difference what they do; women church is coming through; patriarchy got drowned. Oh Margie, don't you weep." I stood up and gave her talk, to remind all present of her words. And over in the corner was her casket, covered with a peace quilt. I quoted her, ". . . I still have that dream. . . .Just do it. Take it." Everybody in the room clapped! The next day I realized that moment was the beginning of our taking church to ourselves, saying to women, "We are church. We are coming out as church."

The funeral was held in the church where she'd been baptized and served as principal. William Sloane Coffin [of Riverside Church in New York City], people from National Council of Churches, Church Women United—her funeral was packed with people of all faiths. Before the Mass the pastor said, "We are all brothers and sisters under the skin. However, I must remind you, that only Catholics can receive communion." I was dozing off. I heard this murmur going around the church and I said to the woman next to me, "What did he say?" "You can't receive communion unless you're Catholic," she said. In a loud voice to all in the pews around me, I called, "That's not true. No, no, no, that's not true. You know that's not true. You're all welcome."

At the consecration, the priest on the altar was surrounded with women. He was trying to elbow them back to give him his sacred space. But all of us extended our hands and said the words of consecration so loudly that you could hear it in this huge New York church. Now we've said consecration at many of our liturgies, in living rooms and smaller places. That's the first time in my life I've ever heard a consecration said from a parish church. Finally, we could really hear it. Before communion, Maureen Fieldler got out of the pew and went up and down the first seven rows saying, "Everybody, please come to communion; everybody is very welcome." And I grabbed the arm of the woman next to me and said, "Are you Catholic?" And she said "No" and I said, "You're coming, aren't you?" And she said, "Yes, of course." At that point we saw William Sloane Coffin walking back from communion, and people who had meetings scheduled—Protestants—all stayed so that they would receive communion. And the pastor had disappeared. He had said his words—he knew the New York terrain. Women-church. . .came into its own at Margie's funeral in the way that Margie wanted.

You know, you can't just bury Margie in a normal parish type of a liturgy. She was too big for that. It was the turning point. . . .That's right. There is a new church emerging. A church of women and men—we shall equal be!

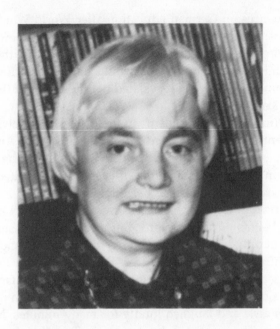

ELISABETH SCHÜSSLER FIORENZA

"I feel my contribution is to provide a critical theological analysis in this struggle to end patriarchy, to help women get in touch with their resources. Church was not made by just men. . . .Today the American church couldn't exist without the work of women. The whole renewal in the American church couldn't exist without women; theology wouldn't be what it is without women; everything wouldn't be what it is without women."

Born in Rumania of a German family, Elisabeth remembers the street fighting in 1944-45 as World War II ended. Her family became fugitives and fled to Austria and ended up in West Germany, where her parents and a brother still live. One of her great wishes as a child was to receive a "care" package, but, she adds, "It never came."

She recalls American soldiers throwing gum and chocolate from passing jeeps to hungry German children, but she was too shy to jostle for her share. Elisabeth also recounts that American influences on German education after World War II were enormous: German history was redirected to create new heroes like George Washington and his "cherry tree," rather than Hitler and his henchmen. She would be a typical Reaganite anti-communist today, she says, had not the events of the 1960s in America changed her.

Her "first idea of a problem" in the U. S. was the civil rights movement of blacks. It transformed her image of American democracy. The Vietnam War added yet another enlightening dimension to her understanding of events in the United States and consequently radicalized her thinking.

A "Bavarian Catholic," she was raised in the strict and traditional beliefs of her religion. But as a youngster she questioned not only why she was obliged to be so quiet and stiff in church, if indeed church was the "Father's" house. One day she dressed in a Mardi Gras costume and painted her face. Proceeding alone to the empty parish church, she stood in the middle of an aisle and laughed loudly for many minutes. Nothing happened. The ground did not open and swallow her as she had anticpated.

The experience stimulated an intense questioning of church teaching on what God was like. As a teenager she often thought of becoming a nun. But her pastor whom she admired and trusted always told her, "Elisabeth, don't do it." He was convinced that she had no vocation to obedience and would in fact "Go in the front and just as quickly come out the back door." She considered becoming a celibate pastoral assistant for a parish. Such women wore small modernized veils and blue dresses, possibly patterned on those of Protestant deaconesses. But after finishing an extended education, most of these pastoral associates ended up as secretaries. Elisabeth was certain she would never be a good secretary, so she therefore applied to the University of Würzburg and went on to become one of the most important Catholic feminist scholars writing today. A dedicated feminist, she says that we "need transforming moments, breakthrough 'ah-ha' experiences" to pierce the web of socialization. But it is essential, for Elisabeth, to act on these moments of illumination, these epiphanies which come into lives that listen for the voice of grace.

Currently Talbot Professor New Testament at Episcopal Divinity School, Cambridge, Massachusetts, Elisabeth is a distinguished author, scholar, and model for women who want to understand what the fellowship of equality means in a hierarchical church. *In Memory of Her,* one of her many books, is a feminist hermeneutic of the New Testament. She has received many awards, including the 1987 U. S. Catholic Award.

In this interview Elisabeth shares both her understanding of feminism and her views on the creation of women-church.

As a woman and a Catholic feminist scholar, you are perceived by some women to be working on a very "heady" level. How do you respond to this perception and how do you make your thoughts as a feminist scholar and theologian accessible to the average woman?
Schüssler Fiorenza: I doubt that all women have this reaction. However, I'm deliberately intellectual, yet I don't like the presupposition that "heady level" is something men can be, but for women it's not quite acceptable. There is a great danger in the women's movement of falling into this trap, and to say that thinking is masculine; women are not to think. It is a trap. The culture has always maintained that thinking is man's work. I was fortunate to be invited to the conference at Grailville on "Women Doing Theology" in 1972. It was a very decisive conference for the development of feminist theology. I remember exploding at one point because in my group they were saying "ministry" is fine for women but "theology" is a male head-trip.

All my life I have been told that because I'm a girl I ought not to read or to study, but to do all the household things that *real* women do. All my life I've rejected. . . .So very deliberately I am on a heady level—an intellectual level—because I think our culture allows only a very few people from a certain class background to learn to think analytically, and to define and name the world. Women are usually not among those people. If women move into the intellectual sphere, then women are allowed to do the legwork for the men who provide the theories, and so on. But women are not then seen as *authorities* in scholarship.

Do you feel that this view is changing?

Schüssler Fiorenza: Only very slowly. . . .Although some of us have moved into the academy, because of this ambivalent relationship of feminism to scholarship and intellectual work, we have not emphasized sufficiently that feminist work needs all the intellectual work that we can do. We must, therefore, be able to disagree. We must explore theory for the sake of developing a better understanding of our world, of the church. Feminists in general have not sufficiently worked through the anti-intellectual cultural prejudice, but feminists in religion have done even less.

Recently, for example, I was at a dinner for my school. Someone from the board, very well intentioned, talked about the last years, and how the school has moved forward. He announced that they were able to hire some women faculty with great scholarly potential. Now, I and the other women on the faculty are not twenty-five. If he had a man on the faculty of my age and stature, he would never say that such a male scholar had great potential.

Did you correct him?

Schüssler Fiorenza: Oh, no, it was a big dinner event. He would not have understood what I meant. I'm sure he thought it was a great compliment to point out the women faculty had potential for scholarship!

Because of pressure by women students, the liberal academy has recognized that there must be women on the faculty. But to have women on the faculty, and to acknowledge them as *shaping* the discipline, are two different things.

You feel that while many women look on you as having made great headway, you in turn look on the academy as having a long way to go.

Schüssler Fiorenza: I *have* made great headway, and I do not want to detract from that. In 1959, I was the first woman admitted to the full course of theology for the master of divinity in Würzburg. I had no idea that I wanted to be a theologian; it was beyond me. I wanted to become a pastoral assistant! That didn't work out, for good reasons, and I'm glad. I am very proud when young women come to me and say, "Oh, when I was finishing college, you gave a talk. You were the first woman theologian I ever heard, and that really influenced me to do theology. Suddenly, I too, imagined that *I* could be a theologian."

This is an accomplishment, but whether or not feminist theology will shape theology as a discipline, or shape church policy, that's a quite different issue. That requires struggle; it requires much broader support among women who will not say that it's a head-trip. Rather, they might say it's good that she's doing this; it's a part of our struggle.

TOWARD A FEMINIST THEOLOGY

Mary Hunt, among others, constructs feminist theology. Are you encouraged by that?

Schüssler Fiorenza: Yes. Feminist theology is the most exciting area in theology. The question is: How much impact does it have? I am on the editorial board of *Concilium*, an international theological journal, and, many of my colleagues such as [J.-M.] Pohier, [Edward] Schillebeeckx, Hans Küng, Leonardo Boff or [Gustavo] Gutiérrez have had trouble with the Vatican. When we sit down for a glass of wine, they will express their anxiety about their situation and troubles with Rome. In response, I always point out, "Look, if they were to invite me to come to Rome, to defend points of my theology, it would be great progress because they would have to acknowledge that a serious feminist theologian exists. What you are all bemoaning, what is tragedy for you, that would be progress for me!"

Theresa Kane noted at the Women's Ordination Conference in October 1985 that ten years ago women were not really an issue of concern for the Vatican. Yet, five years ago women became part of Rome's agenda and in 1984 Catholic American women, in particular, were perceived as problematic. Do you agree?

Schüssler Fiorenza: That might be Theresa's perspective. Coming from Europe, and having done a book in the early 1960s on ministries of women in the church, I don't see the Vatican as just recently concerned about women's issues. There was a motion for women priests at the Second Vatican Council. Many books in the 1950s and 1960s were written on the issue of women in the church. What concerns the Vatican most now is that the "good sister" are no longer just faithful daughters of the "fathers." This is very troubling to the Vatican.

Could you elaborate . . .?

Schüssler Fiorenza: A recent conference in Washington D.C.

was called "Women in the Church." I am told that around two thousand five hundred people attended, most of them "nun-women." What happened is the conference was allegedly organized by men. Men defined it; women paid for it.

The participants were interested in the issue of women in the church. But it needed to become a safe issue. [In my view] they were looking for a middle ground where they could be secure, and not have problems like the twenty-four nun signers of the ad in *The New York Times* [See Appendix A]. This conference communicated, "You're not on the radical fringe here; you have center stage; and it's acceptable to the 'fathers.'"

Excluding the keynote speaker, there were four major addresses. Three of these were delivered by men. What is your view on this?

Schüssler Fiorenza: It is important to view this event as a "political conference." Most women—and perhaps also the organizers—do not understand politics, and that's why it's necessary to have a critical analysis. This brings us back to our starting point.

The Vatican and the bishops are nervous about the nuns. There needed to be a conference where the nuns could feel safe and still address the women's issue. You see, the "women's rights issue" in this country is already very much in the consciousness of all Catholics so that you cannot any longer exclude women simply on the grounds of sex. To do so is sexist; even conservative women will not deny that.

There are certain moral realizations in a culture. . .and even though people reject them, they still are affected by them. The people who came to this conference—in my analysis—needed to get a middle-of-the-road feminism, which, of course, is a co-opted feminism.

CO-OPTING FEMINISM

Can you explain what you mean by co-opted feminism.

Schüssler Fiorenza: Co-opted feminism is defined by men. At the same time, it upholds the exploitation of women.

There are numerous women, sisters, who are socialized into the system that if "Father" says it's okay, then fine. But to get women together, especially from women's canonical communities, is dangerous in the eyes of the Vatican. Permission [however] was given by holding this conference, and it let the bishops off the hook, because they did not need to officially sponsor it. At the same time most of the people present have probably never read much feminist theology. Consequently, women participants might receive a reinforced message that they could believe what was said because "Father told them."

Don't you think that's sad?
Schüssler Fiorenza: It's sad, but it's part of the struggle we are in. To deny it doesn't help. Feminist theologians have said all along that the issue of women in the church is an issue especially for middle class women. Working class women, black, white or Hispanic, and lower class women have neither the time nor the energy to organize and fight for their rights in the church. They need all their energies to survive. They don't have the money to go to Washington, or to a conference anywhere.

It was very important for me to learn of differences between the American church compared to the German and European church. You still don't have a women's movement within the German Catholic church, for instance. The nuns there did not have the sisters' renewal movement.

Did European nuns not renew after Vatican II?
Schüssler Fiorenza: Not quite. They are not as highly educated as the Americans nuns. The sisters' renewal movement in the U. S. advanced a group of middle class, educated women—even if they came from lower classes. Convent living socialized them into the middle class. They are [comparatively] highly educated women. . . .The renewal movement then raised issues of cloister, dress and governance—modern versus medieval questions. Still, it was not consciously conceived of as a feminist movement. True, there are pockets in sisters' communities who have raised women's issues, as well as issues of the poor, peace, and all those "acceptable" things. But, on the whole, nun-women have not defined themselves in terms of women's communities not controlled by men. They are all still canonical communities. Canonical status means they are controlled by the hierarchy—the bishops or Rome. For over ten years I have been saying to the Women's Ordination Movement, "Let's get together and talk about the structural issues that divide us, so we can do something about them. Let's not just wait for the men

to decide whether or not they will ordain some of us. We don't want ordination under these conditions."

But as the controversy surrounding *The New York Times* ad showed, even the leading feminists among the nuns have deeply internalized the patriarchal vision of authority and that is why we were so affected by Rome's clampdown. Asking nun-women to question their superiors, or co-ordinators, requires a feminist process. Had analysis been done, it would show Rome's reaction for what it is. But the nuns focused on Rome, and so superiors could all fall back into the old game of secrecy.

In light of all that, what do you think of Barbara Ferraro and Patricia Hussey?
Schüssler Fiorenza: I admire them. I have great respect for them because they are the only ones who have not recanted. All the others tried to assure us that they didn't think that they recanted. But Rome knew that it got what it wanted: the nun signers [who withdrew their names] accepted church teaching on birth control and abortion. It's no accident that Ferraro and Hussey have stuck with their decision, because they work with poor women.

Margaret Traxler, one of the twenty-four ad signers, is grieved that her order, the School Sisters of Notre Dame, thought her expendable after forty-five years.
Schüssler Fiorenza: I would have been ten times more hurt in her place by what the women in the community did rather than by what was done by men in the Vatican. I admire sisters who try to stand up to Vatican patriarchy, yet look at what happened not only to the signers of the ad, but also to Liz Morancy and Agnes Mansour. Why has nobody the courage to say what actually happened, namely, that the congregations are prepared to sacrifice their own members in order to continue canonical status? They have let their own members go, their very own sisters.

MISSION AS A THEOLOGIAN
How do you perceive your mission as a theologian?
Schüssler Fiorenza: I am a very churchy person because I was born a Catholic. I come from a section of Catholicism which is anti-Roman; I am not a Roman but a Bavarian Catholic. It's not Roman because German Catholicism is culturally very anti-

clerical. It was so difficult for me at first when I came to this country to keep my anti-clerical tongue in check. Because of the immigrant American church situation, the clergy has had a much different relationship to the people. For me the Second Vatican Council was not so decisive; I grew up with. . . [a different kind of] theology. I never made sense out of catechism, but I was fortunate to have had a pastor who otherwise was pretty conservative, but biblically and liturgically he was ahead. I was a child after the war—I have no direct experience of Nazi Germany—but this pastor always spoke of the failure of the church to stand up to Hitler.

My first publication was in second or third grade. We had to write an essay with three wishes. The teacher selected and published wishes like "no more war," "some chocolate to eat," or whatever. My third wish was that one day I would be pope! I'm not too sure whether I still wish it.

I enrolled in the university to study theology, German literature, and history to become a "lay" theologian. I also worked part-time with the diocesan youth office. Because of this work I found out that the clergy looked down on the "lay" theologians as having only some theology but not "the real thing."

Although it then took six years in Germany to earn the master of divinity, I decided to apply, and to seek the bishop's approval for my state scholarship. The bishop looked at me and said, "Elisabeth, I don't think I can approve it." I told him I could not understand. He said, "Elisabeth, I don't really think you should work for the church because you see its wounds. Rather than spreading a blanket or a mantle of love over them, you point at them with your fingers." I never forgot [that]. Afterward I was shaking. . . .But, I looked at him and I said, "Your Excellency, if I thought that a patient was dead, I would bury him with all the love I have. But as long as there's a chance for survival I think you need to operate." He gave me permission.

Were you therefore an anomaly in theology?

Schüssler Fiorenza: After I got permission to do theology, I realized that theologically I was missing my vocation because, according to modern progressive theology, the vocation of the laity was the mission to the world. My thesis, therefore, was on the mission of the laity in the church and I took women as the test case since women by law were always "lay." I was best in my class, and I believed them when they said, "We don't know if you can do it." It cost me six years of life, but I finished the thesis and it was published as a book.

My thesis tried to prove that the [traditional] theology is wrong. I looked at all the places where women were working in the German church. Male theologians at the time argued for the permanent diaconate because grace was there and the church should confirm it and ordain married men. What I tried to show was that the grace was where actual women and lay people were working in the church and that's why the theology was wrong. I was not interested in "clergy" because I grew up with the notion of "people of God." I was not interested in women's ordination, but I took women as an example since in the church they are always lay people. I thought women working in the church was a case illustrating lay ministry. That to me was the problem—the issue of laity working in the church. The time was 1961 to 1962 and I did not have a feminist analysis. In the process of doing that thesis, I became aware that the women's issue was a special theological issue separate from the lay issue.

So you were a pioneer already in 1961. . .
Schüssler Fiorenza: I found that in all theological discussion [women] were perceived as essentially different from men. In Germany, all the priests were educated in the "eternal women" theology which was full of this romantic glorification of women. It was a reaction against a negative or misogynist traditional theology; positives were "motherhood" and the "veil." Whether you had children or not, motherhood was your special vocation. . . . But I never bought into the Catholic woman notion of either being a spiritual mother, [either] as a nun or as mother of ten kids.

To find support for my contention that there was no theology of women, no "special nature" of women, I found no help in psychology. Freud and Jung did not help. Sociology too had the same kind of family and vocation pattern for women: motherhood.

After finishing the thesis I began a doctorate in New Testament [studies]. The two best teachers in Würzburg were Rudolf Schnackenburg in New Testament and Alfonse Auer in moral theology. Schnackenburg asked me to do a thesis on the "priesthood of all believers" and that's how I ended up in New Testament studies. I hoped to combine my training in pastoral theology and New Testament so that I could become director of the oldest seminary in Germany for women. But I met Francis and we got married. That's how I came to the States.

When did you come to the United States?

Schüssler Fiorenza: Notre Dame invited us in 1970, and assured us they had no nepotism rule. Then came the first American Society of Biblical Literature meeting in 1971. It was very hopeful [to see that] Carol Christ initiated the women's caucus. I came away from the meeting with two new insights. First, I, a foreigner, barely a year in the country, found out that I was the only *married* woman who had a full-time academic theological job. Even though in the 1960s the academy needed qualified people and the job market was really wide open, there were no women, no married women, full-time at least, at this meeting.

That said to me that the academy hired men and it really helped me to understand my subsequent struggle at Notre Dame. The university hired men as scholars and expected them to have the support system of their wives. Therefore, the great scholar is a male scholar who is married and has his family support system; or a celibate who has a community support system. That's what I learned not just in terms of Catholic circles, but in terms of the structure of the academy. And feminist analyses of the academy have documented this!

Is this still the case in the United States?

Schüssler Fiorenza: There's no question about it. It has changed somewhat, but it is still the case at social functions. You are stereotyped as a wife. I was giving a lecture at a nearby school not long ago, and I was introduced as "wife and mother."

You object to that?

Schüssler Fiorenza: Yes, but you have to realize what you're dealing with. You're role as wife is still more highly valued by the institution. The *second* insight which I brought from my 1971 American Academy of Religion/Society of Biblical Literature meeting was that I was the only woman of biblical literature willing to get involved in the caucus. Therefore, I became the co-chair of the caucus with Carol Christ. In fact, my colleagues in biblical studies told me that to be associated with any woman's issue was to put myself in jeopardy. Now that's another success story because SBL [Society of Biblical Literature] has just elected me president.

How did these incidents influence you?

Schüssler Fiorenza: That caucus gave me the opening to [contact] feminist groups like the Grailville Conference. From then on I became involved with the feminist movement. Because of this, I was able to meet practically all the feminists who later published great materials.

I was lucky to be involved in that learning experience. To be part of a movement for change was one thing, but to understand myself as shaping a discipline and a system was another. Meeting feminist scholars in religion who argued that women had a special nature forced me to articulate my own understanding of feminist theology. My article [1975] on feminist theology as a critical theology of liberation expresses my position for the first time.

DIRECTIONS IN FEMINISM

How did you articulate your disagreement?

Schüssler Fiorenza: Within feminism in religion there are three different directions. One is the so-called equal rights feminism striving to incorporate women into society in general. My first book, *The Forgotten Partner,* describes this approach. There is a second direction: a strong understanding of feminism in terms of gender-dualism, the domination of men over women. It presupposes women to be less damaged by patriarchal structure, and therefore they have more possibilities of creating a new world. Mary Daly's understanding of exodus and new women's community is representative language here. Since this theological direction was for me reminiscent of the "theology of women" that gives women a special nature, I looked for a third approach.

We cannot assume that there is a special nature of women, or a woman's way to do things, unless we are socialized to it. That means we are part of the problem; not just part of the solution. Therefore, I put *critical* before feminist theology, because a *critical* reflection and analysis of systems and structures is necessary. This third approach is the approach of feminist liberation theology on which I have been working ever since. Feminists in religion are in danger of falling back into a kind of dualism: a "we" and an "other."

In 1975 someone in the Women's Ordination Conference asked me to participate in their first meeting. "Are you," I asked, "going for ordination at any price? If so, I don't want to have anything to do with it." They assured me it was not the case and that they were serious about "New Church: New Priestly Ministry." I did not want to get involved in the movement for ordination because I was convinced it could lead to the exploitation of women, and make married women fourth class citizens.

Because of my speech at the conference, Notre Dame got some flack. My chairman became upset about my feminist theology article and he called me to his office three times to inform me that someone who writes such an article ought not to teach at Notre Dame. "But what are you going to do?" I asked. "You just gave me tenure. Are you going to give me a research professorship or what?" This started all my problems at Notre Dame. I share this in order to point out that you cannot do feminist theology without ramifications. You have to pay the price.

Did that injustice change you?
Schüssler Fiorenza: Notre Dame helped me clarify my notion of feminist theology both as a critical and as a liberation theology of struggle.

Feminist theologians insist that feminist theology is based on women's experience. Now if women, as well as men, are socialized into a societal system which is patriarchal, then we must know what kind of status to give such experience. Phyllis Schaffly, for example, can do theology reflecting on her own experience, which I venture might not be a feminist theology. That's why I needed to clarify what was meant by women's experience.

Secondly, I needed to define that experience. I needed to hear what black and Hispanic women said in terms of the white women's movement. The experience also pushed me to analyze more carefully the structures of oppression. As a result, I have redefined patriarchy, not just in terms of gender analysis, of the domination of men over women, but in terms of Aristotle. He articulated a complex notion of patriarchy: only freeborn, propertied Greek male heads of households were free citizens. My books, *In Memory of Her* and *Bread Not Stone*, developed an analysis of patriarchy, not just in terms of gender, but in terms of class, race, and colonialism. These oppressive structures are all part of Greek democracy. I showed how Christianity was not the originator of patriarchy, but its mediator for Western culture.

Classical Greek democracy originated the notion that citizens define and control their destiny and their city. Theoretically, every Greek citizen ought to have been participating in public, political decision making. Since *de facto* freeborn women and Greek-born slaves, as well as non-Greeks, were excluded from citizenship, Aristotle fashioned a theory [that argued] that they are excluded because of their "deficient natures." This Aristotlian philosophy has influenced the New Testament, Augustine, Thomas Aquinas, and Christian theology on the whole.

Free women and slaves were excluded in a classical, patriarchal structure of society. Aristotle argues that the dominant thing in being a human, as distinct from an animal, is the capability of speech and rational thought. This deliberative part, he claims, is decisive. Freeborn, propertied men have this quality in its fullness. Theoretically, women could also, but they are debilitated because of their accident of birth. Further, slaves, women as well as men, are on the whole, rational. But you need a deliberative part, not just a rational part, to be human. This deliberative part, according to Aristotle, is lacking in slaves. Slaves, therefore, cannot participate in decision making. And of course the people at the pinnacle are the philosophers. But we must see how Aristotle developed his theory of different natures for women, free women, slaves, rational *man*, and philosophers in order to argue why some can, and others cannot, participate in political action or decision making.

His understanding was revived in the first century and used against emancipatory movements when women and slaves tried to gain greater freedom. Unfortunately it found its way into the New Testament. The so-called Household Codes of the Post-Pauline writings say that wives should be submissive to the husband who is the head. These codes strongly influenced Augustine and Aquinas, and were not objected to by Luther and the

Reformation. They shaped Christendom and are still shaping it.

In the Roman Catholic church we find the classical form of patriarchy as it was embodied in those societal structures. It is still in other church polities, but not as blatant as in the Roman church. This analysis of patriarchy, which can be applied to society, church, and academy, places all kinds of arguments in perspective. With it you can look at why women are defined as having a special nature. You can understand the class structure in Roman Catholicism between nun-women and lay women. That's what I mean by critical analysis and critical reflection. It is what enables women to do such critical analysis because women are not trained to engage in a critical analysis of society and church but tend to personalize issues.

WOMEN AND *ECCLESIA*
What is your place in this Catholic church?
Schüssler Fiorenza: I don't know. I say this Roman church, because the model I just outlined is typically Roman, derived from Roman imperialism. The Catholic church insists on Roman patriarchy, like the Anglican Catholic, for example, insists on the Commonwealth and colonialism of the English empire.

But I think of *ecclesia* in terms of the assembly of adult women and men, responsible decision-making citizens, which is. . .not yet realized. That's why I coined the notion of "Women-Church." Remember, Mary Daly understood, in *Beyond God the Father*, sisterhood as anti-church. Rosemary Radford Ruether's theology is strongly influenced by Exodus theology that seeks to leave behind patriarchal structures. There's also another type of theology which says the church is good; the church is our home; the church is the ideal, and so on. What I try to do with the notion of the *ecclesia of women* is take "ecclesia," which comes from the democratic Greek tradition and is not a biological family term like sisterhood, and then take "women," and put the two together. I say women are church; always have been church. But because of our language, women as church is not even in women's consciousness. Just as I put women and *ecclesia* together, I also put nun and women together. It is an attempt to say to the church that all is not well. This house of authority is not our home, but neither is it exodus which suggests that we can leave. Remember, we women also are a part of the patriarchy. We must therefore engage in a struggle for the church of the poor, the church of the Third World, the church of women. Unless all these elements of church come into full bloom and become conscious, we will not have the Catholic church. The fullness or the Catholicity of church is not possible.

You feel, then, the current church is a "starved" one in the sense of being a patriarchal system?

Schüssler Fiorenza: It's a diminished and oppressive church. As long as the patriarchal hierarchy is taken as the *whole* church, the catholicity of the church is diminished. But I refuse to participate in an exodus. I say, reclaim the center, a center in which *everybody* can be included with their rights, their say, their vision, and their decision making.

In terms of theology, everybody has a gift from the Spirit, and ought to participate. Gatherings of women who are women-church are not representing the fullness of church, but gatherings of [the] hierarchical [element]—the patriarchal church—does not represent the fullness of church either.

Are you talking about a "new" church?

Schüssler Fiorenza: That's exactly what I'm *not* saying. I am not opting for a new church on the fringes that just repeats the pattern of the patriarchal church.

But how can women formulate their own theology in a masculine setting, where they're not even allowed to preach?

Schüssler Fiorenza: You have to find spaces where you can do that, but it doesn't mean you go aside. You still claim you do it as central for theology and church. I would never say that what I do—feminist theology—is a "fringe theology."

Also by Catholic I do not mean Roman; by Catholic I mean what is usually understood today as *ecumenical*. The fullness of church does not exist as long as other churches haven't come to communion in the "church" in terms of ecclesiology. What women in all churches have in common is that we are women-church. Even the Protestant churches which ordain women today have done so for a very short time. Being ordained (any feminist ordained woman will tell you) does not mean that you participate in the decision making and shaping of church. Ordination is one way, doing theology in a patriarchal institution is another; neither means that women are at the center of the patriarchal institution. What I try to say is that for the transformation of the patriarchal church the struggle must place us in the center of the *Catholic* church. We cannot give up this claim.

WOMEN AND ORDINATION

How would you respond if you read in *The New York Times* one Monday morning that twelve women were ordained by a U.S. bishop?

Schüssler Fiorenza: These women would, I think, feel [that it would be] a great success. In terms of the theological analysis of patriarchy, I wouldn't be impressed. What it would do, as it has in the other churches, is incorporate women much more strongly into the system. Ordination vows and the whole ritual is quite different from becoming a professor, or having a ministry in the church. Vows and ritual do something; the church won't ordain one who does not fit the clerical pattern. It is much more difficult for Roman Catholic women to do what our colleagues have done in the Episcopal church, namely, try to become irregularly ordained. The Roman Catholic church does not have a minimum of democratic government. Roman Catholic women have different kinds of possibilities than women in other churches, however.

How do you communicate your sense of vision to others? Are you hopeful about women? I meet many discouraged women in the Roman church.

Schüssler Fiorenza: I've coined the expression "*ecclesia* of women," or "women-church" to give us a different vision of being church that can claim our freedom and spiritual energy. I, for instance, could not do my work if I were defined by the patriarchal hierarchy either as a theologian or as a feminist. There is no intellectual work of integrity possible if you must look over your shoulders and think about what the "fathers" tell you. Yet, that is now the great problem for men, especially ordained men; there is too much control exercised over them. One reason why I moved here [Episcopal Divinity School] was because I did not want to spend my life in a futile struggle. At Notre Dame, the right wing had already asked why the university retained me as a feminist theologian. The only answer my former chairman could give was because I had tenure. So they rightly asked, "Why don't you remove her from the faculty, because the new code of canon law demands it?" My chairman's response was that one signature in *The New York Times* would not be enough to fire me, but the university might consider it in other circumstances.

So you signed the "Catholic Statement on Pluralism and Abortion" printed in *The New York Times*?

Schüssler Fiorenza: I signed the ad. But the ad was only an occasion. The major concern for the right [wing] was my feminist theology. I don't say my choice is the choice for every Catholic woman, but I do not want to spend my energies being ground down into the system. I came to Episcopal Divinity School because the former dean told me that the issue facing the church (and he did not just mean the Episcopal church) in this century was the "woman's issue." He believed it is not just a question of ordination, but is [also] a question of theology. I came here because I could not teach feminist theology at Notre Dame. I was not even allowed to use my book *In Memory of Her*. I got into trouble when I assigned my book as reading in a Luke-Acts class. I was told I had to teach "straight" New Testament exegesis.

How were you able to cope with this?

Schüssler Fiorenza: A Catholic colleague in another Protestant institution was very helpful to me. He said, "Elisabeth, in the next twenty years or so, however long the pope lives and the reaction lasts, nobody will be able to do Catholic theology with integrity in a Roman Catholic institution." This was another major reason why I moved. The move allows me for the next twenty years of my teaching life to teach women—and other students who are interested—theology as liberation, as critical thinking, and as an approach to New Testament studies. I teach more Roman Catholic women here than I could ever teach at Notre Dame.

What I want to say to every Roman Catholic feminist is you give the system too much power if you knock your head on the wall and you think that's the only way of being and bringing about church. If you take seriously what women-church says, then you have to define where your allegiance, your commitment, and your vision lies. For me, my allegiance is to women in the Catholic church, because that's where I've grown up. But it is also to women in other churches and to all women in society. I do theology, I shape theology, and I shape ministry in the tradition of women-church. That's why I'm a very traditional theologian.

Where did the term "women-church" originate?

Schüssler Fiorenza: Actually, the first time I used the expression was at a meeting of "Women Moving Church," where twenty or thirty people analyzed responses to questionnaires. One response came from a woman who said, "I'm over sixty. Yesterday I wrote you a response that said I'm very happy with my church. Today, this morning some man tried to rape me. Suddenly, I realized that it's my church which promotes a rape culture." That's where we were at the conference: divided. Going home I thought, "What are we going to do with that woman's response? How are we going to shape the conference in light of it?" I realized then that we still work only with the vision of "push and push." But if we would move the Cathedral of St. Peter one inch, that would be a miracle, wouldn't it? Yet it wouldn't make any difference.

Instead of hitting our heads against the walls, we women must conceive of ourselves as "church on the move" into the future. You do not change structures by begging them to let you in. Rather, you try to change structures by redefining the issues; then let the structures react to you, rather than the other way. So if Roman Catholic women say, "We want ordination," they have two choices: one is to go to other churches and be ordained there for parish ministry. . .do it as Catholic women, and make the hierarchy realize what the consequences of their policy is. Secondly, do not hide in the closet. Make it public that Catholic women move to a church which accepts women in ministry. Were I convinced that I wanted parish ministry, I would go to the Episcopalians or Presbyterians or whoever, and get ordained and be a parish minister in the church. And nurture women-church. Why not? Vatican II admitted that other Christian churches are church! A lot of women do it, but they must make it public. I suggest that [this] would make the Vatican and especially the American bishops really nervous. If the nuns had gotten together and declared, "Either we are getting ordained or we are no longer doing any work for you," the American bishops wouldn't know how to run the church!

If women withdrew all their work, the bishops and the Roman church could not exist. Another way is not to take the patriarchal system too seriously. Every time Women's Ordination Conference contacts those who are called to be ordained to the priesthood, I write back and ask when are you going to do something for those of us who feel called to be pope or bishop? Theresa Kane also feels called to be bishop. Womens Ordination Conference should argue [that] since all bishops are men, all cardinals ought to be women. Cardinal is not a scripturally based office. Until the last century laymen could be cardinals. Not that I think we will be cardinals, but just to expose the system and the flimsiness of the theological arguments.

SOLIDARITY AMONG WOMEN

Are you concerned about women not sticking together, about disunity among women?

Schüssler Fiorenza: I'm very concerned with that. I have no traditional loyalty to the pope or to anybody in the patriarchy, but I have a lot of loyalty to women: be they Phyllis Schaffly, Mother Teresa, or Theresa Kane. My problem is not how to motivate the patriarchal church, but rather how to engage women in this struggle to end patriarchal structures.

Do you have an answer?

Schüssler Fiorenza: I don't have an answer for everyone. Just a commitment. I feel my contribution is to provide analysis in this struggle, and to help women get in touch with their resources. Church was not made just by men, even though they are on the top of the pyramid. Today the American church couldn't exist without the work of women. The whole renewal in the American church couldn't exist without women; theology wouldn't be what it is without women, everything wouldn't be what it is without women. I say we must reclaim our tradition, and define where to place our energy in the struggle. We must get away from being passive victims, and decide when something seems to be just. When it's time, we must shake the dust off our shoes and move on. Now the patriarchy defines us, rather than we, women, defining the church.

How can you get women to come around to your vision?

Schüssler Fiorenza: I don't know. I've done a lot of writing, speaking, sitting through committee meetings, conferences, strategy sessions, all those kinds of endeavors. I started the *Feminist Journal in Religion* with Judith Plaskow. I initiated the program for feminist liberation theology at EDS [Episcopal Divinity School]. I serve on all these male theological boards, and I have worked for a feminist theology section as one of the theological areas for *Concilium.* I have worked to get feminist Catholic groups together to pool our energies, rather than every little group having their own office and no money. I have failed in that. I believe women must rethink how they spend their time and energy in terms of women-church. I don't say to Episcopal women here, "You shouldn't get ordained." I say, "Get ordained, but you better define what feminist ministry is all about." And we need to do much more thinking and strategizing in such terms.

Men are freer not to buy into the patriarchal model. . . .If I say something is so and so in the New Testament, they go along with it. Women have not learned how to handle and recognize our gifts. There's a great tendency, especially among Roman Catholic women, because of our spirituality and socialization, to say that all women are the same. It is exactly the opposite. I have privileges and possibilities because of my theological education denied to a working-class woman. On the other hand, women in the parish have possibilities for change denied me. It would be foolish for me to try to do what a woman in a parish, a full-time homemaker can do better. Likewise, in the struggle it would be foolish for a woman in a parish to try to do what I do.

The issue is: do not give too much power to the patriarchal system. At the same time, take it seriously in order to change it.

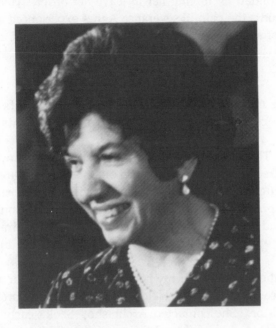

AGNES MARY MANSOUR

"I asked what options were open; it seemed like none. I asked how much time I had. . .the bishop had to leave that evening. . . .I asked if I would be in definance of the Holy Father if I resigned. And he said 'no.' In fact, he had the dispensation papers with him."

A Sister of Mercy for thirty years, and President of Mercy College in Michigan for twelve, Agnes Mary Mansour decided to change her career in 1982. After prayerful and communal consideration she moved into political ministry. She was appointed Director of the Michigan Department of Social Services by Governor James Blanchard, and secured the approval and blessings of her order and her archbishop. She is currently with Mercy Health Services in Michigan.

Because a miniscule portion of the department's budget was allotted to Medicaid funding for abortions, rightist pressure was brought to bear on the archbishop and on Rome. They, in turn, responded by forcing her to leave her order. This interview recounts the painful severance Agnes experienced and the implications her experience holds for women and for the church.

GOVERNMENT AS MINISTRY

You have made a public statement of your beliefs about what the church should be. What prompted this statement?

Mansour: The necessity for a public statement was not my doing. It came directly from my acceptance of a position as Director of [the] Michigan Department of Social Services. I had received all the appropriate prior approvals of both my religious community and the hierarchy of the church. The withdrawal of hierarchy approval came after two months into my appointment.

When the possibility of my being appointed director arose, I communicated with Sister Helen Marie Burns, our provincial administrator. She contacted Archbishop Szoka early in December 1982, and he indicated there was no problem as long as the cabinet position was in keeping with the propriety of religious life. I had, moreover, made known my position on abortion.

What is your position?

Mansour: I'm opposed to abortion and consider it a violent solution to a human problem. I don't consider myself pro-choice; I am pro-life. I also recognize that those who are pro-life need to be more convincing in changing attitudes than in controlling what is done in a pluralistic society. Living in a morally pluralistic society, one must respect the fact that other people may conscientiously come to other decisions regarding abortion. We should not attempt to control their decisions through public policy when no consensus exists. Neither do I feel it would be appropriate to withdraw resources for the poor as long as abortion is legal in our society. It would be illegal to withdraw Medicaid funds for abortion. Yet, that became the main issue in my case. . . .When you live in a morally pluralistic society, you need a consensus in order to legislate restrictively. We do not now have such a consensus. On the other hand, I don't want to return to pre-legal abortion days, because I think there was a good deal of abuse of women. Those who are pro-life need to work more toward a consensus through means that do not alienate. The means currently used create greater alienation.

AN ARCHBISHOP UNDER PRESSURE

You had the approval for your position from the archbishop. What happened to change his opinion?

Mansour: He changed his tune saying that he told me I must come out publicly with a statement opposed to Medicaid funding for abortion. . . .What happened was the publicity surrounding my appointment, and the concerted effort by conservative Catholics and others, pressured the Holy Father and the archbishop to remove me, or to request my removal from the position. In February 1983, the archbishop told me he was very concerned. He said he had been bombarded by various groups who indicated that I was creating a scandal. There were ads in *The Wall Street Journal* and in *The New York Times* opposing my appointment.

You became famous overnight?

Mansour: That's correct. At that point the archbishop attempted to get me to change my position. I said I could not. I had made a conscientious decision and I would stick by it. I was very consistent in my position. He knew it, he also knew the Holy Father's stance on religious life and political ministry. Yet he had supported me. Quotes in the local papers referred to his support, because initially he saw, as I did, the Department's very extensive responsibility and that Medicaid funding for abortion was a very small part.

What percentage of your overall budget is allocated for this measure?

Mansour: Our budget is over four billion dollars; we spend five to six million dollars on Medicaid.

That's not even one percent.

Mansour: No. But conservative pressure grew. [The archbishop] then indicated during one discussion that he might indeed have to request my superiors to ask me to resign. I acknowledged he had to do what he had to do. I had to do what my conscience approved. I then gave my first press interview. Up to that point I had been shying away from reporters, because I didn't want to focus on the controversy. I wanted to take time to learn the department and prepare for confirmation hearings. I did not want the main concern to be Medicaid funding because it was totally inappropriate to slant the agenda, to distort my role and my qualifications for the position. This interview in my opinion came out very well. In fact, one bishop called me and said that it made an excellent article in the paper, and that probably it would help to dissipate any concerns of the archbishop.

The following week, however, on February 23, the archbishop, without notifying me, contacted the provincial administrator, Sister Helen Marie Burns. The very morning he was having a press conference he requested her and my superiors to withdraw their support for me. He then held his press conference requesting that they ask me to resign. He never came directly to me. The religious community did not ask me to resign. But these superiors met with me and decided they would dialogue with the bishop, seeking reconciliation in some way. They had not fully concluded what they wanted to do. But the Detroit Province of the Sisters of Mercy issued a statement, prior to the confirmation hearing early in March, indicating they saw no reason for me to resign.

But at the same time you read in the newspaper that you must resign? How did you feel about the archbishop's intervention.

Mansour: I considered the approach of the archbishop totally inappropriate. I thought it was a lack of respect for the religious community especially not to contact them prior to a press conference, not to dialogue with them about his concerns. To inform them in this fashion was inappropriate. Possibly, something might have been worked out, that I don't know. But to go out and make a public statement created a great deal of public interest.

It became a media event.

Mansour: Absolutely.

ROME'S INTERVENTION

Mansour: I know I became a media figure unable to move without reporters cornering me, wanting to know what was going on. But there was nothing ever to report. After my confirmation hearings in March, the Mercy superiors were still in dialogue with the archbishop. In mid-March when I was in Washington, Sister Emily George, Vice President of General Administration, called me to say that the Apostolic Delegate was in the United States. [The papal nuncio representing the Vatican in Washington, D.C.] Archbishop Pio Laghi, had contacted Sister Theresa Kane asking the general administration to request me to leave my position. In other words, the archbishop did not get any satisfaction from the provincial administration in Detroit, so Rome moved to the general administration. The general administration, of course, wasn't about to ask me to resign. Besides, Sister Theresa Kane was going on retreat, and she didn't really want to address the matter. I suggested requesting a leave of absence from the community until my term was completed. . . .It would be unfair to the government and the people of Michigan to just to get up in the middle of my work and leave. Not only was it inappropriate and unfair, but I had done everything possible to request *and* to receive prior approval. Consequently, I saw no relief except to request a leave of absence on April 10. My superiors granted it; later Rome found out and overruled my superiors.

Who was Rome?

Mansour: Rome, the Congregation for Religious and Secular Insititutes (CRIS), evidently with the approval of the Holy Father. Theresa Kane, Helen Marie Burns, and I then met. I noted that Helen Marie began to shift her thinking. Initially, she respected the authority of the archbishop. Although she had not asked me to resign, I think she was leaning in that direction. But when she saw how Rome bypassed the local community, she began to switch her thinking. At the generalate level, they felt my appointment had had all the necessary approvals. They would never request resignation under these circumstances. They simply backed me. Theresa had earlier requested a meeting with the Holy Father while in Rome with other general superiors. It was never granted.

She wanted you to take a leave of absence?

Mansour: Correct. In late April—you see how fast this moved (you know how slow Rome is usually)—Rome had moved with unbelievable swiftness. I received a call from a priest in the marriage tribunal in Detroit. He indicated he had a letter for me from [a New York] bishop and wanted to deliver it. He was asked to deliver. . . .

A kind of a Federal Express. . .

Mansour: A pontifical express. . . .This priest gave me three dates to meet with him, I could not make any of them. He wanted to deliver the letter. I asked him to wait a minute and I would call back. I at once called Theresa Kane and Helen Marie Burns to ask what was going on. Had they known about this letter? They knew nothing. I called the tribunal priest and gave him a date. The poor priest! I could tell he did not want to be the messenger here, but he had the responsibility to deliver the letter. He didn't even know what was in it.

He must have known it wasn't good news.

Mansour: That's right. He delivered the letter and gave three dates for the bishop to meet with me. I called this bishop and arranged a May meeting. The letter indicated it could be immediately.

There was a sense of urgency.

Mansour: Yes, and I could bring *any* other sister. He didn't even mention I could bring a Sister of Mercy. That's a bypass of my religious community.

Did you feel offended?

Mansour: Absolutely. . . .I think again it's a lack of recognition of my religious superiors and their authority. I had been a sister in the Mercy community, and my colleagues were the Sisters of Mercy. My vows were taken and accepted in a religious community. That's a community I selected to be a part of for thirty years.

Do you feel there's something going on. . .a vendetta against the Mercy order? It sounds very peculiar.

Mansour: It's hard to know whether or not there was a vendetta. We know, of course, the lack of acceptance of Theresa Kane in Rome and the concern that she possibly was not giving the kind of direction and leadership the Holy Father and Rome wants for religious in America. But whether or not it made any difference, I just don't know.

What I do know is that the religious community was bypassed. But I brought with me my provincial, Helen Marie, and Emily George who was the assistant to Theresa Kane. Theresa Kane was in Rome on May 9, our meeting date. The bishop had two other people with him; one was a sister from the Detroit area, and the other person was head of a tribunal in Pennsylvania.

A woman?

Mansour: No, one woman, one man (one sister, one priest). The bishop said he had a mandate from the Holy Father. He had a letter indicating I resign my position, or be subject to a process of dismissal.

EXPERIENCING CHURCH PATRIARCHY

You were in a room, one of six people. How were you feeling at that moment?

Mansour: Resentful. I did not cry, but Sister Emily did. The dialogue was so one-sided. It wasn't a dialogue, it was a monologue. And it wasn't really open to any views. To my mind it already had drawn its conclusion.

So essentially the bishop was there to deliver an ultimatum?

Mansour: That's correct. There was no due process; there wasn't even a full understanding of my rights. The fact was that it had been handled in such a secretive way, completely ignoring a willingness to dialogue. It made possible negotiation of some sort of compromise out of the question. It was just. . . . It was an environment that you felt you had nothing to say that was going to be heard. There was no openness whatsoever. Questions were asked; we left to discuss them. My concern was that I did not want to be dismissed from my religious community. Nor did I want to be in defiance of the pope. I did not trust Rome, though I really worried that if we left that room without some action I was going to get a letter of dismissal. I did not want that. I did not want such a thing to happen to the Sisters of Mercy. Nor to myself. Nor did I want to be in defiance of the Holy Father.

So you really were then back to the obedient religious of earlier days . . .?

Mansour: Well, that's right, according to my sense of obedience. The request came by virtue of holy obedience. I did not consider my position a disobedient act at all. In fact, all of us. . .nuns should have moved beyond how we previously defined obedience. We should define obedience, especially after Vatican II, as a sincere attempt to discern what God's will is for us.

And had you nuns achieved that aim?

Mansour: What these people asked of me was compliance, not obedience. I never considered a vow of obedience to just do what others tell you to do. Seeking the truth, seeking God's will, is for me obedience. It must be much more communal than this awful experience. I asked what options were open; it seemed like none. I asked how much time I had; the bishop had to leave that evening. I asked if I would be in defiance of the Holy Father if I resigned. And he said, 'no.' In fact he had the dispensation papers with him. I could leave—voluntarily. He came out later with his description of what happened, saying I had immediately requested a dispensation from my vows, which is absolutely not true. That statement of his I resented very much. I did not go to the meeting thinking I was about to leave the order, or be dispensed from my vows. I knew the situation was serious, but I had no idea that I was going to be forced to separate. Of all the alternatives open to me—all undesirable options —this was the most offensive. One option was dismissal; the other was to resign on my own. In that way I could make the choice myself and sign the dispensation.

And did you sign?

Mansour: He had the papers.

You were a member of an order for thirty years, a religious order that nurtured you and was your cradle, and by evening, with this ultimatum, you are ripped out. Could you talk about how you felt?

Mansour: It's very hard to talk about. I was really numb. The impact of it did not sink in until later. I suppose there was anger. I'm not a person to hold grudges or wishes for retaliation. I don't think it an appropriate way to drain my energies. There was definite hurt, there was real resentment. And not only for myself, but for the Sisters of Mercy.

And for women?

Mansour: Religious women particularly. Again, it just reemphasizes the lack of respect and consideration for the contributions of women religious. Or for women in general, and nuns in particular. It was a very paternalistic approach. We as a community had moved way beyond that sort of posturing. It was foreign, something that my own community would never do— never, ever did, even in pre-Vatican days. It was a very un-

pleasant, unbelievable, first-hand experience in church patriarchy.

**At four o'clock on May 19, 1983, you, after so many years,
were no longer a nun. When did that reality hit you?**

Mansour: Slowly. I had been very active in the community, as
well as in my ministries. My ministries had been very time-
consuming. As college president I had been living alone, although close by the nuns. Those things did not change. I didn't
know exactly what would change. Sister Emily made some
comment that there would be change. I knew my life would
change, but I was sure it was going to be gradual. The sisters
have always been supportive, and continued to be very supportive. They still are. But, something does happen formally,
there's no question. Although there's still very good friendships there, it's not the same. You don't belong. That is understandable from both sides. It was slow moving both in my
thinking and my acting. I still contributed my salary for a
shorter time.

So you kept on sending your check. . .?

Mansour: Yes.

Who decided you should start taking care of yourself?

Mansour: Well. . . the sisters did. I knew I had to start planning for myself.

Could you sleep? How did you function?

Mansour: Well, I'm not the best sleeper in the world, that did
not change. The change wasn't all consuming. I can cope very
well. I always have been able to cope even with suffering. You
simply move on, you don't dwell on it, you don't let it take negative tolls on you. There was too much to do. I just moved on.

**Did you notice any perceptible change in your relation-
ships in the department? One day you were a nun; the
next you are a lay woman.**

Mansour: No. In fact, it's very interesting. People still call me
sister, not necessarily in the department, but when I go out to
speak. As college president, I had been very active in the Detroit community and in the state for twelve years. I was well
known.

**Is there anything else you want to add about this inci-
dent?**

Mansour: I know it was very, very difficult for the sisters, especially Sister Emily George, who was a very dear friend of mine. We were in the same group with strong bonds. She told me that she hadn't felt so much pain and suffering since her mother's death. . . .She started crying, but I was not going to give anybody the satisfaction of those tears.

What Sister Emily George was expressing was that she had a death in the religious community?
Mansour: That's right.

POLTICAL MINISTRY
How did you come into political ministry?
Mansour: I've had a very unusual background. I graduated from college before I entered the Sisters of Mercy. I was interested in a health career. I have a graduate degree in medical technology and chemistry. Through the Sisters of Mercy, I received a doctorate in biochemistry from Georgetown University. As a scientist, I taught at Mercy College in Michigan. I received an education fellowship in higher level administration at the University of Kentucky. I then applied for and was selected to become president of Mercy College, Detroit, in 1971. I was president until 1983.

After [Ronald] Reagan came into power, I became very concerned about his lack of sensitivity to domestic issues. I felt his policies and budget cuts were very detrimental to the needy and vulnerable in our society. Being interested in social justice issues all through the 1970s, I was interested in moving on a different career path. I wanted to combine my professional life with social justice issues. I wanted to try a form of political ministry with emphasis on serving the poor more directly. The Mercy community was really open to political ministry. Liz Morancy and Arlene Violet were also interested.

I ran for elective office in 1982, against several good people. It was a trial run, and defeat was expected. But I wanted the exposure to let politicians in the state realize I was interested in public life.

Some of these good people recommended me to Governor Blanchard. This gave me a good opportunity to explore the new ministry of Director of Social Services and to be in a position that will have a more direct service impact on programs to serve the poor.

"A HEAVY AND SKEWED CHURCH"

You were interested in this ministry of service to the marginalized and the poor. Would it not seem that a Christian church would support you in this?

Mansour: That was one of the comments that Archbishop Szoka made in the newspaper right after my appointment. He commented about it being a most appropriate position for a sister. One of the major contradictions so obvious to me was that I had to leave a religious community in order to actually carry out the special mandates of both the church and this community to the poor and needy. It just never, ever should have come about.

Part of the church mission is to have a preferential option for the poor. The gospels imply this. The church should indeed be grateful to have somebody with my values and my experiences, perspective, energy and commitment in such a position. But all of that seemed to fade into the background, with the issue of Medicaid funding for abortion. It became terribly slanted and inappropriate in my mind to mask the impact of everything else. It showed a very heavy and skewed church approach.

In a way, an un-Christian church. You're talking about the hierarchy. . .?

Mansour: That's right. Church to me is the people of God, not the hierarchical church. They should not control as much as they control.

What do you think is going on in the hierarchal church?

Mansour: Two issues: one is obedience, and the other is human sexuality. They seem incapable of handling those two areas well. They want a controlled church; they want a nonintellectual church. They're back to the days where people were not educated. Nor do they want the people who are educated to think for themselves. That I find very disturbing. I don't know what they expect to get out of it, but they're not going to get this control in our day and age. People are going to make judgments on the merits, not necessarily on the judgments and pronouncements, of a church. I find what happened very disturbing. Not only in my case, but the Charles Curran incident, and Archbishop Hunthausen. They want to control appointments at Catholic colleges and universities, and one must ask, "To what end?" They will alienate people rather than support and encourage an expansive development of people's spiritual and personal lives.

It also alienates women. It truly amazes me how accommodating women, especially religious women, have been to the church. Still more amazing to me is that canonical status is so important for religious communities, seeing the way they have been treated. All I see in canonical status is control.

Are you suggesting that nuns are better without it?
Mansour: It is something the orders have to wrestle with, but something that I supported and proposed prior to my leaving. With the kinds of control they want over ministry, not only choice of ministry, but institutional ministry—I think it's just inappropriate. We don't need them telling us what to do.

But people have to report to someone in a corporation and the church is a corporation.
Mansour: The church is a corporation which can set guidelines, but should not ignore the rights of religious women for self-determination.

Would you discuss the second issue which you feel the church handles poorly?
Mansour: The hierarchy does not know how to handle women and women's issues. They seem skewed in their thinking regarding human sexuality. Sexual sins have always been more horrendous than sins against charity. Almost anything sinful that you could think of is lesser than sins of sex.

The cruelty to you would not be viewed as a sin; but the fact that you rule in a department that has less than a one-percent budget for Medicaid funding, was problematic...
Mansour: That's correct. Reflecting on my own position, my broad mission was totally in keeping with that of the Catholic church. My position on abortion is in keeping with the Catholic church. We always behave as if we possess the total truth. It is an elitist, proud attitude that we Catholics should not have. We think nobody else can contribute to the dialogue, because they don't know as much as we know in moral and theological matters.

THE HIERARCHY'S FEAR
What are these hierarchs afraid of?

Mansour: They want an accommodating Catholic population. They fear that thinking leaders who do not identify with their position will lead the fold astray. As though the fold doesn't make its own choices whether to stay or to leave. I'm still a practicing member, but sometimes, I don't know why. I often find liturgies meaningless. I know that some relationship with God and Christ is important to me; it helps me be a better person. It helps me in everyday life to make my value system stay balanced.

You need to worship?

Mansour: Yes, that's correct. It depends on the parishes. There is such a mix out there, and I'm sure it gets tainted by what is happening broadly in the church. I don't like what's happening in some areas of the church.

A TROUBLED CHURCH FUTURE
What do you think about the future of the Catholic church?

Mansour: [I hope it will be] better off. Troublesome issues are not going away. We saw this with the twenty-four sisters who signed *The New York Times* statement. The hierarchy is becoming more cautious. They were more cautious in their handling of the twenty-four nun-signers than they were in my case. In my case, they were amazed by the counterforce. Even with people who indeed might not support my position on Medicaid funding for abortion. Yet these same people did not approve of the lack of due process and other issues which surfaced. I think the hierarchy learned at least to step back and attempt to negotiate, which is what they did in the case of the signers of the ad. What has happened to Father Curran is another issue that's not going to go away. His stance to pursue his rights will make them pause.

So you think that the church is looking worse and worse in this country.

Mansour: Worse and worse in some respects.

And does the pope have any clue about what is happening?

Mansour: It does amaze me. He is a bright man. I thought at the time of his visit here in 1979 that he needed more time, and perhaps along the way he would see more clearly what he did not see then. But that hasn't happened. I identify especially with many of his statements regarding social justice. But with regard to religious communities, and the role of women in the church, he's just very regressive. He does not understand American religious women at all. There is no way, in my belief, that he can control them. If he attempts it, important members of religious communities, people who are vibrant and committed, will leave.

Are you satisfied with the support the order gave you?
Mansour: Yes. They were very supportive, very sensitive, and very concerned. They continue to be.

Did you receive any support from other bishops or clergy privately?
Mansour: A couple of bishops were very, very supportive. A number of priests, religious, and various formalized groups rallied round me also.

Were you surprised how few really rallied round Archbishop Hunthausen, one of the most Christ-like figures in America?
Mansour: Bishops had so many opportunities to rally forcefully and they didn't. The structure of the church is such that it prevents it. It's self-perpetuating in the sense of who gets leadership positions. Church is not decentralized; the autonomy that's supposedly there is not always there.

If bishops do not rally round one of their own, how will they support a woman whom they look on as a second-class citizen anyway?
Mansour: I think they feel very powerless. Those who want to do something, don't know what it is they can do. And I think it's true, there isn't too much people can do. They certainly can speak out about injustice. Yet, there's an intimidation against speaking out. . . .We need more courageous leaders.

SISTERHOOD
Over thirty years ago you finished college. What prompted you then to become a sister?
Mansour: Those were times when the alternatives to marriage

were few. If you wanted to be a professional and of service in some way, the sisterhood seemed the only way to go. Besides, there was a desire to have an agenda bigger than my own, so I was attracted to the sisterhood, the Mercy nuns.

I am the youngest of four girls, and my parents. . . my mother (still living) is a strong individual. She is a person whose potential I think was never realized. She had the Lebanese ethnic drive and desire that her children have much more than she ever had. My family was a loving one, supporting me in anything I wanted to do. No holding back on women. When my father died, my cousin told me that she learned from him that it was all right to be a girl. He always paid as much attention to the girls in the family as to [the] boys. My cousin's statement says something. My desire now is to devote my energies and experience to work with the poor, the sick and the uneducated.

What are the roots of those desires?
Mansour: It's a combination: the family impact, schooling, early formation of the church, as well as a family value system. It was a very simple, unsophisticated, supportive life. Being a Depression baby enters in too. I don't want to see those times again.

Now you are in your fourth year of the governor's administration. It seems like it could be a tortured kind of job. . .?
Mansour: That's a good way to put it. I don't regret it at all; it's been a marvelous experience. We've done many good things, made an impact, had a good platform to speak for the poor and needy. I would do it again.

No regrets. . .?
Mansour: No regrets. The only regret is I was forced to make a choice that I should not have had to make.

That lingers, that assault on your person.
Mansour: No, it doesn't. I don't dwell on these things. I move on; what's happened has happened.

VISION OF THE FUTURE
You lived during the exhilaration of Vatican II; you may be living in its recall.
Mansour: If Vatican II is recalled, it will be a disaster for the

church. I don't think it can be recalled. I don't think the Christian, Catholic public will let it be recalled. What will happen is we'll get the balance that may be needed.

Is this pope responding to a certain perceived need of the church, or do you think this agenda is really his?
Mansour: I think it's his agenda. He couples it with one he thinks is needed by the church. There's a good analogy in my mind between President Reagan and what he thinks important for the American society in terms of government's role, and the Holy Father and what he sees as important in the church's role. Both have such an impact that it will take a long time to recover from whatever major regressive policies and practices are now occuring. . . .On the other hand, as I've said, I can identify with the Holy Father in terms of this social justice issues. He does speak out.

Yet some might say talk on behalf of the poor is cheap. Actions are another thing: in cases like Charlie Curran and yourself. . .
Mansour: I understand, I understand. The Holy Father, however, plays a leadership role, countering some of those who speak against reform. He speaks for the church and for the poor. As you point out, the church has to be far more credible in its behavior and certainly in its belief in justice.

Are you hopeful, essentially?
Mansour: Yes, it may take thousands of years, but I'm hopeful. I think that what is right will eventually prevail.

What would you like to see prevail?
Mansour: The church must address a number of issues much more honestly. One is that seventy-five to eighty percent of the poor in our country are women and children. They are forced into poverty through divorce, lack of child support, or a violent home from which the spouse is forced to leave. Although the church may indeed want the family to stay together, they don't look at why indeed separation occurs, and in some cases must occur. Few church programs hit head-on the responsibility for child support, and that spouse abuse occurs not just in poor situations, but often in the homes of professionals who supposedly reflect good Christian beliefs.

Do Catholics ever hear sermons on these things?

Mansour: I've never heard a sermon on them. What people look for is religion having meaning in their everyday lives. This is what I find missing in many homilies. The priest somehow does not touch the congregation. Clergy must make it much more meaningful. To make it more meaningful, they've got to be more honest and open to experiences outside their own. They know that real life is out there; they must make the connection . . .with. . .the various forms of violence that we know exist. I see the ravages of it, the toll it takes. An infusion of women also into legislative bodies and board rooms would make a difference in terms of our public policies and our economic policies.

Will women, in your lifetime, find liberation within this church?

Mansour: To a certain extent I see it. The backlash of recent happenings in my case, in those of Curran and Hunthausen, will continue to push for more balance. It does not necessarily mean that all needed reform will occur.

I, myself, have no desire to be ordained, but I support women's ordination. It's nonsensical that the ordination of women is viewed as a major issue when there is such need for ordained ministers. To exclude women is ridiculous. It is an example of concentrating once again on the non-essential and preventing the essential from coming to pass.

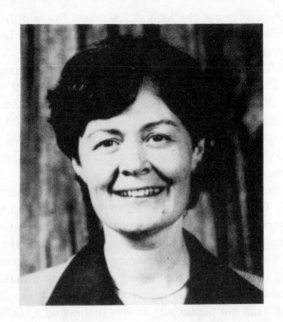

ELIZABETH MORANCY

"Shortly after I was elected in 1978, I attended a lecture by a Boston feminist theologian. She defined ministry as 'making private pain a public issue.' I thought it the perfect definition of political ministry. It is certainly the way I try to operate as a politician. I listen to the experience of people in my district, of women, and other people who in any way are vulnerable. I listen to their private pain and try to get the political system to address that private pain."

Elizabeth (Liz) Morancy is State Representative for the Eighteenth District of Rhode Island. She entered politics as a nun in the 1970s, when political ministry was encouraged by Pope Paul VI. He saw it as one way Catholics could penetrate the power structure at influential decision making levels.

Assuming office in 1978, John Paul II, unlike Paul VI, took a dim view of clerics and nuns in political office. By 1982, Sister Elizabeth Morancy realized that her status as nun in political ministry was being challenged. A fellow Sister of Mercy, Arlene Violet, was forced to withdraw from her order to continue her quest for political ministry as State Attorney General of Rhode Island. The signals from the Vatican became clearer, and eventually, in what she describes as "an act of violence," Sister Elizabeth Morancy was forced out of the Mercy home where she was nurtured, and in which she had served for twenty-five years. Relinquishing her official status as a nun, she made a difficult and courageous decision to pursue her political ministry.

A woman of remarkable vivacity, Liz grew up in rural Rhode Island. Claiming that her attachment to tennis and the water has shaped her, she loves the beauty of her native Kingston. Her parents instilled in both her brother and herself a sensitivity for the vulnerable and less fortunate persons in society. She noticed in grammar school that gifted black female athletes did not have the same opportunities that whites did. "My analysis was not profound; it was instinctual," she said. But her father talked with her about discrimination as well as "every human interest." Looking back, Liz realizes that as a very small child, she, with him, was doing "systems analysis."

In 1959, after finishing high school, she entered the Mercy order at a time when a pre-Vatican II monastic system was in full swing. During the next twenty-five years, nuns' lives took enormous strides toward modernity. She describes in a fascinating, often poignant manner, how her life evolved in political ministry.

EARLY YEARS IN RELIGIOUS LIFE
You entered the convent before many dramatic changes were made in American religious life. What was your entry into religious life like?
Morancy: Like the typical young woman who joined the women's orders around my time, I joined the Sisters of Mercy right after graduating from high school in 1959. I had a different background from your regular high school girl joining a women's order in the late 1950s. I grew up in Kingston, Rhode Island, then a very rural place. My family worked at [the] University of Rhode Island. I went to a public grammar school because

Catholics were the minority in Kingston, unlike the rest of the state. [When I entered the convent]. . .I wore the long black habit, kept the great silence, and did all the traditional things.

Like kissing the floor?
Morancy: No, we didn't do that in the Mercies, thank God. But I found the life difficult. Maybe it was because I was a country girl.

And athletic. . . .Then suddenly you were in a constrained environment. What was that like?
Morancy: I took it so seriously that I hardly ever broke silence. Yet, I had a habit of not conforming to whatever the model of the perfect novice or perfect young sister would be. . . you know, in little things.

You wavered in the little things?
Morancy: One reason I got in trouble was my poor housecleaning skill. It was the one thing [highly] regarded. I found the atmosphere anti-intellectual and, always a student, I liked to study, to read, to be stimulated. Being a good housecleaner was second in my estimation and that's where I got into most of my trouble. I was zero in the cleaning field. I did not challenge the authorities. I just tried to stay out of trouble. After two years novitiate I went to Salve Regina College in Newport, Rhode Island, and graduated in 1964. I majored in history and minored, like all Mercies, in education.

But something spurred the political in me at that time; of course, if there isn't a seed within, then an event doesn't bring it forth. In college, some picture magazine like *Life* or *Look* did a big spread on the new governor of the state of Oregon in 1963. The then new governor—now Senator Mark Hatfield—was profiled in the article as a former political science teacher. I noted that he went into politics and that he was also a very devout member of the Baptist church where he was a lay preacher. He saw politics as a "ministry"; it affected people's lives. I remember that day distinctly. I looked at those words and said to myself: "Isn't that an interesting concept? Political ministry."

Years later when I was in New Bedford [Massachusetts] teaching, I was surprised by an article in *Time* magazine on an upcoming U.S. Senate race in Oregon. . . .Ordinarily, the article noted, Governor Mark Hatfield would be unchallenged because he has been for years a most popular governor. Yet, he was then in a very tight race. In 1966, he became a lone voice, or, in a sense, one of the few prophetic voices in public life. He challenged the morality of the Vietnam War. He did it long before. . .ordinary folks said that [the] war wasn't even our war. But he had a prophetic message, and became not exactly "Mr. Popularity." When I reflected on his situation I thought: Of course Mark Hatfield would take a courageous stance. I prayed that he would win. I remember one sister telling me she was going to keep her radio on during the night to get the Rhode Island election results. I said to her: "Please listen to the results of the Oregon race." At breakfast, next morning, I learned that he had won. His coining the phrase "political ministry" at the time I studied history and political theory for my masters at URI [University of Rhode Island] really stayed with me. It was at that point I brought the two concepts together and said I would do that also. But I had a nun's habit on; how could I do it?

"VATICAN II CHANGED THE NUNS"
But then Vatican II came. . .

Morancy: Vatican II changed the church, but most of all, it changed American nuns. There is a direct line in my life from my childhood to the convent and to my choice of politics as ministry. I taught high school while earning a masters' degree in political science and then a way opened for me.

The incumbent state senator in my district decided to run for lieutenant governor. I saw the perfect opportunity but I lost that race; I ran unendorsed in 1978 and won. I have won every race since.

Several years ago, it seemed that your decision to be in the political field was also regarded as a ministry by Pope Paul VI.

Morancy: When I was elected in 1978, Jesuit Father Robert Drinan was in Congress; there was a priest [Robert Ogle] in the parliament in Canada, and there was a priest state senator in the West. Some nuns served in city councils in many places. Political action for political change was encouraged.

But this has changed recently. In September 1983, you be-

came aware of the fact that your bishop would not exempt you from the new canon law which forbade nuns and priests from holding political office. At the time, you were running for re-election. What happened?

Morancy: Well, immediately I felt that it was a larger issue than my running for re-election as a state representative. I mean, the be-all-and-end-all of my life isn't to be the state representative, so if I didn't think there were larger issues, I would have said okay and retired. Even though the pope [John Paul II] said [that Father Drinan must resign from office]. . .I think it was a woman's question. It was a woman's question tied very much to American nuns. American nuns since Vatican II [have] been operating more and more on a consensus kind of decision making. Superiors were not saying: You do that; you must not do that. Communities were struggling; they were going through processes and pain to really reshape their orders. We were operating on a peer model. We discerned and prayed with others about what our ministry should be, what our lives should be. That was how we would make our decisions about what ministries in this contemporary society [should be and how the] the church [was] calling us.

Vatican II [in my opinion] very clearly said that we had to stand with the poor, we had to bring about change in the structures that are oppressing people. What we did as women from the end of Vatican II to the point of getting John Paul II after us was changing the way we made decisions. We changed the way we saw ministry. We were doing ministry within a contemporary American society, not the European model that this pope comes from. When the pope says you may not run for political office, the larger thing he is saying to the women of American orders is: you may not determine one of the relevant ministries. . . .Consequently, I thought that was really [important] in the framework that I placed my decision within. The other thing I saw was a challenge to try to make women's orders regress. It raised the authority question in the church, which in an ongoing sense is raised all the time with this pope.

It's clear that you did not make this decision only in terms of your own personal life. Rather, you made this decision globally in terms of the American situation, the American nuns who took Vatican II so seriously and practiced their

option for the poor and the marginalized, and so on.

Morancy: Absolutely. In this country, one way to do that ministry is through the political process. And I always say that you have to respect people's experience. I said that to [my] bishop. No one in the hierarchy of the church has ever said, "What has been your experience since you've been elected? How do you see it as a ministry? How can we learn from that?" I told [my] bishop that there are not a million nuns and priests in political office. It would be very easy to tap the experience of the few. No one ever did. And the older I get, the more I value my experience and experience of others—a lived experience—just as I wished that they had tapped mine and valued it and therefore may have seen how, in this country, politics can be a ministry. I respect the experience of Pope John Paul II. He comes from a totalitarian country in which he viewed government as the enemy. He led and rallied his people and held them against that government. All right: that's his experience. I don't pretend to tell him what to do in that experience. It is not mine. He doesn't know the experience of American churchpeople within the political process. Yet, he made decisions which I feel were contrary to. . .our experience. He wants to return the church to its former discipline and uniformity, and that means everybody [has to] get in line.

What was going on at the time you were considering running for re-election?

Morancy: Well. . .Sister Noel told Arlene [Violet] and me in September 1983 [that our bishop would not exempt us from canon law]. I felt my decision should not totally be my own. I was a member of an order, and I had a responsiblity to take in all that data. I did a few things. I talked to my friends, both within the Sisters of Mercy and outside the order, and I canvassed the neighborhood. The Sisters of Mercy were really good and supportive. They brought in a woman canon lawyer in November 1983 for a day of reflection on the political question as it related to the new canon law. The group reviewed my particular situation that day. I also made a retreat to get away and sift out my own thoughts. At some point in November, I decided to seek re-election.

Simultaneously, we had Arlene Violet's [similar] situation.

I do not, and never did, see Arlene much, yet I regard her greatly. Canon law was formally adapted around the last Sunday in November 1983. Everybody knew that and all the focus was on Arlene. It became obvious that she made a decision to ask for a dispensation in order to run. But I made the decision that I wasn't going to do that. I was going to go ahead and see what happened. In January, Arlene made public that again she sought election for attorney general.

POLITICAL MINISTRY IN THE CATHOLIC CHURCH
At a recent point in history, we had a pope who condoned Christians' involvement in political ministry. Yet with this pope the messages had changed...
Morancy: [Approximately twenty years ago, the church began to encourage us] to immerse ourselves in the world, address the major issues, and...take a preferential option for the poor. The Second Vatican council was calling Catholic Christians to a truly systemic change, in other words, to global justice. Paul VI was superb and consistent in his papacy, in articulating this major concern. His two most important writings for our purposes were *On the Development of Peoples*, or *Populorum Progressio* and what came to be called "The Eightieth Year Letter" [*Octagesima Adveniens*]. This latter one was a call to action, written on the eightieth anniversary of the encyclical *Rerum Novarum*, (the great labor enecyclical of Leo XIII). I consider *Populorum Progressio* to be Paul VI's greatest encyclical. Paul repeatedly spoke of the empowerment of the poor. He urged penetrating the economic and political places of power because that's where the decisions affecting people's lives...were made. He urged Christians to get into those places, and effect the decisions that mandate global justice.

"The Eightieth Year Letter," on the other hand, was written in 1971. In this letter it was observed that politics was a demanding way to live out the Christian message of service to others. The pope was picking up the theme that through the political process you had the opportunity to make decisions and to effect change.

Americans nuns in particular took up that message and in December 1971, Marge Tuite gathered forty-seven of us in Washington, D.C. to ask how we, as American churchwomen, were going to respond to the mandates of *Populorum Progressio*. Out of that weekend was born Network, the organization that [now] is so well known nationally. It's the national Catholic Social Justice Lobby Group. It originally was just forty-seven nuns; it is now several thousand people, from all kinds of religious denominations. It has become an effective tool of lobby for change in the political process. As one of the original founders of Network, [I was able to see] very clearly the need for political involvement.

Is this organization also in jeopardy with the present pope?

Morancy: It hasn't felt any pressure directly, so far. . .

Does he know it exists?

Morancy: Possibly. And some of the issues that it espouses are issues of the institutional church. Network takes far more action than the hierarchical church on the massive military buildup in this country, the weapons systems, economic justice, feminization of poverty—all the budget priorities which are so [unjust] under the Reagan Administration. The institutional church would certainly come out "verbally" on the same side as Network.

Getting back to the issue of your re-election, when did you notice trends changing in the Vatican?

Morancy: The year I was elected [1978], there was an. . .attempt to restore law and order and discipline and a far more conservative stance on the part of the hierarchical, institutional church. It was apparent by 1980. Scarcely was [John Paul II] installed (I was seeking re-election [at the time]) when he demanded that Jesuit [Rev. Robert] Drinan not run again for Congress.

Did Drinan not run?

Morancy: Absolutely. He quit. He was told to and he did.

What do you think of that?

Morancy: Well, I think there are a lot of us wishing that he had stood his ground more. Certainly some people think that if he had, things would have been different. He was a very powerful Congressperson. He had a very influential, wealthy constituency who certianly admired the great work he was doing. I think he would have. . .had tremendous support. I don't know what went on behind the scene. Yet many of us women felt that had there been more of a fight, then things would be different.

But you know, a dominant theme in the Jesuit order is obedience to the pope. How could he reconcile that dilemma and stay still a Jesuit?

Morancy: Well, I think you have a key point. Father Drinan is a member of the clerical system of the church, and the canons then applied only to clerics. Secondly, because he is a member of the clerical system, he certainly doesn't feel the oppression of the hierarchical church that we women do. [As a male] he would never feel as so many of us do, that we are outsiders and not valued for our gifts and contributions to the institutional church. Father Drinan was therefore coming from a far different stance within the system.

UNDERSTANDING THE AMERICAN CONTEXT

You think it's different for women than for men? Please explain.

Morancy: I have a lot of responses, some of them incomplete. The question is a larger one than just participating in politics, although I do think that is a factor. We have to keep in mind that we are all products of our experience. [As I said] the experience of John Paul II in Poland is that government is the enemy. You work against it; you rally the forces to stand strong and stalwart and unyielding. And that's his experience and I respect that [but] it's not my experience and I can't relate to it. But neither can he relate to the American experience of democracy and participation bringing about change.

The larger issue is the authority question in the church where women are shut out of any kind of participation. When women orders say we are going to determine our own ministries and we see politics as a ministry, the males, church males, don't want us to do those kinds of things. The larger issue, therefore, for me and for other women, is the authority question—really, self-determination. The nuns' orders have the right to determine our own ministries within the process I've mentioned before: discussion, consensus, and so forth. I always characterized what happened to me as a real act of violence toward me and toward the order. The violence that I felt was [based on the fact] that at no point has anyone, [including my bishop], in the institutional church ever asked [me about] my experience.

From a political ministry viewpoint?

Morancy: Yes. No one asked: How do you see your position in the legislature as a ministry? Do you think it's valid? They said, when I first ran in 1976, it was fine. Suddenly, it was prohibited, without anyone seeking my experience and my input. Secondly, everything they said was just a dictation of policy. They didn't want to listen to what the Sisters of Mercy collectively were saying about the order's experience or the chapter's decision about policial ministry. Finally, the lawyer hired by the Mercy Order had a very difficult time [establishing] any kind of communication [with the Vatican]. All the Vatican wanted to do was hand down their prohibitions. They did not want to listen. When, finally, they said, "This is what you have to do," it was without [my] input, dialogue, or an opportunity for me to share the experience of my ministry.

You mention the canons. What does the new canon involve? You noted it covers clerics, but was later changed to incorporate lay women.

Morancy: The canon is church law. Every group has regulations or laws by which they govern, so that's what they call the canon law of the church. Prior to Novemeber 1983, the canons, laws that dealt with politics prohibited priests from elective office, except where it was seen to be a "good thing." What that meant was that when you're in situations or locales where you really don't have anybody else or there's unique expertise that a priest could bring, it was always allowable to seek office. In the Canadian Parliament, there was a priest, Robert Ogle, recognized as a great authority on the Third World. He had served in Latin America for many years, and he was [widely] recognized as giving that parliament a unique expertise. Unfortunatly, he was told at the same time I was that he couldn't run again and he didn't. Yet, he had a real contribution [to make].

The prohibition, with its flexibility, was for priests. It was never clear to the hierarchy whether this canon law applied to nuns. Certain sections dealt with priests, others with lay people, and the nuns, as always, had no identity. I think when it came to prohibitions, they lumped us with the clergy. But when it came to rights, such as sacraments, etc., we were lumped with the laity and therefore prohibited from that ministry. Canon law was revised under the guidance of the present pope and went into effect in November 1983. And when it did, it said clearly that nuns and priests could not seek political office— elected office—or appointed to office if [it involved] the exercise of civil power. It also said, however, that local bishops could exempt persons from that canon.

How and when were you affected by new canon?

Morancy: Indirectly in 1982, when Arlene Violet stepped forward to run for attorney general and our bishop immediately reacted and said she should not run. His statement was mixed. It was mixed with reference to the canon that was not clear whether or not it applied to nuns. He also mentioned that [he saw] the role of prosecutor [as] problematic.

When the canon was unclear, he backed off. In 1982 she lost the election. From 1982 on, I suspected the Vatican would clarify and make sure that the prohibition against nuns was inserted in the canons.

The next time I felt that was in September 1983. The Provincial Administrator of the Sisters of Mercy, in separate meetings with Arlene and myself, told us she had met with the bishop. She said to him, "I know the canons go into effect in November 1983. I know they prohibit nuns seeking elective or appointed office involving civil power. I also know the local bishop has the power to exempt from that canon." He said: "Yes." And she said, "I'm asking you to exempt the two sisters in my community." "No," he told her, "because I know that the pope does not want that. I will not exempt them." Well, I went through a period of prayer and discernment, myself personally, and also with other support systems, other Sisters of Mercy, some of my neighbors, my constituents, other friends who have always supported me. And at the end of that I came to the conclusion that I was going to seek re-election. I saw this as a ministry and as I mentioned. . .one the church had never asked [me] about.

And this ministry constituted a real human contribution to the marginalized and the poor, as you keep saying. Could you describe your district while we're on the subject?

Morancy: Oh, sure. I represent a district that is probably one of the most multi-ethnic in Rhode Island. It's about forty-five percent white, thirty-five to forty percent black, and then Hispanic and Indo-Chinese principally. The Hmong [Laotian immigrants], and the other people in it, range from working class to the homeless. Significantly, McCauley House, a hospitality house for the homeless, is in that district. We definitely have a population needing a representative who knows their experience.

VATICAN CRACKDOWN

You saw the handwriting on the wall, you prayed, you sought a support system, and you checked with your voting district. It came time to decide. What was happening at this time?

Morancy: In January 1984, it was clear that the bishop was not about to exempt me. I remember the interesting dialogue that took place. At one point he said that I would be violating church law if I sought re-election. I saw politics as a ministry, and one of the ways that we should be living out the gospel, living out the gospel call of justice in contemporary times. He made it clear that if I ran when the church says I shouldn't, then I'd be violating church law. If I violate church law, then I'm in violation of the church. I said to him, "Sometimes church law violates the gospel." And he said, "Never." I said, "Well, let us start with the Inquisition." He said that was an aberration. It was interesting. In the middle of our conversation, my voting record on abortion came up.

I always voted pro-choice. Regardless of my personal feelings on abortion, it is my obligation not to vote for unconstitutional laws.

Do you feel that your voting record on abortion may have influenced your bishop?

Morancy: I think that certainly was part of it. Later in March 1984, the General Chapter of the Sisters of Mercy met and invited me to attend. They asked my permission to appeal my case to the Vatican. Because I had been in office for six years, and the office was part-time, they considered these extenuating circumstances. I knew an appeal would be very long and exhausting. But I agreed. They hired lawyer Peter Shannon of Washington, a former priest and a canon lawyer.

[He] was from Chicago [and] he attempted to see the Cardinal there, but was turned down. He tried to get church people of note to back up his case. He didn't get anywhere. He and Sister Noel met with our bishop and it was another dead end. He wrote an excellent brief to the Vatican. We waited; we waited a long time. Finally, toward the end of April, at midnight the day before I was to announce for re-election, the day before a fund-raiser, Rome's "no" arrived.

It is the last minute, one minute to midnight. Next day you are to hold a fund-raiser, and still you did not know if you are in violation of church law. Was that conflictual?

Morancy: Ah, yes! Originally I said I'm going to run, and if they want to throw me out, they can come after me. But when I got down to the wire, that midnight, I was exhausted. Often, during the wearying process I received calls at 6:30 a.m. or at midnight. I was so tired; besides, I had to get re-elected. When Rome said, No, you can't run, I reflected: "If I have to leave the Mercies to do this ministry, I will leave." And I did.

Do you feel that the Mercies put up a good fight for you?

Morancy: I think they did absolutely everything possible. They did the same for Arlene, and yet, they did it with respect for our ministry. Arlene pursued her course of action. The previous year the Vatican had, in a very, very violent series of events, forced out Agnes Mary Mansour. . .

Who is also a Mercy nun.

Morancy: I was the third one. It was a time of great pain for the Mercies. Every nun in the order, of course, did not agree with me. I got letters from people telling me not to dare defy the pope. But the leadership of the Sisters of Mercy, and, of course, the majority of the members, gave as much support as they could.

Will you talk more about the "violence" you mentioned earlier, and if you are still suffering?

Morancy: No, I don't think I am still suffering. I think I got beyond a real anger. On one level, at least, I experienced a feeling of relief. There was a finality to it. Being so tired, I don't know if I felt anything, because I knew the inevitability of the outcome. The conflict for me was the fact that I was a member of the order. I felt a certain responsibility which I would not have felt if I alone were in conflict with the Vatican. Besides, several years ago, I told myself that the church, the institution and its attitude toward women, was hopeless. Long before this personal 1983-84 controversy, I realized that there was no way the hierarchy, the power people in the church, were going to recognize women. Within myself at that point I responded spiritually. I felt drawn to feminist spirituality and alternative styles of worship. That is why the feeling of violence was stronger than the anger. I had already gone through the anger realizing that the church didn't value its women and their contributions. I felt much more strongly the violence of the Vatican. I was a member of an order—the Mercy order—under fire and I felt a responsibility to these women.

Under the present pope, our leader Theresa Kane was also under fire. Hence, there was always a tension: wanting to do and say things as an individual, and feeling a responsibility to the nuns. Remember, the Mercies were trying to get Rome to recognize one of their ministries. I was the person who was the instrument for them to try to do that. It was difficult for me. But while I had long ago given up as far as the institutional, hierarchical church and women were concerned, I knew the order had not and I was a member of that order. I was so appreciative that they were willing to go to the wire for me.

VALUE OF PEOPLE'S EXPERIENCE
You said you were already interested in alternative forms of worship. In light of that, how do you get spiritual sustenance for your strong principles of justice and fairness?
Morancy: I have learned to value people's experiences. I describe my representative district as "the many faces of God." It is multi-ethnic; [there are] so many different backgrounds. People there come together to pray and to reflect out of their experience of God. When they reflect on life's deeper meaning, I find it very, very important. Also, I am sustained by my love of the countryside, its natural surroundings. Once in a while I go to Caratunk Wildlife Refuge in Seekonk [Massachusetts]. I walk and restore my need to be alone and to reflect. I need time and space because my life is cluttered with issues and people, with meetings and work.

Now that you are in office, where do you see your future since you have sacrificed so much for political ministry?

Morancy: This will probably be my last term in the Rhode Island Legislature. After ten years, it is time to move on. I want to run for major office. Politics, however, is timing, and who knows what [the future] will bring? At present, I work at The Rhode Island Protection and Advocacy System. Rhode Island legislators need full-time jobs because the legislature pays only three hundred dollars a year. Yet the work load is enormous, and I hope our system changes. My full-time job is advocacy in behalf of developmentally disabled people. The work is a human service for those who, for whatever reason, are the most vulnerable of our population. I bring their experiences into the political arena where the decisions that affect their lives are made.

Are there clerics in the state of Rhode Island in powerful positions?

Morancy: I mentioned that canon law prohibits clerics holding elective or appointive office when the exercise of civil power is involved. Yet in 1984, when all this was happening to me, there were two priests who came under that category of appointive office exercising civil power. One sat on the Parole Board and exercised far more power over people's lives than I did. One of these, a member of a five-person panel, is required each month to vote whether an incarcerated person is to go free or be held in jail. That is a pretty powerful position. I'm not sure I'd even want to have [such a] position of judging people. Another priest served on the Conflict of Interest Commission, and held the appointed post for years and was there in 1984.

What are your current reflections on your political ministry?

Morancy: Shortly after I was elected in 1978, I attended a lecture by a Boston feminist theologian. She defined ministry as "making private pain a public issue." I thought it the perfect definition of political ministry. It is certainly the way I try to operate as a politician. I listen to the *experience* of people in my district, of women, and other people who in any way are vulnerable. I listen to their private pain and try to get the political system to address that private pain. When one does that, one is making private pain a public issue.

Let me use an example. In my first week in office, a woman, head of a household in my district, told me: "I need to move. My house is a mess. I've got an absentee landlord who won't fix the property. I'm afraid for my two little children. But no one wants me because they say, 'You've got children? I don't want to rent to children.'" Simultaneously, a young attorney. . .moved into Rhode Island to take the bar examination. He needed to settle his family quickly. He and his wife had one child. No one wanted him since he had a six-year-old son. During the same week, both told me that other states can't discriminate in renting to families with children. [In] Rhode Island, however, [people] could do it and they were doing it wholesale. It took me five years to bring a new law into the legislative arena. Actually, it took me six sessions because there was such opposition to the bill.

Has it become law?
Morancy: Yes. It is one example of taking private pain. . .and bringing it to public exposure. The best testimony came from those people who shared their experience. The awful experience of not being able to find a decent place to rent because people had kids! Imagine, triple-decker [house] owners not wanting to rent to kids. And the whole history of why Rhode Island has double and triple deckers built in the 1920s was because these houses were filled with families and children. These kinds of laws tie together the private and the public, and that's what I think political ministry is all about.

THE CHALLENGE OF POLITICAL MINISTRY
Are there other laws you have been able to get passed in your political ministry?
Morancy: I'm very proud of a major piece of legislation enacted last session. For eighteen months I chaired a landlord/tenant commission. I brought together every side of the issue. I don't think there is any issue more volatile than landlord/tenant relations. The concept of property versus personal rights, of injustice and profit motives, all enter into landlord/tenant relations. I brought together the developers and realtors, the tenants, the civil rights attorneys, and the code enforcement people. Polarization between these groups took years to overcome. Finally, I got the legislature to completely rewrite and

revise all the landlord/tenant laws of this state. Now the fifty-two-page law is just a marvelous tribute to my commission. I am really excited about it.

And a tribute to your leadership. . .

Morancy: I was a moderator and sometimes a referee in the process. I've worked in the housing field, and I also work for victims of sexual assault. My experience on the board of the Rape Crisis Center showed the need for changing laws in that area.

These laws as well as those on the handicapped address very Christian concepts. Why then, in your view, is the church against this kind of ministry?

Morancy: I think a wonderful response is to quote someone else. At the sisters' chapter in 1984, when they decided to push my issue, the nuns discussed political ministry. One of the chapter members said, "I can see how you can effect change and how good it is. But I'm really worried that our sisters, if they get into the political arena, are going to compromise their values. We all know of the compromises that take place in politics. It really worries me." Sister Theresa Kane rose, and said very simply, "I think our sisters who go into political ministry have to keep that in mind. That is why justice is so important. I don't recommend that every nun be a teacher, or a nurse. I don't recommend that all of our sisters be politicians. But," she added, "regarding this fear of compromise, I worry far more about our sisters who are working in Catholic chanceries. . . ."

Recently we saw an example of what Theresa was saying. A group of women outside the Providence Cathedral held a prayer service protesting some priest being made a monsignor. These women and a few men were praying out of the pain of what happened to Mary Ann Sorrentino and out of pain for women in the church. The prayer service seen on TV showed a reporter interviewing a nun who worked officially for the diocese. She stated, "I don't think women should be priests." So, you see, if you work for the diocese or the chancery, you have to take certain postures. I also believe that the men around the bishops have to compromise far more than I do in the political arena.

You don't want to be ordained a priest?

Morancy: I would never want to be a priest in the present system. The important thing for me is to be open to life. I'm a great lover of sports, tennis especially, and music. Somebody gave me a sign once, "Only one thing matters, wherever you go, whatever you do, you hear the music of life." And I think that that's an important thing—to be open to the way God reveals herself.

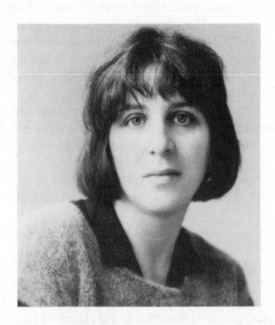

MARY GORDON

". . . I actually think [we] Catholic women, because of the experience of having nuns who are at least in a somewhat powerful position. . .are better at seeing women as authority figures. . . .It's easier for Catholics in that there's a notion that there was 'Sister' as well as 'Father.' . . .The problem with Catholics is we want to obey somebody, and we're not really so particular whether it's a man or a woman."

Mary Gordon, a novelist whom Catholics claim as one of their own, is the author of *Final Payments, The Company of Women, Men and Angels,* and *Temporary Shelter.* Mourning what she perceives to be a loss of beauty and majesty, she describes the present barren church scene as agitated "busyness," banners with banal statements, and ill-prepared strummers playing on loud guitars. Her view and vision of both women and church is indeed bleak.

Despite her pessimism, she cherishes the Christ figure in

Christianity because Christ represents a vision which no other religion possesses. Her ideal of a fully Christian human being is Pope John XXIII. Believing that he—unlike most church leaders—was unafraid of learning, she yearns for his vision of church and of all people. She, nevertheless, remains in the Catholic church (albeit on the periphery) for her children's sake. The fellowship of left-wing Catholic groups also attracts her because, as she wistfully notes, "They are my people."

Mary Gordon is an ardent admirer of Virginia Woolf and claims, "The beauty of prose and the beauty of appreciation of nature, and the tremendous rhythmicity of her prose was a real inspiration." These words aptly describe Mary Gordon's own artistry.

THE CHURCH AND THE ARTIST

Where are you in relation to the church?

Gordon: The institutional church is not at the center of my life. I come in and go out of the institutional church as I have more or less patience for it. I have periods where the whole thing makes me so impatient that I lose hope. I feel so alienated. I feel like these bishops and the pope have nothing in common with me; they have nothing to give me and I leave. It's not a great cost to me to be in or out of church. But I was impressed with these women for whom the church was at the center of their lives—the sisters—they had really taken very courageous stands. But for me it's not such a courageous stand.

Some of the characters in your novels, especially in *Final Payments* and *The Company of Women*, have certain Catholic underpinnings.

Gordon: I think my characters do, and I do. The underpinnings are certainly there. What I'm not sure about is whether the church that formed me even exists any more so that some of the things that were terribly important to me in the church are aesthetic memories.

Such as?

Gordon: Memories of a kind of silence. The ritual provided a kind of solemnity in the sense of formal beauty—the beauty of the prayers, the beauty of the music.

You're talking about the pre-Vatican II church?

Gordon: Yes. I find very little in the current church to feed me aesthetically. I think the ritual, at best, is nondescript. Sometimes it's actively ugly. And so much of what was important to me was that sense of silence and solemnity that I think is gone now. That doesn't mean that I'm going to go back to the silence and solemnity, because the people who seem to be still holding onto the ritual which I liked are politically abhorrent to me. And that is a real problem for me. I'm not going to go into some church where they're suggesting that we send money to the Contras [U.S.-backed rebels in Nicaragua] and, you know, excommunicate anybody who uses birth control, so that I can hear "Pange Lingua." So I feel very lost in both camps because I'm a person for whom beauty is very important. That's my life. I am supposed to create beauty and to be constantly in the midst of ugliness or mediocrity. . .is to me a grief. It's really a grief to hear ugly music, to be in ugly buildings, to hear ugly or stupid or hackneyed language. It hurts me.

You feel quite alienated, then. . .?

Gordon: Oh, yes. And a lot of people whose politics I love and admire don't seem to have the same aesthetic and ritual and formal sense of beauty.

Who are these people you admire?

Gordon: Well, people very much on the left, and very much concerned with social justice [even though they] seem to put together rituals which to me are quite thin, and, therefore empty. And so I feel lonely within them in the same way that I feel lonely if I were ever to approach the people on the right who have a more formal ritual. I find a kind of physical repulsion to [those on the right]. I feel no ambivalence in relation to them. My ambivalence is to the sort of people on the left whom I admire, but who have lost the sense of solemnity.

REJECTION OF MODERN AESTHETICS

So what's the cure for that?

Gordon: I really don't know. I think it's over. I feel very sad. I don't think that we're in an age that can create great public art. We're not in an age of great architecture; we're not in an age of great communal music in the way that either the Middle Ages were, or the German Protestants in the eighteenth century.

Modern aesthetics. . .are on the level of the high, very privatist, and on the level of the low, very jangling—there is no religious expression. The *zeitgeist* of the age is not religious. I think
we're not going to come up with any more great religious art
that I can see.

**And are you saying this for the Catholic church or for
the whole of Christendom?**

Gordon: The whole world, I mean, not just Christianity. But
certainly for the West.

You're very pessimistic.

Gordon: I'm very pessimistic, and I really don't know what to
do about my children.

**How do you feel about having your children participate
in a church whose ceremonies have little meaning for
you?**

Gordon: The children go and there are people jumping around.
Nobody's very quiet and nobody's saying anything that has any
depth or richness. The language is ugly. The music is exceedingly ugly.

Better that there be no music most times, because it's so bad.
Much of what formed me as a child was a reflective spirit, a
spirit of reflection and spirit of contemplation and a sense of
seriousness that I was participating in something quite ancient
and quite solemn.

Can you give me an example of . . .

Gordon: I remember Holy Week as a child.

Ah, yes. Tenebrae. . .

Gordon: . . .Absolutely.

Even James Joyce went back to hear Tenebrae.

Gordon: That's right. And Christmas midnight mass. I can't
even go now. It's too painful.

**Do you think that some of those sentimental memories
are exaggerated?**

Gordon: I don't think so; I really don't. Because I can hear the
music—I have to hear that music which they played then—on
records now. I hear those records and they trigger in me tremendous memories. When I was in London I went to the Brompton
Oratory. They were singing "Pange Lingua"; they were doing
the Gregorian Mass. Before the sermon. . .before I could hear

what they were talking about, I just experienced the old ritual. I was flooded with those very potent memories. I don't know what there is in the church now that is valuable for my children in terms of ritual. There is a kind of spirit of Catholicism. I think I'll keep them in it, because there's nobody like John XXIII anywhere else. There's no image like that in the world, that I can hold up to them as an image of goodness and open generous love and concern.

Do you resonate with any other figure around, for example like Mother Teresa.

Gordon: Oh, no. She just irritates me, quite frankly.

What about figures like Flannery O'Connor, whom we think of as totally Catholic. How do you perceive her?

Gordon: Well, she's a great artist. I personally don't care what it was that made her able to write those stories. I thank God that those stories exist in the world. I think she had a singular experience. Remember she was stricken with a crippling disease at age twenty-four. Who knows what would have happened to her had she moved out into the world. Maybe she would also have been the way she was. But, I don't care. I honor her art. And if it was that strictness of the church that created it, fine. I'm glad of that accident. I have no quarrel with her. I don't want her to be any different, I don't need her to be different. She is genius.

You described many church flaws in your novels. Do you see yourself as a Catholic?

Gordon: It seems to be who I am; it seems to be who my people are. When I go to Catholics for a Free Choice conferences, those are my people. And I see these people have tremendous ideals. The figure of Christ and that kind of love are very, very important to me. I could not give that up. Catholicism and Judaism seem to me the form of continuum to which I'm very attracted, because of the kind of richness and openness to the world which [I feel] Protestantism lacks.

Judaism, I feel, is blessed in not being cursed with the dualism that is so much a part of Christianity, which I guess is the legacy of the Greeks. There is that figure who gave everything, even unto death on the cross, that I think is unique to Christianity.

But all the first Christians were Jews. Rosemary Ruether suggests that one group pushed the other out of the synagogue.

Gordon: It was a tragedy. It was a terrible tragedy. But I am not convinced that one can be a Jew without having been brought up a Jew. I think it is something much rooted in the family, in the community. It's a much less privatist experience than Christianity. My father was a Jew who converted to Catholicism in a very thoroughgoing way.

What was growing up with two different religions like?

Gordon: Well, my father was more Catholic than anybody. . . . He was extremely anti-Semitic. He was the most anti-Semitic person you'd ever meet. Nevertheless, every night he said over my head a Hebrew blessing. So it was very odd. I did have a slight oral Jewish memory. But in terms of being brought up with a Jewish feeling, it was Irish Catholicism all the way.

MALE DOMINANCE IN CATHOLICISM

In *The Company of Women*, you say you were fascinated by the way women are dominated by men in the church.

Gordon: I'm fascinated, appalled, horrified by the way. . .by how hard it is for women to be powerful without appealing to a male authority, and by how easy it is for us to give that over—how the instinct to submit to a man is so thoroughgoing and so deep.

But that's not unique to Catholic women.

Gordon: As a matter of fact, I actually think we Catholic women, because of the experience of having nuns who are at least in a somewhat powerful position. . .are better at seeing women as authority figures. I think the whole authority problem is harder for Catholics than for other people. But it's easier for Catholics in that there's a notion that there was "Sister" as well as "Father." The presence of the Virgin Mary and the female saints, the presence of nuns who had a powerful position in one's life, which was removed from the domestic—they were not like your mother—I think that gives Catholic women actually more access to female community than other women have. The problem with Catholics is we want to obey somebody, and we're not really so particular whether it's a man or a woman.

Are Catholics, therefore, good candidates for the women's movement?

Gordon: Yes, I think we are. Actually, we're quite overrepresented for numbers in NOW [National Organization of Women]. There's a disproportionate number of Catholic women in NOW compared to our presence in the general population. I think we are good candidates for the women's movement if we can get over our stance of general obedience.

People who know the women in this volume of interviews feel that Catholic women are up against an impossible task. How can women change the Roman Catholic church?

Gordon: I think if the church lasts, then women will prevail. I think the problem with the church is its insistence on a celibate clergy. It's going to run out of clergy. And I think that's what will do it in. And so if the church endures, it's going to have to be very different within forty or fifty years. You're not going to have these celibate males around running things from Rome, because they're not going to have any audience. And so I'm not sure if it will exist. I'm not sure if the church can exist without a powerful hierarchy and I just don't see young people flocking into seminaries.

As a matter of fact, in 1986, there were 1,847 parishes without a resident priest in this country. Mary Hunt feels that ten years ago, had the bishops put stoles around the nuns, walked them two-by-two up the aisle, and ordained them, they would have stopped the clergy shortage. So now she feels women can create a new church, a women-church.

Gordon: Except, what would be the meaning of this church? Mary and I diverge on these things, too. She is more forward-looking than I am in some ways. What would be the meaning of the sacraments that women-church create?

She's talking about women doing what American blacks did in the 1960s. Many of them in colleges and universities withdrew to be by themselves.

Gordon: And, where are we now? They came back into the mainstream, but, you know, the situation of blacks is worse [now] than it was—economically. I mean blacks are still the underclass, the impermeable underclass. . . .If you're a black child, you still have an infinitely smaller chance of a healthy, productive, safe life than a white child. Infinitely. That's not a model that gives me very much hope.

You are pessimistic about the possiblity of women constructing their own theology.

Gordon: The point is very few people want it. For the majority of the people who are still in the church, it's because they want to be attached to the church of their forefathers and foremothers. I mean, we can't even pass the Equal Rights Amendment in this country. And if we think we have problems, what are you going to do with the Third World? If the hope of the church is in Latin countries, what are you going to do with their ethic of machismo? They're going to accept the ordination of women much more slowly than we are. I've talked to women who work in the church in Latin America. They don't see it happening very soon. If it does, it will be because of weariness on everybody's part. Maybe the women will be the only ones left.

In the church?

Gordon: Yes. Like what's happening to the Episcopal church. Practically the only Episcopalians you know are people who want to be ordained themselves. They have no congregation. The congregation is of twenty-five priests and two people who do not want to be priests. I don't think we're in a religious time. I don't know what that means. I cannot prognosticate in that way.

Theresa Kane has said that although there is much talk about faith, we do not live in a faithful time.

Gordon: No. If you hold up John Paul II and Theresa Kane, people are not going to flock to Theresa Kane. They're going to flock to "big daddy." People in the Third World—I was once in El Salvador—had pictures of John Paul II on every street corner. I'm sure these base communities in Latin America are very moving. The idea of having women leaders are fine, but they don't have that mythical power that the great white father has.

And the women going around doing something informal. . . ? Even if those women are there for the people, and with them, and living and serving with them, they don't have that mythic appeal. The mythic, the irrational appeal of the church is very, very strong. And I don't see what's going to replace it. I don't *like* it, but I see its importance, and that's what keeps people in, that sense of the irrational. I really think it's over.

You feel that sense of the irrational is appealing to people's unconscious?

Gordon: Yes, I do think that.

What does this have to do with God?

Gordon: One does not go to God for rational reasons. There's no rational reason for belief. Obviously, even if educated people choose to believe, it's not because there are better reasons for belief than for disbelief; there are much better reasons for disbelief than for belief. The whole posture of being a religious person is a posture which you weigh in on the side of the irrational. I think that the new church does not tap deeply enough into the unconscious.

So you feel that the irrational sense is what's missing in the renewed church?

Gordon: Yes. I never thought of that until just now. I think that that's the whole problem. The present church is working on relatively superficial levels of human activity. But the activity that is touched by prayer are beauty, reflection, and a kind of race memory. We've jettisoned all that. And then what do we say to people? What do we give in their place? Try to love Jesus. Give yourself up. Lay down your life for your friend. . . .*Why* lay down your life for your friend? Why should I? Is there a good reason?

CURRENT DIRECTIONS

Where is your art leading nowadays?

Gordon: I'm writing a novel about Irish immigration. I've thought a lot about the Irish. I'm reading about their history and thinking a lot about them. I love and I feel very drawn to them. At the same time, I find them appalling at some levels, particularly in America. So I have a real love/hate for them. I think that there is an Irish attachment to both language and nature: the beauties of language and the beauties of nature that is quite extraordinary. And that makes them a very special and different situation from a lot of people.

Certain pagan cultures were never totally permeated by Christianity. Do you think that your attraction to Irish culture stems from its earlier system of belief?

Gordon: I'm not someone who romanticizes paganism. I think paganism is quite cruel. I get really crazy when people talk about the great matriarchal religions. They were very cruel religions. I'm not saying that patriarchy is not cruel, but there is something about the ideal of justice which is terribly important to human beings. It is something that entered the culture when the mother religions went out of it. Now, a lot was lost, a lot of our connection to the earth, and to nature, and to the moral unconscious was lost. Nevertheless, we don't want to be at the mercy of the unconscious. I don't see nature as a benevolent force.

When did this element of justice enter our cutlure?

Gordon: I don't know quite enough about it, but certainly the notion of justice was very much of the Jews. With the Greeks also, as they progressed. You can see the difference from Homer's *Iliad*, which is a bloodthirsty, cruel work. The difference between that and the later Greek Tragedies is extraordinary. I would much rather live in the world of the Tragedies than the world of the *Iliad*. I would rather live in the world of the prophets than in the world of Baal any time, because you have no recourse if justice doesn't have some sort of sway. Not that justice has not been perverted—it has—but unless you introduce that notion of justice triumphing over nature in some way, I think we face a very merciless prospect. Nature is very bleak; nature does not protect the weak.

Many of the women represented in these stories feel that justice is precisely the element women will bring into the church.

Gordon: Because we have been victims of injustice, I think we would be more sensitive to justice. I don't think justice, however, in any deep way is gender-related. I think that there are people of good of both genders who will suffer a great deal for justice. I think it's too hopeful, because the just man or woman is a very rare animal. I don't think there's any magical thing about having ovaries and a uterus. I think there are some things that women are better at. Woman are better at having that sort of third ear, alert for the needs of other people. I happen to think that women are very happy because we're trained more sociably; we're rewarded for that more. But I don't think that women are of necessity more just than men. I don't think they're less just than men. I think to be a just human being is difficult and rare.

WOMEN AS ORDAINED PRIESTS

Therefore it would not make much difference if women became part of the Catholic clergy?

Gordon: It would make a difference in other ways. But I don't think it would necessarily create more justice. It would create more understanding, and it would erase a particular kind of injustice practiced against them. The fact of that bar being lifted would be a triumph for justice. But I certainly don't think that there's any magical way that if there are more women, there will be more justice. You've worked in groups of women, and so have I. One of the things you find out is that there are some ways in which we work together very well, and then one is constantly disillusioned. I always expect women to be better than men.

And some women do not want to be liberated.

Gordon: That's right. And morality is a very difficult thing, we're all very selfish. People like power; men and women. People like having their will; men and women. And I don't think anything magical happens because you put women together. I wish that I thought that but I don't. To be a moral and a decent person is a very grueling thing and a very rare thing. There are ways in which women together act better than men because they are not acting for the approval of men. They can sometimes be more natural. But I've seen women be perfectly terrible to each other.

I mean the cruelest people in my family are women. They are more powerful than the men, and they are very cruel. I've always found women more interesting than men; my closest bonds are with women. But I have no romance that they're necessarily nicer. I have a son and that has really changed me completely about men.

How did he change you?

Gordon: I have a son who is by nature much more loving, much more generous, much warmer than his sister. I adore my daughter; it's not that I love one more than the other. My daughter is a very tough girl. And she walks into the room, takes what she wants, and if she happens to knock somebody over in her path, "toughie for them." But my son worries; if David thinks that

I'm not feeling well (he's only three), he says, "Do you have a headache? Are you tired?" He's much more vulnerable than she is. He's much more easily hurt. If you correct her, she will fight you to the death to prove that she's not wrong. If you correct him, he literally lies down on the floor. If you say, "That was naughty," he cries. My daughter wasn't allowed to touch the hi-fi. I said, "Don't touch it." She touched it and I spanked her. She went over and touched it again saying, "I know you're not going to spank me twice. Since I've already been spanked, I might as well do it again." She did that at three.

Where did she get this from?

Gordon: Genes from my grandmother, my mother. Now I'm going to be the tough woman in my family for many generations.

Your mother is a strong woman?

Gordon: She's tough; I don't know how strong she is. She's a combination of being very dependent and rather aggressive. But my grandmother was very tough and very strong. Not a nice woman. Not a tender woman.

Do you think that women who came from oppressive situations are more understanding than women who do not?

Gordon: I don't think so. I'm writing about immigrant women who could not afford to be too understanding because life was very hard. The message they had to give to their children was, "Life is very hard. Better be ready to stand up for it and protect your flanks. Because they'll get you." I think there is a sentimentalism about women. I think that the women who survived were very tough. Particularly the Irish. I didn't know a lot of very tender Irish women, but there was a lot of very tough, admirably strong ones. I didn't get much sense of the tenderness you indicate. Irish men were much tenderer than the Irish women, if they weren't drunk. And I think that's important with the Irish, because so many of the men were alcoholics and walked away. The women had to take over. I also think that Irish women tend to "infantilize" their men.

DEFINING A "GOOD PERSON"

Who is the opposite of Margaret in *Final Payments*? What is your ideal of a good person?

Gordon: I go back to the image of John XXIII, who seemed to me to enjoy life, to be very open to life, and to have virtue which did not exclude generosity and openness and a kind of pleasure. It's a liveliness. My idea of the good person has to be a lively person who embraces life, as well as being able to deny himself or herself for the sake of others who might be in need. If Christianity could somehow rid itself of this hatred of life, hatred of the world, hatred of the senses, then the ideal of virtue would be much richer and fuller and come closer to my idea of a good person. The good person ought to like to laugh, and ought to be not be so exclusionary, so willing to judge and to damn. I think of the face of John XXIII was a wonderful face. A face—it was a peasant face—the famous picture of him when he was a cardinal, with a drink in one hand and a cigarette in the other. Generosity is the virtue that is the linchpin of my system of virtues.

So this is the opposite of Margaret in *Final Payments*. . . . Do you feel that Margaret is a harsh character because she is a woman?
Gordon: I don't think there are male Margarets. I think that because women have a smaller arena of power, their cruelty is more pointed. When men are cruel they hit you; they steal your money; they kill you. So it's very different. One does not choose one over the other. They're both terrible. The "Margarets" don't rape and beat you up and set your house on fire. So their arenas for cruelty are more pointed and in some ways more pernicious. But obviously they are people who steal lives.

Men and Angels does not focus on the church as much as your earlier novels. Have you moved away from Catholic issues?
Gordon: I am writing about the Irish now, so there is perforce an inclusion of Catholic issues. But I never know what will be next with me. For the moment I'm very involved with the Irish; so it is also the church [too in my novel]. But my Irish people are not very religious; they're kind of angry at the church. They were involved in the labor movement and they feel that the church sold them out, which in fact it did. One of the truly depressing things is to look at the early labor movement and see the number of Irish women who were the "heroes." Mother

Jones was an Irish woman, as was Leonore O'Reilly. The early labor movement started with the mills in western Massachusetts which were largely staffed by Irish women. So the heroes of the early labor movement were largely Irish and the church just stomped on them.

Wasn't the church afraid of losing its laborers, as was the case in France?

Gordon: The church was pro labor as long as labor didn't go too far left, as long as it could keep labor within the rubrics. Any hint of socialism and the church became really scared. The fact is that there were no Irish women, very few Irish women in labor history after about 1910. Then the field goes to Jewish women. And it's because the church really moved in. Priests gave sermons about how unwomanly it was for women to be involved in these things.

THOUGHTS ON THE IRISH

Have you visited Ireland?

Gordon: Yes, I've been six times. I wouldn't want to live there. I find it very magic. And I'm very drawn to it. Very special, a most sacred, magic place. But I know that if I lived there, it wouldn't be very nice for me. There's some wonderful spirit, but I think the Irish are very tricky. People think that they are openly warm and intimate. But I think the Irish really use language to steel [themselves] against [outsiders], and to distance themselves. And they are very clever at it. Because there are a lot of words coming out, and they're put together very well, you think you're getting information, but you're not getting any information.

Do you think the Irish know themselves?

Gordon: No. I think there's a real premium put on not knowing. But if you know, better not tell. Do they know themselves? Very interesting; I hadn't really gone on that level; it's a very good question. . . . .

I think one of the interesting things most Catholics think is that Irish Catholics are from Mars. It's such a different model from the model of either Jews or Protestants that they find them really alien. There's the guilt, but there's also a tremendous idealism which both ennobles the Irish and drives them nuts, or causes them to commit suicide. They're always stepping on their own feet. They're always snatching defeat from the jaws of victory. And I think—well I have a lot of thoughts about the Irish—but I think they love the invisible more than the visible.

The United Nations' ten-year study of the major health problems of the world in the 1970s revealed that the worst international problem was depression. Whether countries are rich, poor, underdeveloped, or developed, they have depression as a major health problem. But two spots are particularly depressed: one is the west coast of Ireland.

Gordon: But there is some real sense of the spirit there, nonetheless. There's a way in which I like the Irish for not running after success and progress. I can't defend that; that's an absolutely indefensible position. They are receptive. And it's funny [in] a new book—Herbie Miller's *Exiles and Immigrants*—[the author] gives you the idea that he's angry at Irish immigrants because they weren't pulling themselves up by their bootstraps. One reason is because generosity and hospitality was such a big ethic that they spent a lot of money on funerals and weddings and parties. That is what makes him angry. They're not with the program all the time. There's something in the Irish not being with the program that I like.

WOMEN ARE PEOPLE

What would you say to women like Theresa Kane, Mary Hunt, and Bernadette Brooten?

Gordon: Courage. Better to try than not to try. I don't like to give the idea that they'll win without a fight. What is that phrase, "If we lose hope then all our fears will come to pass." I think they probably have more hopeful natures than I do, and good for them. I genuinely think they're doing a good thing. I don't have much hope and I don't put my energy there. But I'm moved by their spirit and by their energy. I don't exactly understand anybody still wanting to be a sister. What do they get from that communion that they couldn't get elsewhere? What is the official sanction that they see? I can certainly understand it for those who have been in it for a long time and that's who they are and that's how they define themselves.

The reason that some sisters may stay is, let's face it, social security.

Gordon: That was one of the terrible things about those twenty-four nuns who signed the ad facing the threat of being thrown out.

Were you surprised by public reaction to Geraldine Ferraro?

Gordon: I was tremendouly excited when she was nominated. But I'm real mad at her. I think that if she didn't know her husband was involved in those kinds of things, then we'd have to say she's a fool. A public figure has a responsibility to know where her money and her husband's money is coming from. If she doesn't know where her husband's money is coming from, she has no right being vice president of the United States. And she made women look very stupid by saying, "Oh I didn't know where my husband's money comes from." I mean she's not any ordinary housewife. She's a lawyer. She has a responsiblity. Also. . . .There's no such thing as clean real estate money in New York. . . .She should have known that. Mondale should have known that. And her defense, "I didn't know where my husband's money was coming from," made her look like a dumb broad.

So you're disappointed?

Gordon: Very. And I feel quite betrayed by her. She set us back. Women as political figures will be less credible. It will be a long time before we get a woman vice presidential candidate. Unless someone like Jeane Kirkpatrick turns up. I'm not going to be excited if Jeane Kirkpatrick is nominated. But to be a woman who says, "I can do the job that a man can do," and then fall back on, "I didn't know where my husband's money comes from," was just ridiculous. And she made us all look ridiculous.

How did you become this person who you are?

Gordon: I had this sort of magic father. I had a father who loved me above anything else in the world. And thought I was the most important, wonderful, miraculous thing in the world. Even though he died when I was seven, I always had that. It was an incredible strength that he gave me. He gave me literature and languages and music at a very early age, and talked to me seriously. And that was a richness that I'll never lose. The other thing is that I met my two best friends when I was thirteen years old, and these women and I have gone through life together.

Like Liz and Isabelle of *Final Payments*.
Gordon: No, they're not like that; they're very different. One is actually teaching at Notre Dame, where she is a medieval historian, and one is a doctor. But we gave each other courage as we went out into the world.

It seems that there was something very important in that early love and cherishing with your father and friends. . .
Gordon: And the fact that it did not matter to my father that I was a girl. He never said to me that there are things that you can't do because you are a girl. He taught me Latin at five, he taught me French at four. I certainly didn't get from my family the idea [that if] there was anything that I wanted to do, I couldn't do because I was a girl. Luckily, I didn't want to be an architect, or a neurosurgeon, or something where I needed training. I just needed to read and write, which I could do in private.

You were only seven years old. . .did he die suddenly?
Gordon: Yes. Terrible. Terrible. I mean I had five years of my life which were a total daze after he died.

Why did you become a writer?
Gordon: Well, my father was a writer. That's what I was trained to be. It wasn't really a revolutionary act. I was brought up to be that. I never got to be anything else. I was really educated only with women until graduate school. I went to Barnard [New York City] and then I went to Syracuse [New York]. And that was the only place that anybody said you might be as good as a man. It hadn't occurred to me before. Because I'd only been among women.

But he encouraged this world vision and scholarship.
Gordon: Absolutely. I think that was very Jewish. I would not have got it if I were only Irish.

Do you think you have inherited the love of learning from your Irish roots?
Gordon: No. I think that the Irish love of learning was always tainted by the fear of learning. For the Irish, and for Catholics in general, learning, secular learning, is what will push you out of the fold. Therefore, reason is the enemy. Imagine a Jewish *Index*. Imagining the whole idea is incomprehensible. The *Nihil Obstat*, the *Imprimatur* of Catholics—there is always the notion that learning is dangerous.

Whereas for the Jewish person everything is open and one makes a judgment on its merit.

Gordon: But I think we can be romantic about that. Those of us who love Jews can be romantic about Jews. . . .There's a sense for Catholics that learning is a danger. Not only that you have to stay away from anything with sexual content, but anything that talks about freedom of thought is a danger in itself.

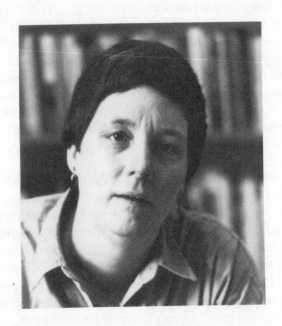

MARY E. HUNT

"I'm. . .absolutely sure that history will read that this was the time, the first time in the history of the church [and] in Christian tradition that women, through [their] experience, saw the fullness of what it means to be a part of a discipleship of equals."

Mary E. Hunt, founder and co-director with Diann Neu of Womens Alliance for Theology, Ethics and Ritual (WATER), is a Visiting Assistant Professor of Religion at Colgate University [New York]. A highly educated feminist and theologian, Dr. Hunt lived and worked in South America, where she mingled with liberation theologians who, she claims, have deeply affected her own development as a Christian.

"I come," she states engagingly, "from a white, middle-class Catholic family in Syracuse which is a real bastion [of progressive Catholicism]. One of the best. It must be in the water in Syracuse: Dan Berrigan, Phil his brother, and quite a load of us come from Syracuse. I am quick to add, it's the only city in the country that has a traffic light with the green on the top, and the red on the bottom, by passage of a special federal law. Otherwise, the Irish would throw rocks to put out the red light. . ."

Accepting and delighting in her heritage, Mary realizes that with it comes a deep sense of Catholicism's values of love, justice, and community welfare. Her sense of humor, she claims, helps her to cope with incredible church goings-on. Her vision of the church acknowledges a long haul, and as this interview shows, constructions of her vision, her image of a new church, pour forth to engage the reader.

In the late 1960s, she entered a Catholic high school and then went on to pursue a college degree. Her entrance into the university educational system coincided with the civil rights and womens' liberation movements which were gripping America. Yet, she states, at that time she had no sense of herself as a woman. In 1972, she went to Harvard Divinity School because Bernard Lonergan, S.J., one of her great heroes, had been there. When she arrived, she realized no one could even spell his name: "He was gone, leaving the most minimal trace. . . .He sort of paled. . .next to some overblown egos still roaming Harvard yard."

On the positive side, she found at Harvard the prolific scholar, Rosemary Radford Ruether, and the Uruguayan liberation theologian, Juan Luis Segundo. Mary Daly's *Beyond God the Father* had also just been published. Together these scholars helped her to overcome her sense of alienation as a Catholic, and she then went on to Berkeley [California] for her doctorate. By 1980, she had completed her education and had come to a realization of herself as woman. She spends no time or energy on what she visualizes as a currently perverted church which has lost its sense of justice and love. Rather, her creativity and lucidity is focused on constructing a theology for the future, a new church, women-church.

Do you take exception to being described as one who says "no" to the church?
Hunt: People in larger number are seeing the limits of the institutional church. This is nothing more and nothing less than

what we as women feel, and what the feminist theologians have been saying for the last ten years. I think it would be a mistake to construe women-church as women saying "no" to the institutional church because it gives the institutional church too much power at a time when its power is on the wane. It is a redundancy to say that women are saying "no" to the institutional church.

VISION OF NEW CHURCH
Explain what your vision of the church is.
Hunt: As a theologian, I have the obligation to call things by their name, and develop some clarity in these things. Theologians do this kind of work. It is not a question of saying "no" to the institutional church; it's a question primarily of trying to live up to our responsibility as baptized Christians to be church. That I do it in the context of women-church. And obviously one has to explain women-church. I start with the understanding of church that Edward Schillebeeckx used in his book *Church with a Human Face*. The Greek words. . .is where I start. *Ecclesia* is the regularly convoked assembly of free male citizens who make decisions; that's what it means to talk about the institutional church. It does not have anything to do with people of God. It has less to do with the women of God.

The only way, then, I'm interested in being church is the way that Schüssler Fiorenza talks about: a discipleship of equals. I want to be part of a community that is what I consider the early church's model of equality, mutuality, and inclusivity, based on the gospels of love and justice. Hence, to enter freely into a pyramid structure, a hierarchical structure as a Christian, much less as a theologian, would be a scandal. So, the only way that I, as a person, can be church is to be a part of this movement we call women-church. Whereas taking [the definition of] church as the regularly convoked assembly of those who gather to vote, namely everybody, is a lie. Using the word "church" only means men. We affix to that the word "women" in order to say that it is only in the context of women-church where in our time as Christians the gospel values are lived out, perhaps for the first time, between men and women as equals. That is what it means to talk about women-church as a movement.

When you talk about women-church, you're not talking about excluding men then.

Hunt: No, I'm talking about the movement of women-church. The women-church movement grew out of the ordination movement. We began, in 1975, to look at the question of ordination in an organized way, with a first meeting in Detroit. In 1978, when we looked at ordination in terms of a renewed priestly ministry, we began to see the development of a movement of Catholic women focused on the question of ordination. Between 1978 and 1982 with the Women-Church conference, there was a proliferation of women's groups around the country, and [a] deepening of the understanding and a broadening of the agendas of those groups. We had groups like National Association of Religious Women (NARW), and National Coalition of America Nuns (NCAN), and the Quixote Center, the Center of Concern, all working on women's issues. Las Hermanas, Black Sisters Conference—all these groups together were part of what was at that point called Women of the Church Coalition. Then Women's Alliance for Theology, Ethics and Ritual (WATER) came along, and a few others. What had begun with ordination as a focus opened up many doors. Ordination wasn't going to happen, so people who were trained for ordination had to look to other places for our work and for our development. The agenda broad-ened. . . .if the institutional church had been smart, they would have ordained us all ten years ago, co-opted and assimilated the whole question.

I always say they should have put the stole over the veils and sent the nuns, two by two, up the aisle to solve the priest shortage. Clerical, celibate, hierarchical nuns to the fore, you see, and they would have become the clerical, celibate, hierarchical priests. And it would have all worked in terms of the system. But, in fact, what happened was that the agenda broadened. . .and so by 1982 you have not so much an interest in ordination on the part of most women, but [an interest in] the questions of ministry, and what it means to be church. That is a significant shift, and out of that in 1983 came the conference in Chicago, *From Generation to Generation: Woman-Church Speaks*. In that conference, what you had was a primary agenda to be church, in other words, to be the discipleship of equals in a regularly convoked assembly. To be church was the primary agenda there. The secondary agenda was institutional and structural change.

You see, the focus has shifted from knocking on the door of the church, even to say "no" to it, to being church. That's a significant move and I think it would be well for this work to reflect that women are no longer saying "no" to the church. It's somewhat anachronistic at this point because people like Elisabeth Schüssler Fiorenza, myself, and others. . .

. . .You're past this issue?

Hunt: We're long past [it] and we're urging other people to bypass [it], and to move right along into the primary responsibility of any baptized Christian, which is to be church. That means to form a small, local community of solidarity and celebration. That's what I mean to be church, to be part of a small, local community of solidarity and celebration, which at the same time is connected to a global, historical, and transcendent movement of those who have been church throughout history and who will be church long after we're gone. It's that dual notion of solidarity and celebration.

There are now hundreds of women's base communities around the country, as well thousands of other small groups of people who are not connected to a parish. There are mixed communities with families and dogs and cats, who are trying to be church in this way. Solidarity with those people in the concrete struggles of economic, political, and social change, it seems to me, is what we're called to be. At the same time, because we are church and not just a political movement or a social club, we are called to celebrate both the sacramental life of the church in terms of being a eucharistic community as well as the varieties of ways that women, particularly now, are developing feminist liturgies in their church. I think that that's what I mean by "church" and that's where I locate myself. That' where I work, that's where I live, and to say that I've said "no" to the institutional church is really at least of much less interest. It doesn't describe what I think.

WOMEN-CHURCH TODAY

Where is the movement now?

Hunt: It's important to take the movement where it's at, and even let the way in which you look at it be shaped by what the new reality is. That's feminism, and what we meant by feminism in 1970 was a very different animal from what we mean by feminism [now]. For example, in 1970, few white middle-class women were putting parameters around their [interpretation] of feminism in terms of how conditioned their understanding was by their being white and middle class. Now we know. We talk about white, middle-class experience of what we call feminism, and what happens for women of color, for poor women, for women outside of the U.S.? These are all quite different things and we don't have any more monopoly on the definition of feminism than anyone else does. To make a feminist contribution [today], one begins with an understanding that racism, classism, heterosexism, and ageism are all part of what we mean by feminism. We had no sense of all this when we said "feminism" in 1970. When we talk about church moving ahead, those of us who are trying to push this thing mean certain things that we didn't mean in 1978. We have a different understanding of what church is and secondly we have a strategy, conscious or unconscious. It is a strategy to try to transform what we mean by church.

[As] I was saying earlier. . .it's important not to buy into the old definition of church in order to enhance it in any way, even by refuting it. But at the same time, one can't be naive about the fact that the word "church" and the reality of the institutional church are really quite powerful. So at the same time I'm trying to develop a new understanding of church and be church as the primary goal of what I do. The secondary goal, and it must be both secondary and a goal, is to transform the institutional church. Because what happened, what is happening to Barbara [Ferraro] and Pat [Hussey] and what has happened to Charlie Curran and what has happened to Agnes Mary Mansour, and the list goes on, are real things that have happened at the hands of the patriarchal, hierarchical, institutional church. And those are things that must be stopped. And so it becomes a part of the strategy.

CHURCH TRANSFORMATION
Could you talk about a strategy for your two goals.
Hunt: I talk about a four-part process in terms of doing the the-

ology and the transformation of structures from a theological perspective. It has four elements: experience, analysis, celebration, and strategy. These are the four elements of doing the kind of theological change that I work on, and my experience is obviously a kind of praxis based [on] liberation theology. One is involved in the doing of it; one isn't just talking about it.

The notion of praxis is the Marxist understanding which is really helpful in terms of looking at the way in which we do things. It asks how the work we do informs even the theory that we choose, and how the theory informs the work that we do. There are a lot of people for whom praxis is kind of a dirty word. It has a certain red tint around the edges, but in fact what it means is that we do a certain kind of work for social change. We do it out of a faith commitment, for example, and the work itself strengthens the faith commitment. On the basis of that work we have a new way [of] looking at Scripture, our own tradition, and re-understanding the history and community out of which we come. It is a particular set of perspectives that are informed by the work we do.

For example, if I'm going to work on reproductive rights, I do so as a Catholic. I do it not simply out of a notion that the Catholic church is opposed to abortion, and opposed to certain forms of birth control, but I do it in spite of that, and with the firm assurance that the church is committed and has been historically committed to justice.

Further, love and the integration of love and justice, particularly in its most embodied form through sexuality, are values that come from that tradtion. But because, for certain historical and ethical accidents, there happen to be misunderstandings and perversions of some of [these] values at the moment, does not in any way lessen the fact that I do [this] work as a Catholic.

But going back to the other question: I think once you have the experience, there has to be some kind of analysis which is the reflective, theoretical component. There also has to be some kind of celebration within our community. It's not simply solidarity, as I said before, but it's also celebration. There's some way in which our work, our commitment, the lives of the people, are brought to public expression in what we traditionally call the sacramental life of the church. That's what I call celebration. Out of the grace of the sacraments, and you'll see a very traditional understanding of grace, out of [an] understanding of shared experience, of tough critical analysis, of celebration in the sacramental sense, can emerge, and must emerge, certain strategies for doing that work better. Certain ways emerge both from the norms of the tradition and from the necessity of the work itself that take us to something new. Think of a circle that takes us around to yet another new, deepened, fortified kind of practice. Hence strategy, and strategizing, "seeing a vision" is what Jóse Míguez Bonino talks about as a historical project of liberation.

The strategies, in fact, emerge out of an historical project. A historical project is a vision, but at the same time a plan. The historical project of liberation is not just a vision of what liberation might look like, but it also includes some ways of getting there. The historical project of liberation that I see is the bringing about of the reign of love and justice. Bringing about what has been called the Kingdom of God or the Queendom of God. I talk about it as the reign of love and justice, making love and justice normative. That becomes for me the vision. The practice for doing, or the strategy, or the plan which is part of this historical project of liberation, is changing the social, political, economic, and ecclesiastical conditions. What's important is that it gives you a glimpse of the vision.

But I am also realistic enough not to think that we're going to bring the vision into existence [right away]. Yet, it gives one a concrete way to say that what I call a precondition for the possibility of the reign of love and justice can be brought about in my lifetime, and the preconditions are overcoming racism, sexism, heterosexism, and the structures of economic domination. These are preconditions for the possibility of love and justice. I'm not convinced—and here I do not part company with liberation theologians but I clarify what has been misunderstood in terms of the word. . .I believe that bringing about these kinds of changes are preconditions for the possibility of the reign of love and justice but do not in and of themselves bring about the reign of love and justice.

Why not?

Hunt: [One] critique of liberation theology is that people think that bringing about a socialist social order is somehow commensurate with the reign of God. I say, no, that's a mistake. Liberation theologians are not saying this, but [this] is the conservative critique against liberation theology. If, for example, I were talking as a [particular kind of] feminist theologian, if I were talking about the reign of God or the reign of love and justice as I'm talking about it now, then. . .I [could say that] overcoming sexism. . .would then be the reign of God or the reign of Goddess. And I'm saying no; it would not be. I'm not claiming that. What I am claiming is that without that happening, there's no [possible way] to talk about the reign of love and justice. Consequently, the overcoming of concrete social problems is a precondition for the *possibility* of the reign of God.

Will you briefly review these four steps?
Hunt: Let's review briefly. First, the experience or the praxis is the working on an issue of justice. Second, the analysis is the critical reflection. Third, celebration is a way of bringing this to public expression so as to fortify and enliven the community. Fourth, out of this experience we come to some strategy. Now what's important is to challenge how the celebration component is prevented or prohibited.

HANDLING HIERARCHICAL EXCLUSION
Could you talk for a moment about how celebration is circumvented?
Hunt: Let me give a concrete example. When women are prohibited from being ordained, and this is the most profound problem with ordination, the four-part cycle of change is stopped. Most people express it simply in theo-political terms, as a question of women's rights or whatever. I am suggesting that it's even more profound than that. The extent to which women are prohibited from celebrating, you see, means that you can short-circuit the whole process. Women can have the experience of ministry and be involved in transformative, social, theological, and pastoral ministry. We can do a kind of analysis that will lead us to the strategies. But we're short-circuited [from] the possibility of being agents and subjects of celebration. We're really domesticated at that level. And so it becomes very important to say that because we are short-circuited at the celebration point, legally and canonically, we can't get to the strategies. Even within the church's own understanding of how the

sacramental life of the church fortifies and strengthens and gives certain meaning and dimension to things, we can't become celebrants because that dimension is cut off. A whole process is short-circuited so that women's energies can't be put into full service of the church.

What do you suggest women do about it?

Hunt: Well, I think there are two options. One option, of course, is the one that we have pursued to a certain extent, which is to work on women's ordination within the institutional church. I have been a part of that. I have written some of the background work and I think there have been some very fine efforts and steps made in that direction. A second option is to develop new ways of being church. For a variety of historical reasons, [especially] that the Vatican is not moving in the direction of ordained women in the foreseeable future, we have realized that the institutional church's model of ministry is inadequate to the needs of most of the church.

We have chosen, as women, to take a different tack. It is to develop new forms of church, namely, women's base communities. There are hundreds of those around the country. I participate in one called SAS (Sister Against Sexism), which is a very well-known one in the Washington area. [It has] a mailing list of probably sixty-five people and [on] a typical Sunday evening maybe twenty meet on a rotating basis at different people's homes [for a] potluck dinner and worship. The person in charge of the liturgy or worship is the one in whose home we meet. Forms of liturgy are quite varied, depending on the season of the year, the mood, the occasion, the group. There can be anything from a quiet prayer service to Scripture sharing. Often there is something like a blessing or sharing of particular experiences, using symbols and music or poetry from women's experience.

Where does the bread and wine fit in these celebrations, or does it?

Hunt: Sure. The bread and wine are traditional elements of the Christian eucharist, particularly in the Catholic tradition. The bread and wine are something that go without saying. In these experiences, there are times, not always, but there are times when we choose to have a eucharistic celebration. We now name it as eucharist. We don't call it Agape or Love Feast or Birthday Party. We call it eucharist because that's what it is. It is eucharist, celebrated by the group gathered. We sometimes use the words of the institutional church, sometimes not. Sometimes we have a Scripture reading; sometimes we have an even more informal sharing.

I emphasize that it is the fullness of eucharist as we understand it in the sacramental terms of the church. We do not always feel ourselves obliged to use the eucharistic form in order to worship. So let's say those two things at the same time: it is the fullness of [the] eucharist in the sense that it is the church, the discipleship of equals gathered to share and to remember and to look ahead in a fortified way, and we don't need to do that every time we get together. And so we feel very free. I think we've come to this over time. The SAS group has been together since the late 1970s.

Is this a group of men and women?
Hunt: No, all women. And it is intentionally all women until such time as the group decides that it's time to invite men. We've had that discussion on a range of occasions. We meet twice a year to set up our program for the next six months, and I'd say almost every year that question comes up, and is discussed and debated. Every time it has been decided, up to the present, that the group will be all women for reasons of preference of the group. But what's important is that the model of church I operate from is both a local experience, mainly SAS, and a global sense of church, which means that SAS has no meaning outside of a network or a way of being connected with a variety of other base communities which have met. So it is not a separatist movement or a separatist group; it's simply a group.

Or an exclusive group. . .
Hunt: . . .No, no, no. Some may argue that it is, functionally, and it is at some level simply because, given our experiences, we have chosen at this time to maintain this group as it is, namely, all women. But it is neither my vision nor my preferred future to have either a group or a church that's exclusively women.

You will recall that in the late 1960s and early 1970s blacks sought liberation in this country. In places like

Brown University these black students kept totally to themselves. There seems to be less of that type of separatism now.

Hunt: Yes. I think that what you're pointing out is the importance of understanding the difference between separatism and discrimination. Discrimination is where we're talking about what I call theo-politics or the power dynamics involved. We're really talking about power when we're talking about church. Discrimination means we are told we cannot join. Separation means a previously excluded group decides to meet alone for support and nurture. We're talking about a situation in which unequal power relationships [dominate], which is the pyramid model which essentially has a very small little peak at the top. . .

You're referring to the pope?

Hunt: Meaning the hierarchical, institutional, patriarchal church as it's set up with the pope on top, a few cardinals, a few more bishops, a few more priests, and then a vast majority of the rest of us below the line. I draw you a picture that would look like this:

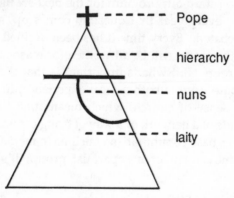

Above the line is the clerical part of the church; below it is the massive lay part of the church. The lay people will never get [above the line]. You see, this is an absolute separation. Even the nuns are only the half circle beneath the solid line. They're never going to be clerics, which means they're never—even Mary Linscott who's been a part of this Congregation for Religious and Secular Institutes (CRIS) business with Barbara and Pat—going to be real decision makers. The first situation is that [a woman is] never going to get up above the solid line, barring a sex change operation. It is just a structural reality.

DISCRIMINATION, SEPARATION, AND CHURCH WOMEN

Now, your clerical model is very similar to the medical model. One side of the medical pyramid represents hospitals and agencies of the conglomerate; another side is the medical profession. Both sides rest on the backs of the nurses who form the base of the pyramid. Yet these nurses carry the health system and yet make only four cents out of the health dollar. It's the same power structure.

Hunt: [That's] exactly what I'm talking about in terms of power. In this kind of a model, we are talking about discrimination and separatism. In this kind of a model, discrimination is at play when those on the top tell those on the bottom what they can't do. Separatism is when those on the bottom say to those on the top, this is what we ourselves will do. Discrimination [means] to be put aside as women, to be told, "No, you can't be priests." Separatism is to say, out of the position of an oppressed group struggling to find its own identity and its own liberation. . .for the time being at least, we don't want to be a part of such a structure.

Do you see a need for the church to be purified before women can return to it?

Hunt: I don't think it's a question of going back any place. I think it's a question of seeing several things converging. The issue is how do we move toward it. I think it's going on right now, where we see enormous numbers of people in this country who do not have anything to do with the institutional church. Attendance at mass is down, reception of the sacraments is down, all of the traditional ways of talking about church participation indicate that there is an enormous fall-off. That's one thing. The second thing is there is a money crunch, both for the Vatican and for individual dioceses. A money crunch means that people have seen the situation, they're not going to worry about it, and they're not going to put the money into it. And a third factor is that simultaneously there are—and I happen to think that if there's any proof of the existence of the Holy Spirit it's the proliferation of these small groups—these communities that we call women-church.

So you have these things going on at the same time and I think it's only a question of time and energy and some well-drafted strategies before we can say that what's going on here is a new ecclesiology, a new way of being a church. And what we're seeing, I think, in some of these things like the [Charles] Curran case and [Agnes Mary] Mansour case is really the last wag of the dog's tail. It seems a very decided, deliberate move to the right, digging in of the ecclesiastical heels, attempting to rein things in when, in fact, the genie's long since been out of the bottle.

The problem I see is, frankly, that many of us who are involved in things that are new, that are ironically quite traditional (forming small communities and worshipping is all quite traditional), run the very real risk of being assimilated by the institutional church. And I say that I worry much more about being assimilated than being declared a heretic. The genius, what I would call the sinister genius of the institutional Roman Catholic church, has been its ability to capture those things which are new, those things which are taking it in a new direction, and to claim those things for itself.

Which is why Rosemary Radford Ruether feels women's stories have to be told over in every century; their theology must be repeated century after century.

Hunt: That's right. And women have to tell those stories on their own terms. And that's the problem. It's like the ordination question. Although it was a smart strategy to start talking about ordination, it would at this point be an experience of assimilation if women were to be ordained. Now the institutional church can only ordain women to shore up its own clerical model.

You feel that this would be a mistake?

Hunt: I think it's a crucial mistake. I think women who take either diaconate ordination which might be offered sooner or later, or women who will take presbyteral ordination when it's offered, will make a grievous error. We've seen that in other churches, particularly the Swedish Lutheran church, and most of the mainline Protestant denominations. What we've seen is the ordination of women has not meant any structural change at all, in fact, on the contrary. It has shored up the clerical model in those churches. If I were giving advice to the bishops. . .if the bishops would ask me the way to solve the problem of priesthood, or a way to develop more adequate pastoral models, I would say ordain women in a minute. They could capture and assimilate all those good energies, that terrific preparation, and the wonderful clarity of women. They could take it, box it, and it would keep that pyramid in place for another two thousand years. Whereas if women can only resist the temptation, even the most well-intentioned women who are engaged in, say, in a prison ministry, or campus ministry, or a place where they see the need for ministry—if these women can resist the temptation for ordination, they could do what Rosemary Ruether and I concluded at a recent Women's Ordination Conference (WOC) consultation. We suggested that women forego ordination for the sake of *ministry*. And that doesn't mean any lessening of our pressure in terms of institutional change, but it means resisting the potential to be assimilated very, very quickly.

BECOMING A FEMINIST THEOLOGIAN
How about women who want to be ordained and be part of the structure?
Hunt: I think they need education to see the bigger picture. And although I have a number of colleagues in the movement whose work I respect deeply, I happen to think they are making a terrible mistake at this point to accept ordination. On the other hand, I have sufficient savvy. I am resigned to admit that probably both things are necessary for some time yet, because none of us are in the danger of being ordained. But when the time comes that we are in the least danger of being ordained, I think we [will] really need to talk long and hard about it. And I'm afraid at that point our strategies will be quite diverse, and so I pessimistically predict that the institutional church will finally come up with a co-optation once again.

I'm sorry to have to say that. I think that's the case, but I'm working quite hard now to prevent it. I'm not optimistic, just because I know that these hierarchs are masters of the art of assimilation and co-optation. . . .And to think that we as women are going to be able to resist is something that I want to think and something that I will work for, but I wish I could say I was confident. I had had an initial sort of rejection of feminist issues in theology because I thought they were somewhat trivial and a sidestepping of the major issues.

Issues such as heaven and hell?

Hunt: Yes . . .angels dancing on the heads of pins were then thought crucial, central themes. But I realized why I had rejected women's issues. They hit too close to home; they were too important. At the same time I had been deeply influenced by [Juan Luis] Segundo [a liberation theologian from Uruguay], and I had realized that both he and Ruether were treated equally shabbily at Harvard Divinity School. Neither one of them were perceived as doing the real thing. Neither one of them were doing theology with a capital "T." Ruether as a woman and Segundo as a Latin American man, were equally marginalized by the great capital "T" theology. The awareness that came to me was, in fact, that theology was a rather domesticated discipline. There were those owners of the discipline who gave it its name and its shape and its color, and who claimed what was and what wasn't theological. And so for them the challenge of [accepting] women's experience on its own terms, or [accepting] the experience of Latin Americans. . .on their own terms was simply more than they could take.

In the same way that originally you couldn't take women's issues?

Hunt: Right. And I knew why. Because it was too close to home, and it was pushing me in ways that would force me to change as a human being. What was going on theologically [meant that] the discipline would have to change as a discipline. It could no longer be talking about God in one voice, but in fact it would have to be what I call the theological chorus of lots of people trying to find their note, and to stand and to communicate. In fact, one "sacrifices" from the point of view of the pure real thing, but one gains by having a diverse kind of chorus in motion. I think this is an essential power question in that it is the one we struggle with even today in theology. The questions become: What is it to do theology; who is able to do it?

My perspective as a graduate student was to begin to investigate what were the differences and the similarities between what Latin Americans were doing and what North American women were doing. I wrote a doctoral dissertation at Berkeley [California] entitled *Feminist Liberation Theology: The Development of Method in Construction* in which I compared Latin American liberation theology from the point of view of its methodology with white North American feminist theology. I discovered they had many points of comparison. . . .In fact, what both of them were doing was actually challenging the discipline to open up and to begin to talk about theologizing. They engaged a number of people in what I call organic, communal sharing of insights and stories and reflections—questions of meaning and of value. It is a definition for theologizing which I think is adequate and meaningful in our time.

At the same time I was intrigued and seduced by the questions of ministry and ordination, not simply as an academician, but also as a practitioner. I did a Master of Divinity at the Jesuit School [of Theology, at Berkeley]. It enabled me to do clinical pastoral education in a women's prison, and to develop myself as a pastoral person. Eventually, I finished my education in 1980.

That was seven years ago. What did you do next?

Hunt: I then had an opportunity to join Frontier Internship in Mission which is a program loosely affiliated, kind of a cousin of the World Council of Churches. It sends so-called creative young people to ideological frontiers where progressive Christian churches want to be. My ideological frontier was Women in Theology in Argentina. I always say they could have put me in a cage in Buenos Aires and charged admission to see a Roman Catholic woman prepared for priesthood, who was also a theologian talking about liberation theology and feminist issues. For two years I learned Spanish, and taught theology at ISED-IT, which is the ecumenical seminary in Buenos Aires.

Simultaneously, I worked with Adolfo Perez Esquivel's Peace and Justice Service. It is a movement for non-violent social change whose director, Adolfo Perez Esquivel, won the Nobel Peace Prize in 1980. I learned about non-violent social change, particularly about the situation of human rights and disappearances in Argentina. *Servicio* at that time was connected closely with the mothers of the disappeared, so I really received an eye-opening in Latin America. I also worked with a group called the *Centro di Estudios Cristianos*, another ecumenical agency in Buenos Aires having a project about women. I helped them to set up women's groups, with church women initially from Argentina, in Buenos Aires and Cordova and Mendoza and in Montevideo, Uruguay. We set up these groups so that women could begin to reflect. There was no such thing as feminist theology in Argentina at that point.

I finished my assignment and came back to the States in 1982. On the way I spent some time in Europe doing therapeutic work, helping European audiences, particularly in Scandinavia, to understand the connections between feminist and liberation theology. I have been invited back to Argentina for a month every year for the next three years to continue working with the women's groups.

At that point when I was looking for a job, I discovered what I really wanted to do. It was to do what I had been doing: organizing and developing strategies, and working on women's issues. With Diann Neu, who works with me in WATER [Womens Alliance for Theology, Ethics and Ritual] now, I started thinking about setting up something for women in theology here in Washington, [D.C.]. It came from the fact that I didn't find an appropriate job, and because of the need here in Washington. I came up with the idea of a woman's alliance for theology.

THE CREATION OF WATER
This was your idea of WATER?

Hunt: Well at that time it was WAT. It occurred to me, it was sort of in a dream, not a real dream, but kind of waking up one morning. . .I said, "Wouldn't it be funny to add ethics and ritual, the 'ER,' and call it WATER." It was sort of a joke. . .yet it stuck. We got a group of about twelve women, including Elisabeth Schüssler Fiorenza and Mary Collins: a good group. I wanted to set up a collective because I knew that there was nothing in Washington schools or seminaries for feminists in theology. Diann Neu was finishing at the Center of Concern. Diann has a Master of Divinity also from the Jesuit School of Theology in Berkeley, with specialization in literature and ritual. Wouldn't it be great, people said, if Diann did the ritual component, and I did the theology and ethics. In fact, it worked out in a very happy way. . .both of us had done all three. So, we started WATER in 1983; now in our fourth year, it's really been a very exciting and diverse kind of experience. Starting from nothing; we found an office and have since expanded.

What exactly do you and Diann do?

Hunt: WATER is actually what the letters convey. We pull together women and men who are interested in theology, ethics, and ritual from a feminist liberation perspective. We bring them together for programs, for example a weekend. One with Elisabeth [Schüssler Fiorenza], for example, deals with ministerial models in women-church. We have had other weekends with Elisabeth and Rosemary Ruether. We've had workshops with Beverley Harrison and others. We do programs which no one else in the Washington area does. We have two publications: one on feminist liturgies for the Lenten season; and one *Seder for the Sisters of Sarah*, both of which have been enormously popular. We have projects like *Women Crossing Worlds*. My work in Argentina became a part of WATER. . . .[I wanted] to develop the relationships with groups of women, here and in the Southern zone. I've just come back from a month in Buenos Aires [Argentina], Santiago, Chile, and Bogota, Columbia. We had, for example, in Buenos Aires the first *Women Crossing Worlds* international gathering with women from seven countries coming together for a week-long workshop. We worked on the development of feminist spirituality in the southern column. So, at WATER, we do a lot of consulting, we do a lot of writing. . .I'm finishing a book on friendship. It is called *Fierce Tenderness: Toward a Feminist Theology of Friendship*.

One senses your fulfillment. . .

Hunt: I love my work. The only problem. . .a major problem. . .is economic. It is enormously difficult to fund something like this and yet the need is enormous. Just this afternoon we have a brochure being sent which lists events coming up. One is a liturgy class which will meet four Wednesday nights, taught by Diann Neu from our staff, Barbara Cullam, Ph.D. from Notre Dame in New Testament, and Ronnie Levin, a Jewish woman, a doctoral candidate at Brandeis. It will focus on Jewish and Christian women developing new liturgies and rituals.

We will have an evening celebrating *Succoh*, the Jewish festival where we will construct a tabernacle outside, and women will come, bringing with them stories of their foremothers, the ancestors. It's a Jewish ceremony, which is done at the time of the Feast of *Succoh* when people go and sit in their tent for an evening, pass stories and reflections on their grandmothers, and their great grandmothers, and so forth. We will begin the season with a weekend retreat for women—a Friday to a Sunday experience—at a retreat house where we will have some quiet reflective times, celebration, and a time for women within a feminist context to be together and to reflect.

Are there things that surprise you in your work?

Hunt: Well, I think that one never knows what the next day will bring. Yesterday we were tearing our hair around here, because a particular piece of work that was supposed to be done while we were both away didn't get done. And yet, while we were tearing our collective hair, we found hidden in one of the envelopes a wonderful note and a large check from someone who had been here. She was an elderly woman who had found something very special here and wrote a very, very moving note about what was going on at WATER. She saw it as the future and it was quite surprising.

You seem to be moved to tears by this. . .

Hunt: Oh, deeply. Even when thinking about it, it was wonderful. Those things happen all the time here, and they give me a sense in my work, that something very important is happening. Other women who have children instruct their friends at the children's baptism, rather than sending gifts, to make donations to WATER. This is very hopeful in terms of what the new church is going to look like, that people can see the power and can see something very important for the church. It takes us right back to the earlier conversation that if you see this and say "no" to something, it almost cheapens it beyond the richness that's there. It's trivial to say that people are saying "no" to the church. It's much more profound to say—and I believe that the historical reading of this time will be that our great grandchildren will look back and say [this]—what happened in the history of Christianity in the late twentieth century happened with women. I don't think it will be the Second Vatican Council.

Why do you think feminism will take precedence over Vatican II?

Hunt: I'm convinced, I mean I'm absolutely sure, that history will read that this was the time, the first time in the history of the church, in the history of the Christian tradition, that women, through women's experience, saw the fullness of what it means to be part of the tradition of a discipleship of equals—that possibility of being brought to life. I think that is what history will say about this time. And it's only because women, not because we're great, or wonderful, or unusual, but because, following and plodding along in the footsteps of our great-grandmothers, we tried to do something that is possible due to the historical convergence of this time. It's possible in *this* time, and therefore there's nothing else to do but to do it.

HISTORIC MOMENT

So you feel we're at an important historic moment?

Hunt: There's no question. There's absolutely no question and I think that we can see a glimpse of it now. What the great-grandchildren will see is that at this time in history the point is not the destruction of the church, or saying "no" to the church, or leaving the church, or any of those things. But it will be a new way of *being church*. And that I think is quite different. It's being church and that's a substantially different thing than saying I go to church, or there's a church on the corner, or I've left the church, or I don't want any part of the church. To be church is a much more substantial experience, and that is what women have never been able to be before because of the structure.

And you feel the convergence of other things. . .?

Hunt: Yes, the convergence of feminists, of feminist movements, technology and communication, and particularly the education of women have made it possible. However reluctant the participation of women in the structures themselves, women have made it possible for some of us to look at these things and say these are unjust. Now the fact that. . .certain women. . .participated in them is not to me any great step forward, although historically it will be seen as something that certainly made a difference. That women could participate in oppression, I don't happen to see as progress. I happen to see that as novelty, but not progress. It's like saying that having Margaret Thatcher in leadership in Great Britain is novel. True, but I don't consider it particularly progressive, given her position, her politics. But it is novel. No one will dispute that it's novel to have a woman, just as to have a woman Prime Minister or in the White House would be novel. It would not necessarily be a step forward in terms of human history.

It's no different to have a Latin American go to the Gregorian University [Rome] and study to become a priest. There is nothing great in that. That is just taking the same old content and putting it into a different genetic mix. The sending of women to the Gregorian is no step forward, because, again, all you do is put the same content into a different genetic mix. But when people. . .and women begin to do theology out of our experience as women on our terms, on the basis of our experience, then you have something new.

And that is happening?

Hunt: That is happening. And that's being repressed and I think you need to really emphasize the fact. I talk about this as having three and a half stages. The development of theology and the same progressions we have seen in liberation theology are being repressed. There's a *period of preparation*, which in the case of women in theology would have been from the turn of the century through the early 1960s. That was the period of preparation when women started to go to theological school, when some of the nuns' communities began to open hospitals and schools and one thing or another. It's a period of preparation for women's participation.

The second period would be the *critical period*, which began in the late 1960s with the publication of the early works of Mary Daly and some of Rosemary Ruether's books. During that critical period, which went through the early 1980s, everything was thrown up in the air: church history, systematic theology, language, symbols, rituals. Everything was. . .criticized. Some people fell out at that point. Some people fell out along the lines of an evangelical feminist perspective to look at the issues. Some people fell out on the Goddess side, deciding that Christianity was basically and inherently corrupt and bankrupt, and there was no reason to deal with it any longer. I have a great deal of respect for both of those [positions]. I'm not in either of them but I respect them. Others fell out in the middle. These others do this theo-political work, like myself, Ruether and others with a liberation feminist perspective. The critical period really came to an end in the early 1980s, particularly with the publication of Ruether's *Sexism and Godtalk*; and Schüssler Fiorenza's *In Memory of Her*.

You can begin to see then—some of the work that others of us are doing on reproductive rights, and particularly on lesbian/gay issues—you begin to see what I would call a *constructive phase* where we're no longer spending time on a corrupt church; the same thing happened on your question of women's ordination. We went through the critical period from, say, [the] mid-1970s to the early 1980s, when we talked first about women's ordination to the priesthood. Then, we progressed to women's ordination to a renewed priesthood, still criticizing, still critical in terms of the values of faith. Now, we're into a constructive phase, where we're talking about development of women's ministry in women-church.

The constructive phase in theology, which began in the early 1980s, has been met by an equal and opposite backlash or repression. We're experiencing that now toward the laity, both in the theological world where you see women being hired who are not feminists, and in the ecclesiastical world, where you see things like what's happened to Barbara [Ferraro] and Pat [Hussey], the reaction to *The New York Times* ad, even the silencing of [Brazilian theologian Leonardo] Boff who tends to be rather progressive on women's ordination. There are varieties of problems: Agnes Mary Mansour, Arlene Violet, the problems with the Mercy nuns and tubal ligations. The whole thing is backlash, not just against the *critical phase*, but backlash against *constructive work*. And that's where we are now. And that's how I measure how much our constructive work has been effective because the backlash is getting right up there.

So in a sense you feel this backlash is a good sign?
Hunt: Well, I don't want to call it a good sign. It's like saying it's a good sign that her husband needs her because now she'll leave him. It's not a good sign but it's a sign of movement.

And it's a sign that women are being heard?
Hunt: Oh, we're being heard! It's also important to say that women's issues and women's concerns are not only primary for

the Vatican, but they use them as their litmus test. We know now the bishop candidates in the U.S. are literally tested on the questions of women's ordination and abortion, and where they come down on those questions are a litmus test. On their answers depend whether or not they'll be bishops.

CATHOLIC LESBIAN ISSUES
Could you discuss lesbian and gay rights in terms of your vision for a new church?

Hunt: Sure. I've done a lot of work, as you know, on the issue of lesbian and gay rights, and lesbian and gay participation in the church. I'm on the Board of Directors of New Ways Ministry. And I'm also on the Consultation on Homosexuality, Social Justice, and Roman Catholic Theology. I have been very active in the Conference of Catholic Lesbians. As a Catholic lesbian—and I feel very strongly about the need to include the questions of sexual preference as part of a liberation agenda—I see this as fitting into the larger picture that I've been trying to describe in this interview.

Quite obviously, we're talking about the reality of a certian percentage of our population who are homosexual persons. We are proud of ourselves and our way of being in the world as responsible, loving persons. We see this as something that the church must recognize in the same way that the church has to rethink birth control, abortion, divorce and remarriage, masturbation, and anything else that has to do with the real lives of most people.

The church in its theology has erred in a grievous way on its treatment of homosexual persons. As a theologian, as a feminist, and as a lesbian, I think it is incredibly important for me to use whatever platform I have, to use whatever skills I have, to work on this issue as on any other. I've written some fairly tough things that make clear the basis of women's experience, particularly lesbian feminist experience, [and] that the institutional church doesn't know what it's talking about. It will not know what it's talking about until those of us, for whom this is a primary experience, express ourselves and make it known. I wrote an article recently that appeared in *Concilium*. There was an enormous debate over it in Italy. I just received a letter of apology from *Concilium*. They did not publish the article in the Italian version, and the Board of Directors has written a formal letter of apology, begging my pardon for their error. They assured me that in the future lesbian issues will be treated with the utmost respect.

What happened was that we saw, once again, the long arm of Rome. It may have happened in the form of self-censorship on the part of the Italian publishing company with whom I had already published a book.

[In the article] I argued that a change in the model of moral theology has to be made, so that those who are most deeply affected are those who name the tune, really. I used lesbian experience as one that men cannot claim. [I think] it was just terrifying to them. Their terror is symptomatic of the extent to which lesbian experience unnerves them. I'm very careful not to fall into the trap that lesbians are—as the patriarchal understanding has it—women who hate men. That's not the question at all. Lesbians are women who love women. I talk about the potential for every woman to be a lesbian. I did a presentation—using [a] Sweet Honey song: "Every woman who's ever loved a woman stand up and shout out her name." This marvelous song by Sweet Honey continues: mother, sister, daughter, lover. Well, every woman I have ever known has loved her mother, or her sister, or her daughter, or her lover, maybe even herself.

This is, of course, what patriarchy can't tolerate—that we as women would love ourselves. The lesbian experience, in terms of a love experience between women, is something that is so antithetical to the perpetuation of patriarchy that it becomes one of those things about which people become totally irrational. [I feel] it is quite different from gay male experience, because it's women loving women with an emphasis on the question of loving and not so much an emphasis on genital/sexual experience, as tends to be the case with gay men. Therefore, you have an even more profound challenge. Where I am at this point, particularly what I'm writing about, is that this is such a new phenomenon that to talk about it in plain English and to learn from women is novel. It is. . .revelation to talk about women's friendships. They have never seen the light of day before on their own terms.

The ways in which we conduct ourselves sexually and otherwise, the ways in which we carry on committed love relationships, are simply unknown to humankind because of the way in which patriarchy has erased those experiences, blotted them out, acted as if they didn't exist, given them other names, tried to ruin them. This is simply a new moment. It has come to my generation to work on this issue. It certainly emerges out of the necessity of my own life, loving women, and living in a committed relationship with a woman. These are happy things, these are things to be celebrated. I do a lot of work on this issue. I know that it's terribly risky and I'm not in a tenure-track academic position, not because I'm theologically disabled, but because of my theo-politics. That's as clear as the nose on your face.

In other words, because of your theo-politics, Catholic universities won't invite you to teach.

Hunt: I don't think I have much of a chance of being hired in a Catholic school at this point. I'm teaching at Colgate University, as Visiting Assistant Professor of Religion. But it'll be interesting to see whether or not I want to keep a foot in academia for a while. I have some ambivalence about it. WATER is so exciting, yet it's hard to make a living at this sort of thing. A Catholic school is where I most belong, given the training I have and the kind of interests in the work I do. I think it will be quite unusual, and a long time from now, when an acknowledged lesbian who is pro-choice will be hired. That, we just acknowledge. It also means that I've made some choices along the way in terms of being "out," and in terms of taking the responsibility for that kind of information.

And in terms of defining yourself?

Hunt: Oh, yes. I would prefer to [do menial work]. . .than prostitute myself theologically, or ethically, on any of these issues. I have a very small tolerance for ambiguity in this sort of thing; I have a very small tolerance for people whose ambiguity is much greater than mine. For example, I'm not edified by colleagues who refuse to sign declarations or documents for fear of losing their tenure or their job or what-have-you, particularly people in the field of ethics. I had the experience during *The New York Times* ad of calling up a colleague who was tenured in an academic Catholic faculty, and being told that she couldn't sign the Declaration of Solidarity [see Appendix B] because she felt that she would lose her tenured job. It could be taken as doctrinal irregularity if she were to sign. I understand her position and I know she has to pick her own battles. But I'm quite dissatisfied by the fact that she would call herself a theologian, or an ethicist. . .and still proceed with such behavior. I consider it totally bankrupt. There was one gentleman who signed the Declaration, and then took his name off. He told me in plain English that he totally agreed with it, but that he just didn't have it together at that particular point in his life to fight it out. You know, that's his option, his choice. I'm totally dissatisfied by it and I lose complete respect for people of that sort.

But the world, the church, is full of people like them.

Hunt: Sure. But it doesn't mean I have to approve of them. The contrast is not so much condemnation of such people, but simply saying that I hold myself to a higher, more rigid standard of behavior. If those of us who teach these matters, or who pretend to be involved in the theological reflection of the church, can't maintain a more disciplined approach to our own ethical lives, then I don't know. It's a two-edged sword. I'm not falling over myself to teach in Our Lady of the Snowdrop. I think the issue is that persons who represent the kinds of positions I do are prohibited. I would like the choice.

THE HIERARCHY AND FEAR OF WOMEN

One last thing. Do you think the male hierarchy is afraid of women?

Hunt: Well, I think that many of us are afraid of things that we don't know much about, and afraid of things that we have been told stories and myths and untruths about. The hierarchical structure of the church is really a homosocial environment where men have really been with men, to the exclusion of women. They live in abysmal ignorance, with a real lack of care and concern to close the gap.

But they were in touch with women—a mother, for example—somewhere along the line?

Hunt: Sure, but being in touch with your mother is quite different. Having a mother or being a son is quite different from having a woman friend or being a *companero*. This is a quite different experience. You can always look up to your mother, or you can look down on your mother when she's a little old lady. But it's very difficult to have to look straight at somebody who is your colleague, who is your friend, who is your collaborator, who is a sister in ministry, and think of her as an equal, when in fact you've been brought up to understand that there are great women like your mother and the Virgin Mary, and then there are the rest of women who are either like Eve or Theresa Kane. These [women] are evil.

Or Mary Hunt?

Hunt: Or Mary Hunt. It's true, it's certain that they had mothers and that they had some relationship with a warm female body, but that's a very different experience than having a full human body who is a woman, a friend. That's new in our time. That's what I think is so important to emphasize, that it is new for the church to have the experience of full human beings who happen to be women on their own terms.

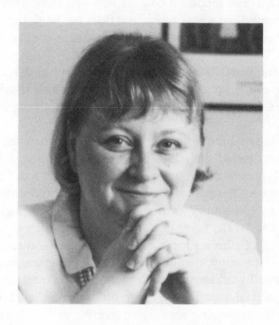

FRANCES KISSLING

"People like me, who [have] returned to the church with hope, [have] also brought a whole set of experiences, new ways of relating to structures which are much more democratic. In my case these experiences come from politics, radical politics. When I say I came back to the church, I never came back on the old terms. . . .I came back to the church as a social change agent; I came back to woman-church."

Frances Kissling is founder and President of Catholics for a Free Choice (CFFC), a pro-choice Catholic organization. Seemingly serene and composed in the political swirl around her, she is emphatic that she, like other women who are culturally conditioned to care for others, must also learn to take care of herself. She also argues that women must face their fear of being called self-absorbed unless they are involved in traditional "nurturing" activities; she feels that women must do work that

147

is fulfilling. She models a balance between self-caring behavior and committed social action and does her work because she likes it, because it rewards her with a sense of control over her life.

Believing firmly in self-respect and sensitive to the economic pressures of her times, she will not employ people unless Catholics for a Free Choice can pay comparable Washington, D.C. salaries.

Kissling is a product of the 1960s, the era when she left the church and tested the edges of societal revolution. Insisting that her return to the church was not to the church of her childhood, she uses her past experiences to move the church in new directions. Her ability to direct an organization which to the hierarchy is "at the heart of darkness" is impressive.

Directing Catholics for a Free Choice means directing her phenomenal energy to educate and lobby Congress, to conduct seminars and workshops, and to publish *Conscience*, the organization's official voice. At a more fundamental level, Frances Kissling is challenging what she perceives as the church hierarchy's battle to control women. In the following interview, she describes this challenge articulately and discusses a wide range of church concerns.

DISAGREEMENT WITH, NOT DISSENT FROM, THE CHURCH

Could you explain your views on dissent and your perceptions of present church turbulence?

Kissling: The word dissent makes me uncomfortable. It is a very formal word and should be reserved for certain legal moments in our lives. Basically, what we Catholics have going on are disagreements and it's not good to raise those squabbles to a realm of dissent. I am calling the church to accountability. The institutional church is using the concept of dissent much too broadly. It takes things having nothing to do with dogma, nothing to do with doctrine, and puts them in a context of religious dissent, when in fact, we're dealing with political disagreements.

Take the issue everyone connects with me: abortion. Whenever a Catholic like myself takes a position on the *legality* of it, which differs from the bishops' position, that difference has nothing to do with dissent.

We have a disagreement because we talk about something that is not in the realm of dogma. There's no divine revelation about certain *legislative* avenues. The bishops have no more right, based upon church teaching, to decide that abortion be *illegal* than I [do]. I have as much right to decide that abortion should be *legal*. It's simply a question that should not be raised to that level in our contact with each other within the church.

What is going on in the church right now, in the broadest sense of the word, is a struggle for political control. The struggles over abortion, birth control, divorce, women's ordination, or any number of other matters, are related to political control, not to church teaching. These struggles have nothing to do with spirituality. It is not a spiritual struggle; it is not a struggle for the heart of the church; it is a struggle over who will prevail in the public arena.

Dissent in the eyes of the institutional church is a very serious thing. People who dissent are marked and marginalized. It is the constant desire of the institutional leadership of the church to marginalize and to cut off people who differ with them. There is a certain value when one genuinely dissents and when that dissent concerns a church teaching. One can dissent on the abortion issue, but that must be done in light of the church's moral teaching about abortion. If, for instance, one believes abortion is morally justified in certain circumstances, then that becomes a dissenting position. It is fair to call that dissent. But, if one simply believes, as I do, that abortion should be legal, that is not a dissenting position. You are dissenting from no church teaching whatsoever, because there is no church teaching on the legality of abortion. That is the reason we must be very careful with our use of language. Further, making people afraid to take positions or to join with us lest they, too, be branded as dissenters, is another form of intimidation.

Having said that, I also believe that dissent is the lifeblood of the church. Without people, without women willing to dissent, to stand up and challenge the church and indeed take a prophetic stance on the issues that affect us, the church will be a dead organism.

THE VATICAN
AND THE REAGAN ADMINISTRATION
Why has control suddenly become a question?
Kissling: I relate what's going on now to Barbara Tuchman's *The March of Folly.* She analyzes the Renaissance church, and it's inability to adjust to the signs of times. There are some obvious differences, of course, but some things are essentially the same.

She wrote about a church very much related to the political structure of its time, and [that] is the same today. Right now, the Roman Catholic church is experiencing a level of political clout and attention in the secular sense that it has not enjoyed since before the Reformation. We see it on two levels: in the Vatican, and in the U. S. church. In Rome the reality is that John Paul II is our pope at the same time that Ronald Reagan is President of the United States. The pope took power at a time of great political crisis in his native Poland, and he played a central role in that secular political struggle. These events came together in a way that made the Roman Catholic church and the pope central figures in political, global, and geopolitical terms. Latin America, of course, fits in as well from what we see going on in Nicaragua. That we have Ronald Reagan and John Paul II in power—two people united in their intense anti-communism—has led to [a] great exercise of secular power by John Paul II with the help of the Reagan Administration.

Do you feel that there's collaboration between these two men?
Kissling: I think that there is cooperation between them. I prefer a neutral term, but I think the reality is that these two men are agreed on their anti-communist mission. For example, one of the ways I see them cooperate is that the Reagan Administration is perfectly willing to give the Vatican whatever it wants on sexual issues: abortion, international family planning, and matters of that sort. It attempts in that manner to maintain links with the Vatican in the anti-communist struggle. Conversely, it hopes that the Vatican, with its conservative perspective, will exercise some control over the U. S. bishops in their [positions]. . .on such issues as nuclear war. We had a situation here, for example, when the bishops were debating a pastoral on nuclear war. . .the initial drafts were [quite strong].

Bishops were called to Rome to meet with the Holy Father, and indeed, as a result of those meetings, the draft was softened.   We do know that the Reagan Administration met with those same people.

And it is these types of bishops one sees rising to prominence in the American church.   They are people who have the ear of the Vatican, and the ear of the Reagan Administration.   I want to point out, there is this enormous public presence and this enormous political power that Rome possesses at the moment. On the other hand, there is a largely progressive power being wielded—except on women's issues—by the bishops in the United States.   They produced a pastoral on the economy, on nuclear war, and a number of progressive issues.   They stand well on Central America.   As a result, the bishops here and the pope in Rome have enjoyed, and continue to enjoy, great political power.   But, in essence, this power is corrupting them.

How does this power corrupt churchmen?

Kissling: To continue to enjoy this political clout, they are willing to subvert every other value in the church to maintain their hegemony over the people of God.   They are perfectly willing to conduct the crackdowns they do on Catholics around the country.   Every attempt is being made to limit the potential political clout the Catholic laity possess.   Indeed, the interesting thing is that in some ways the roots of this political power are in John XXIII.   He opened the doors of the church to modern times and said we had to become involved.   He properly said it was a province for the laity;   but the clergy love it so much that they can't give it up.

I think there is a corruption of the church at the highest levels.   It may not be the venal sort of corruption [which] existed in the Renaissance, in the sense of personal and financial gain.   But it's a profound corruption eating away at the power of the laity.   It can demoralize the people of God and that's a very serious thing.

POPE JOHN XXIII

Could you focus more on John XXIII? How you see his vision being obstructed?

Kissling: I am a pre-Vatican II Catholic, and my formative education took place before then.   I grew up in an era when people bought the whole church: lock, stock, and barrel. If you disagreed anywhere you had to get out. . . .I grew up in a working-class, but not a particularly political, family. My mother was strongly committed, in a very intuitive kind of way, to racial justice. In our integrated neighborhoods, I saw a lot of racial injustice in the church, which [my] mother was very good at pointing out to me. I remember moving from one neighborhood to another, and her calling up the local Catholic school to register me. The principal said, "Come on down and visit us, and we'll see what we can do." We went, we visited, and I was registered. The new neighborhood had a very large black population, and my mother later said to me, "Do you know why they wanted us to come and see them? They wanted to see us to be sure that you weren't black. If you were black, you would not have been admitted to this. . .school."

Does your sensitivity to the powerless stem from these experiences?

Kissling: It's hard to get in touch with exactly what makes us what we are today. A working class background often leads people to an understanding of powerlessness; indeed, people from lower economic backgrounds are powerless. I grew up in a family where both my parents were very, very supportive of my independence. They encouraged me to take charge of my own life, to make decisions for myself. There never was this talk about when you grow up and get married and when you have children; never any sort of automatic assumptions.

Many people like me. . .rejected much of the institutional church prior to the Second Vatican Council. Subsequent to the council, the increased emphasis on the social justice message of the gospels as the root of our faith made an enormous difference in our capacity to return to church. But it also meant that people like me, who returned to the church with hope, also brought a whole set of experiences, new ways of relating to structures which are much more democratic.

In my case these experiences came from politics, radical politics. When I say I came back to the church, I never came back on the old terms. It is true you can't go home again. I came back to the church as a social change agent; I came back to woman-church.

VISION OF A NEW CHURCH
Could you talk about your vision of church?
Kissling: When I talk about coming back into *the* church, I'm not talking about coming back to Sunday mass, confession and all of those things that are the memories of my childhood. I'm talking about coming back to a new vision of church established in the late 1970s by women within the church. Women recapturing the church. I believe what happened in the church was parallel to what happened in the secular women's movement. And indeed, if you examine what is going on in the women's movement and in the church now, it is similar to what went on in the women's movement in the past.

For example, the ordination question—this is where it can be seen most clearly and most quickly. Secular women had to spend time deciding whether they wanted to strike for a piece of the corporate pie. Were they going to become heads of corporations, universities. . .to buy into the hierarchical secular structure and to get their share? Or, were they going to work to transform the structure of society? You find within the secular feminist movement both of those tensions, both desires operating simultaneously, sometimes with tension between them and sometimes with understanding.

The same thing is true in the move toward women's ordination. When that movement began, it was pretty much a straightforward decision for ordination as priests. As it matured and developed, however, some people began to question: Do we want to be priests, or do we want a renewed priestly ministry? Do we want to transform the priesthood into something else, or do we buy into what has existed all along? Around 1975-76, women took their experiences in the secular women's movement and attempted to apply these experiences and values to church. What emerged was an attempt to create a church that was responsive to women, in which women shared power, responsibility, and the obligation to transform the church into an entity that was more sensitive to all powerless people.

Where are we now?
Kissling: We're entering a period of great polarization. The reality is that we are about to go through an enormously painful time in the church. We are into a stage of intense conflict, confrontation, polarization, and challenge. And this is neces-

sary right now in order to grab the base of support for major change within the church. We must find ways to wake up people who don't really see the injustice in the church. To some extent that means pushing against the system and forcing it to respond. I find myself thinking what we now need is to go beyond the point of quietly standing in front of churches, or of the U. S. Conference of Catholic Bishops, or other such places. We need to pass beyond putting on our sweet little blue armbands or our sweet little black armbands, holding our candles, and singing protest songs, or songs of sweetness and change.

REVOLUTION IN THE CATHOLIC CHURCH
You're talking about revolution then?

Kissling: Yes, we really are talking about revolution. You see, when we do this kind of nice resistance, sort of polite, civil disobedience—which isn't terribly disobedient but it's awful civil—we are still treating the leadership with an enormous amount of respect. They don't deserve our respect. Difficult as it is to take it that next step, which is necessary, I would like to see women reach the point where they understood that every bishop in this country should be so embarrassed that he is afraid to show his face in public.

How do you plan to mobilize and bond women together in order to attempt this kind of revolution?

Kissling: First of all, I think the biggest help we have in creating that kind of bonding is the institution itself. This institution—which again speaks to *The March of Folly* philosophy—this institutional church has not learned at all that you can win more people with honey than vinegar. There is this very heavy dose of vinegar that is constantly coming out of the church: in their male rage, and in their fear of losing control, these men behave very badly. They try to maintain their control by repression. Every time something as dumb as stopping altar girls happens, it increases the size of the movement. Every time you have someone like [Cardinal] Ratzinger or [Archbishop] Laghi coming down on a Charlie Curran, you increase the size of the movement.

Our greatest stand right now is in pushing the institutional leadership into corners. We know when we push them into corners, they make mistakes. They don't know how to deal with people who confront them. We're very lucky that they haven't learned as much from the secular world as we have; they haven't sufficiently learned about co-opting. I mean there are so many little things they could do to placate large numbers of women. They make these mistakes of not allowing women to speak at certain meetings, or not allowing their feet to be washed, silly things like that.

As long as we're talking within the context of revolutionary theory, you always have that small segment of the bell curve doing the acting. It does not take a majority of people to bring about change. It takes a minority of people acting with the acquiescence or even quiet support of the majority.

Some historians say less than two percent of a people revolutionize society.
Kissling: I don't think we need to bring everyone to the point where they're on the streets or outside a church. What we need is to create a climate in which the actions of the vanguard, that small group of people who are actively seeking change, [can] be looked on more favorably and kindly by the middle than. . .the actions of the church leadership.

On the one hand, I said the church leadership is doing itself in by the way it is treating the middle. Particularly, when it goes after issues where the middle feels treated unfairly. I say any actions against children are always seen negatively by ordinary people. It's unfair to pick on children. It's unfair not to let little girls be altar girls. You have a situation recently where the priest told a twelve-year-old child that she could not go to Catholic school any more unless she wrote a letter promising not to appear in any pro-choice demonstrations. She must, he argued, confirm that she agreed with the teachings of the church on abortion. Picking on children like this aggravates people, makes them downright angry.

Mothers and fathers find it revolting. . .
Kissling: Exactly. And the people who feel revolted are active in the church. They have a stake in institutional norms and practice within the church. [They are] people who worry about having their kids confirmed, receiving first communion, and being married in the church. Increasingly, I'm hearing stories of women who can't find anyone who will marry them (not men to marry them; they can find mates), but because of their profes-

sions, priests will not marry them in church. For example, we get calls frequently from people who work in Planned Parenthood, or in abortion facilities, or health care facilities where abortions are performed. They tell us their priest said, "No, I'm sorry, we won't marry you. You may not be married in this parish." Those things really mobilize people and that's what the church is doing to itself.

The further question: What can we do, as a movement, to bring people along with us? One thing is certain—something I personally have decided—those of us in positions of leadership in this movement need to put a human face on our work. We must find forums in which to expose ideas and our life experiences to other women. [Then others] can see us as people, not as the stereotypical old bra-burner. They can see us as women who are concerned for the family and for children, and that our lives are intertwined with their lives. We must find ways to show women these connections.

I myself have just begun to understand this place that I and many others in the church are in. We want to be, but are not able to connect with, the church. I have made the conscious decision that I will speak about abortion. It's not just abstract talk about theology and ethics. Rather, I will speak about who I am; how my life experience and the ethic flowing from it is universal. Many people have the same experience. The development of a sexual ethic (never mind abortion) involves getting the institutional church to address reality.

How can the church recognize sexual reality?
Kissling: Church government is not divinely ordained, and I have no particular overriding respect for that government. It is not sacred and should not be treated as sacred.

WOMEN BECOMING AUTHENTIC CHURCH
The hierarchy perceives itself as sacred. That is their problem. That's not my problem. People who simply don't listen to the church do not perceive its hierarchy as sacred. The difference the women's movement and other progressive movements have made in the church is that people have decided not to accept [the insititutional] church. Until ten years ago people who disagreed with the institutional church went about their business and their private lives. They participated in institutional

church, though, without feeling the need to integrate the two. Catholic women, for example, were able to use birth control privately, go to church, hear the priests rail against contraception from the altar, and yet, continue to receive the sacraments. Women did not really see this as an experience of conflict.

But now, we value our personal integrity much more highly. I and many others are not willing to have personal values and ethics lambasted from the altar. It is sheer hypocrisy. We are trying to force the church to a point where pastoral reality becomes consistent with the objective, public, political message.

Similarly, we do not respect the parish priest who privately tells us it's okay to use birth control, but publicly goes along with the positions of the church, even [preaching] the occasional sermon against it. This is not acceptable. A priest who does this is not a person of integrity. Just as he is not a person of integrity, so too if we participate in that deceit, we are not integral. . . .It's a lie; it's living a lie. We don't want to live lives of lies. The commitment to church by women today, particularly women who are seeking to [bring about] change in the church, is much, much higher than that of people twenty years ago.

There is concern in the Vatican that the American bishops may become too strong. But here in the U. S., some feel that many American bishops are weak on women's issues.

Kissling: Well, those different perceptions do apply, but to different realities. One of the distressing sights is the polarization in the church into many separate groups. Each of them fights for its own power, rather than fighting for the whole. Take the American bishops (and bishops of other countries) fighting with Rome over the concept of collegiality. You have theologians, American theologians, fighting with American bishops over what to teach. You have religious communities fighting over who will kick out their members, Rome or the community itself. All of these are just crass, political struggles. These are plain old power games, and totally lost in the shuffle are the people of the church. Nobody is fighting for the people of the church.

What is your role in this struggle and what are you trying to do for the people of the church?

Kissling: We, of Catholics for a Free Choice, may be further along as an organization because we deal with the issue that is most taboo. As Catholics for a Free Choice, our group has dealt with abortion for the past thirteen years.

Abortion has certainly become "the heart of darkness" in the hierarchy's eyes.

Kissling: It has become the test of orthodoxy. Because the church would most marginalize, condemn, and punish any individual of stature who speaks out on the abortion issue, we have been forced to the front. Sooner than any other social group in the church, we were forced to become a lay organization.

GETTING THE CHURCH TO TRUST WOMEN

Do you perceive yourself as speaking for rich women as well as poor?

Kissling: It is the poor and the uneducated who are most marginalized in access to reproductive health care services. Be it contraception or abortion, the constituency most affected by our work are the poor and the uneducated. In another sense, however, we seek recognition of the moral agency of all women through the abortion issue.

Further, it's not the abortion issue that's at question. The question is, how do we get the church to acknowledge that women can be trusted to make good decisions? That is what we're pushing them to do on the abortion issue, to trust women. Women have proven, over the past two thousand years, over the history of the human race, that they are responsible in their childbearing and childrearing capacities. Women who have children today make an enormous act of faith. The faith any woman must possess to bring a child into this world is phenomenal. Phenomenal that any woman has children!

And we do it well. Poor women have children and rear them with the greatest of love and the greatest of care. Women have children under extremely difficult circumstances, especially when their husbands leave them. Look at the differences in the way women and men approach the children they bear. How can you then not trust women to make these decisions? Many men are wonderful. But many men walk out on their children, provide no financial support, no emotional nurturance whatsoever. Do those women who are left alone give up their children? Do they throw them away? Do they run down to St. Vincent's Foundling Home and say, "Here's my kid. My husband just left me, and I'm not going to raise this child?" No. I know this from my own experience. When I was seventeen with three other siblings ages twelve, ten, and nine, my stepfather walked out on my mother. How did my mother, who had never worked, manage? She got a job with the New York Telephone Company on the 11:00 p.m. to 7:00 a.m. shift so she could still care for her children. She worked those hours until her last child was grown.

Are you saying as a challenge: "Point out the men who do likewise?"

Kissling: Point out the men who do likewise! My mother is by no means unique. Most women in those situations do exactly that: scrub floors, anything whatever to care for their children. Knowing this, how can you not trust women? How can you not trust that women will make a good decision about whether or not a specific child should come into the world? When I hear Right-to-Lifers talk about women as selfish, I ask, "Who do they know?" They certainly don't know the women I know. Women do courageous, heroic things routinely to raise their children.

The hierarchy are supposedly not ordinary men. Do you see them as sensitive? What do you think is going on?

Kissling: Well, a number of things. First of all, I do not believe for one instant that the U. S. bishops care at all about fetuses. I do not believe that they care one iota for fetal life. I have seen no evidence historically, or in recent times. Look at the resources of this church. Look at the way the bishops have approached the abortion question. In 1973, the Supreme Court made abortion legal in this country. And what did the bishops do? They immediately launched a *political* campaign to make abortion illegal. Every year the bishops throw in one million dollars on the national level for this campaign, and at least another one million dollars when you count up everything spent in each diocese. My figures are conservative. . . .We all know it's extremely difficult to get good information on church expenditures, so let's be very modest in saying what they spend.

Now they have conducted this campaign for thirteen years. During those years they have not prevented—with all their millions of dollars—those men have not prevented one abortion from taking place in the United States. They are not stupid. Five years ago they could have sat down and said, "Well, we've now spent twenty million dollars in a political campaign to make abortion illegal." If their motive in making abortion illegal is to save fetal life, not to control women's lives, then they could have at that point said, "Our campaign has failed. What we need to do for the next ten years is to commit an equal sum of money to social and economic programs that will [encourage] women to bring children into the world."

You mean developed fetuses. . .?

Kissling: Exactly. That would show that they really cared about fetuses. I challenge cardinals and bishops to show *specific* concern, if indeed they care for fetuses. When the church hierarchy is really concerned about some issue, they allocate a specific sum of money. We are told what the specific sum is. When they. . .say we'll do anything to help you, then I know they really don't want to do anything to help me. When they say we have a fund of fifty million dollars over here, and we can do the following things for you, then we know they mean business.

When I talk to people about programs in two of the largest dioceses in the U. S., both of which publish they will do anything for pregnant women, I get the data. [Through these interviews] what I find is a half-time nun in Catholic charities shepherding women through the government bureaucracy. Therefore, if you come into these dioceses and are pregnant, they'll take you down to the Welfare Office. Well, thank you very much! That's not what I call spending the resources of the church on women and children! This is the kind of hypocrisy that we're dealing with. It's not, I repeat, that bishops care about fetuses.

FEAR OF WOMEN

I come now to my second point. I do believe these men are deeply afraid of women. Deeply, deeply unconsciously afraid of women and the power of women.

The fact is that most of the male leadership of the church has no ongoing, concrete, positive, or personal relationships with women. I'm not talking about sex. I refer to normal friendships and collegial relationships. They do not work with women as colleagues in their institutions. Women are not on the same boards of directors with them, or if so, only one or two. They do not—nor are they encouraged to—have sincere friendships with women. Women who tend to have relationships with priests—be these friendships, confessional, or sexual—tend [to be] unhappy or troubled.

And troubled becomes normative. . .?

Kissling: Troubled becomes the norm. And the clerical conclusion: all women are alike. Most women won't bother to confess the sin of abortion. First of all, they don't think they've committed a sin, and secondly, therefore, it's not a sin.

Women are certainly not going to talk about it with some man, a male priest. Hence, these men have denied themselves sufficient, regularized, normal contact with ordinary women. Therefore, partly they are afraid of us, and partly this fear contributes to their becoming more distrustful. It ends up that they don't know us.

If women really believe that abortion is a great sin which needs special dispensation to be removed, would it not be very worrisome to the church officials if people in their great abandonment, in their great turmoil, just stayed away from the church? It seems opposed to what Jesus stood for.

Kissling: But the good part of it is that women have figured these things out for themselves. I have a deep trust in the common sense and capacity of people to do good. The reality is that there's no reason they should be going to these men about their abortions. There's no reason whatsoever. Women know this, and they stay away. Now, for example, there is this big emphasis within the U. S. church for the various dioceses to set up programs of reconciliation for women who have had abortions. In most places they're called Project Rachel, which I find offensive.

What is Project Rachel?

Kissling: It is named after "Rachel weeping for her children" in the massacre of the holy innocents scene. You see how dumb they really are? They even choose names that are inclined to increase guilt. These projects are touted by bishops all over the country, and by the pro-life offices, as the most wonderful program possible. The interesting thing is the published statistics. Remember this is a big program. How many women do you think call Project Rachel every week in order to be reconciled with the church? Two women a week. *Two women a week!* And the average lag time between the time of abortion and the time they call Project Rachel is seven to ten years. So what kind of program is that!

You have noted two reasons, but is there another reason why the hierarchy is upset about women and abortion?

Kissling: There is also a third reason, a *political* reason. Much has been invested in the opposition to abortion; similar to church opposition to contraception. A Pontifical Commission on Birth Control appointed by Pope Paul VI recommended a change in church teaching in 1968. It was rejected by a minority group and the pope. The minority group went to the pope, and said, "If we change our position on this, then people can't trust us anymore. They won't listen. It will erode the authority of the church." That was the basic reason that Pope Paul VI rejected it.

The same thing is true on the abortion issue. So much has been invested by the bishops in the *political* campaign against abortion that to back off would imply a loss of power. It is the reason the bishops were so angry with Geraldine Ferraro.

FURY OVER GERALDINE FERRARO
Why were they furious with Ferraro?

Kissling: People think it's because she is pro-choice. There is a relationship to the fact that she's pro-choice, but there is something else. Right now, as I noted earlier, the bishops are enjoying this enormous political power. The world is listening to them; they *love* the fact that the world is listening to them. What happened with Geraldine Ferraro is that the Democratic party didn't listen to the bishops, and it drove them crazy. The Democratic party decided that they had a better chance to win with a pro-choice Catholic woman as vice president. They knew the bishops would not like it, but they believed the people would. The Democratic party said in essence to the bishops, "We don't think you're so powerful. Despite your stand on abortion, and what you think about women. . . we're going to nominate this Catholic woman who is pro-choice. We don't think you bishops have political clout." This, in my interpretation, enraged the bishops. That the Democratic party, the party of the blue collar Catholic in this country, would reject the wisdom of the bishops was a bad sign. They had to go after her to prove the party wrong, to try again to control the party.

With Ferraro, some bishops also objected, aside from her pro-choice position, to the reality that if [she were] elected, they were faced with this Catholic woman whom they did not know. Again, you see their lack of knowledge of women. . . . Traditionally, they control and influence male Catholic politicians through the "old boys' network." They find some Jesuit who went to school with politicians, or taught them in college, or a parish priest, or some priest who is their golf buddy. These good "old boy" contacts are then used in backroom politics to influence the politician to do what bishops want. Suddenly, if all these Catholic women politicians come into office, how can they play those "old boy" games with them?

Political power, the theme of our conversation, is really politics: church politics. The reason abortion is central. . .is because the bishops have invested in it much political clout. Another thing we must understand in terms of politics and the bishops is that very often they use abortion as an excuse for other things in the political arena.

ABORTION AS AN EXCUSE
How do you see abortion used as an excuse?
Kissling: Two years ago, for example, the Civil Rights Restoration Act came up for passage a second time in Congress. A section of this act contains an abortion element. It basically says that an institution cannot discriminate in its pregnancy benefits. That means if it gives pregnancy and maternity benefits, it must also pay for abortions. Institutions cannot treat the two differently. Nor can they discriminate against students or faculty on the basis of pregnancy, including abortion. Now this portion of the act never affected the bishops because Catholic institutions already had been exempt. Yet, they sought three amendments to the Civil Rights Restoration Act in spite of the objections of the entire Civil Rights Committee. And the three changes they wanted were: 1) an anti-abortion rider; 2) greater assurance that the current exemptions they have against complying with these laws be allowed to stand; and 3) a change in the number of institutions covered by the exemption.

They wanted these "religiously affiliated" institutions to become "religiously controlled." Everybody focused on the bishops' objection to the abortion portion of the act, but many of us believe that what the bishops really wanted was more freedom to discriminate more broadly against women in Catholic institutions of higher education.

Can you state the ways in which these bishops are discriminating against women in a larger way?

Kissling: In any way: benefits, hiring, all sorts of ways. For example, what they were trying to do in a place like Marquette University was to change it from a "religiously affiliated" institution to a "religiously controlled" institution. The increasing tendency in Catholic institutions is to create lay boards, so they can get federal funds. But if [the universities] want to [obtain] federal monies, then they have to obey the federal rules on anti-discrimination. [The institutional church doesn't want its universities] to obey these laws. Hence abortion was the excuse to sneak through this measure exempting Catholic educational institutions especially from following the law.

CONSCIENCE: CFFC PUBLICATION

Could you talk about the magazine, *Conscience,* and how it relates to the goals of Catholics for a Free Choice?

Kissling: We founded *Conscience* and we concentrate on publication, because as an organization we try to make accessible to the average person the kinds of material appearing in esoteric journals. This goal ties in with dissent. As long as a theologian confines his dissent to a periodical that nobody reads, a theological journal, it's acceptable to object to some church laws. But, if a theologian dissents in *The New York Times,* which is widely read, or speaks in language accessible to the ordinary person, or appears on television, then that's not permissible dissent. There is nothing that CFFC says about authority, dissent, contraception, abortion, or whatever, that has not been published in some prestigious journal by some prestigious theologian.

We bring [theological discussion] to the popular level. The church does not like it. The purpose of *Conscience* is to have a substantial say on many taboo issues. Some Catholics never talk about these taboos. . . .We have situations where even in a house of sisters, [members] have no idea what [the] other thinks about these taboo topics.

How does this situation strike you?

Kissling: It is [an] understandable [situation] when a church deals with something taboo by saying, "no, no, no." Then nobody talks about it because it is too threatening. Catholics for a Free Choice and myself come in for substantial criticism and misplaced anger from people. The reason is that we are confronting the institution. We challenge the limits of debate, dissent, and dialogue. The old reasoning was if you don't relate to, or make up your mind about, a problem, it does not exist. You don't have to do anything about it. A conscientious person, though, figures out what she believes and feels an obligation to act on the conclusion. We are forcing people, whether they like it or not, to deal with the abortion issue. Take, for example, the advertisements in *The New York Times*. People got angry, very angry, because they were forced to deal with abortion. Whatever their distaste, it became a public issue. [In my view] they did not like it because they knew they might come to a point where they didn't like themselves. They had to face themselves, and face the reality of abortion.

IMPOSING CATHOLIC THEOLOGY

Are you tolerant of other positions on abortion that are different from your own?

Kissling: I, as a Catholic, don't want to impose the Catholic perspective on people of all faiths. [For example], the theology of personhood affects the way in which Jews approach fetal life. In Jewish theology, the fetus becomes a person at the moment it emerges and takes its first breath. . . .I must show some respect for people who have a religiously based concern about the fetus.

Do you have any reservations about abortion on a mass scale in this country?

Kissling: Not in a sense of people saying: "Oh! Four thousand abortions a day. This is monumental!" Or 1.6 million a year. Which of those four thousand today, or those 1.6 million last year, am I in a position to judge should not have happened? Which of them didn't I like? Was it [number] "3853"? Or was it the first one? Hence, I have an enormous reluctance to get involved in the numbers game about abortion.

The basic question has got to be *who* shall decide? How shall we, as a society, make this decision? Do I want the state to decide? Do I want the doctors to decide? Or do I want a pregnant person to make this decision? I try to hang on to this last one. I, and others, have not been strong enough in articulating the position that says. . .one should do everything possible not to create life if one is not prepared to allow it into the world. One certainly has the right to bring a child into the world and give it up for adoption. What disturbs me is our unwillingness within the secular feminist community, to have a very, very strong position on women's *obligation* to use contraception. There is too much emphasis in the feminist community on the dangers of contraception. There are, of course, dangers in contraception, but using these as excuses for women not to "contracept" is treating neither life nor women with dignity. And I want to instill dignity [in women]. I do not want to see any of my sisters in a position where they must have an abortion. We at CFFC try very hard to support contraceptive research and education.

A NEW TWIST TO THE ABORTION DEBATE
Your magazine reported new research in this area of conception. What about this pill developed in France?
Kissling: This new drug, RU-486, is a steroid as opposed to a hormonal compound. It can be taken either as a once-a-month contraceptive, or used as an abortive agent to cause a nonsurgical abortion. It has enormous potential for radically altering the abortion debate.

Does not a drug like RU-486 make abortion, in a sense, a non-issue?
Kissling: I don't think it will ever be a *non-issue*. One good advantage, though, is medical: the drug can achieve legal abortion through chemical means with minimal side affects. This is opposed to a surgical intervention. Consequently, we will have fewer complications, less expense for women, and, above all, more privacy. But privacy is a double-edged sword. For the Catholic community, the drug has enormous theological implications.

Many Catholic theologians have taken the position that prior to individuation, or until that moment when twinning is no longer possible, that is, up until the sixth day, abortion is permissible. Even anti-abortionists, such as Peter Steinfels at *Commonweal*, seem comfortable with abortion up until the sixth week. This advance should answer the objection of a number of conservative and moderate Catholics. One argument against RU-486, however, is that some people, some health professionals, will utilize it as a way to *avoid* the issue of abortion.

In what ways, for example?

Kissling: People involved in the research [say that] women won't know whether or not they're pregnant, or whether or not they're having an abortion. But I think this is a degrading way to view women. I don't think women are looking to keep secrets from themselves. Women want to know what they are doing; women want to make moral decisions with full knowledge. I don't think we can fool ourselves with, "Well," "Maybe," "I wasn't really pregnant," or "Maybe it wasn't an abortion." My experience with women who have [had] abortions [indicates that] if they think through their action beforehand, and are comfortable with their decision, then afterwards they do not have enormous guilt feelings.

If we permit women to avoid this step of thinking through a decision to have an abortion, we open doors to confusion, guilt, and unhappiness. While it is a private decision, it is also a social phenomenon, something in which society needs to involve itself. Privatization isolates a person in our society. I worry about a woman who gets a prescription, goes home, takes these pills in the privacy of her bedroom, and lacks an appropriate support system. She is further alienated and isolated from society in her decision. There still is a need for contact, for counselling, for discussion of contraception afterwards.

Do you think the clergy's emphatic stand on abortion will have dramatic consequences for the church's membership?

Kissling: Definitely. This new advance is so closely related to contraception that it will be extremely difficult for the church to speak against it without some kind of response on the part of the people.

Do you think the church will recover?

Kissling: I think, quite frankly, more women would rather

leave the church over divorce than anything else I know of.

THE CHURCH AND THE UNCHURCHED
As women leave the church, they will probably take their children with them. Do you think the intitutional church is aware of this?

Kissling: Apparently [not]. [I think] that the church will be happy writing them off. Rosemary Ruether talked about a historical example in this country. One of the ethnic churches, a group of Eastern Eüropean churches [consisting] of 500,000 to 800,000 Catholics, was totally written off by the church [in the last century]. We just gave them up. We didn't care about those poor people. Look at what the church gave up during the Protestant Reformation because it refused to reform. The history of the church is that it is perfectly willing to lose large numbers of. . . .

In essence, you're saying that the hierarchy would be happy if questioning and dissenting members left their church.

Kissling: They are much happier if many of us. . .if *I* went away. But I'm not going anywhere; I have no reason to leave. I won't give them the satisfaction of leaving. Secondly, I feel an obligation to other women to stick with it. It's not up to me to leave other women alone in the church. I think I'm a good Catholic. They should be happy to have me. My battle has nothing to do with spirituality. . . .I am probably much more traditional in my spirituality than many of my feminist colleagues. Most women call me a traditional Catholic; somewhat Pre-Vatican II. What I'm taking on is the *secular* and *political* aspect of the church. They're spending all of their time dealing with politics, not with the central Christian message. When do you ever hear about spirituality in this church?

Are you optimistic about the church?
Kissling: I'm actually quite optimistic. I don't know exactly why I am, but I believe that we women can change the structure of this church. I just don't see any other alternative for the hierarchy. We are not going away. What gives me most hope is that the will of women to remain within the church is very, very strong, much stronger than people would imagine. Nobody I know is going anywhere else. We're not becoming Episcopa-

lian; we're not going to become Unitarian; we're not going to go
to the Methodists so that they will ordain us. We are staying
right here in this church. I think that that's the key; *we're
not going away*. The institution is going to have no choice but to
deal with us.

THEORY AND CHURCH DEVELOPMENT
What changes do you expect to see in your lifetime?
Kissling: We will see women ordained in my lifetime. Once
women are ordained, that becomes the key to change. Women
will be in the mainstream of the church. Now all the positions
of responsibility in the church are held by clerics. Not just held
by men, but by clerics. Even in political terms, you can't get to be
an ambassador in this church unless you are a priest. I'd love to
be the Vatican ambassador to France. I think that would be a
wonderful job. There are no jobs for women in the church, except
education. The diocesan director of education can be a woman,
but [the position is] very limited in function. To get those
changes we have to become nasty. Then the key question—to
which I don't yet have the answer—becomes: When is the time
to stop being nasty and to seek accommodation? I think in terms
of strategic and political views.

In a political structure you first confront and create polarization. More and more people then line up on both sides. You
must, however, know when in the movement to seek peace. The
biggest problem right now in the progressive wing of the church
is the polarization between men and women. . . .[Male church
members] won't accept women. The source of resistance in the
church now is women's rights. We're the only ones who are out
there fighting, and all our new leadership is in the women's
church movement. . .older men who have traditionally been the
leaders of the progressive movement do not want to accept our
leadership.

I look for ways to bring those two forces together. How can
we accomplish it? That, I think, is the immediate question for
progressive women in the Catholic church. How can the men
and the women get together, because that is what must be done
before we make real and substantive change.

**Therefore you're not advocating an "exodus church"
movement. . . ?**

Kissling: No I'm not interested in exodus church. But, in the meantime, I think it's time to stop being nice. Let me give you a specific incident from the Vatican twenty-four situation [see Appendix A]. We have suffered the death of Marjorie Tuite, one of the ad signers. [Although] her case was settled, many people feel she lost her will to fight for life when she got cancer. Intense demoralization occurred in her through the year-and-a-half struggle with the Vatican. She gave up. Her community betrayed her, the church betrayed her, and she was profoundly affected. It was such an enormous shock when this happened to her. She would muse, "How can they do this to me? I have given so many years." She had been faithful and loyal. They slapped her in the face and threw her in the garbage. It destroyed her, and when the cancer came, she had no will to fight it.

We, women, must call to account the people who did it. We have to [challenge] the organization called the Congregation for Religious and Secular Institutes, CRIS. Two people in that institute come regularly to this country. I don't think they should be allowed to show their faces in the United States of America without the women of this country, and our church, confronting them with their complicity in the death of Marjorie Tuite. This is the level of responsibility to which we must call these individual church leaders.

We women value good manners. But these men don't deserve good manners. We must get to the point where once we know they don't deserve good manners, we're capable—in the same way that [people] in the Vietnam war [were]—of taking to the streets. . . .We have to be able to act similiarly with our church leadership. The other consideration of value in our strategy is that these men take themselves very seriously. They have no sense of humor about themselves, no humility about themselves as imperfect, normal human beings who make mistakes in the world. Nothing will drive them crazier than to be treated without dignity.

How do you relate your strategy to Jesus Christ and his gospel?

Kissling: Jesus in the present church leadership would be in a situation similar to going into the temple: expelling the money changers, and the money lenders, and every other sacrilegious scurrility. If Jesus looked at what the church had become in terms of its institutional governmental character, it would not please him. And he'd throw them out!

Would they do to him what they did to Marjorie Tuite?
Kissling: They would try, they would try. There is always a hope that in each person there can be a moment of transformation. You hope that in the case of Jesus Christ, they might be able to recognize him.

There was a Nicodemus.
Kissling: That's right, exactly. And so Jesus Christ will be with us, plain and simple. It's important that there always be that character, that charism within the church, that kind of countercultural element about our church. One of the things I think is so tragic is that part of me finds that John Paul II has a certain capacity to give a positive message to the world. There's something in his writings and in his glimmers of a mystical spiritual vision which could be very valuable to the church. But that vision is ruled by his need to control. Somewhere in himself, and in our church leadership, [the pope] has lost his ability to trust, not only the people of the church, but to trust himself. I believe that speaking the truth is enough. If we speak the truth, live the truth, and act truthfully, people will rally round. They will become part of that truth.

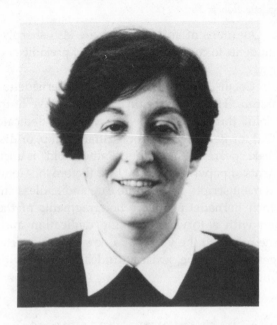

BERNADETTE BROOTEN

"The view that man is the head of woman is the view that keeps the leadership abilities, the intellectual contribution and capablities of women from being recognized, appreciated, and integrated into society. It is an enormous waste for our culture that women's leadership and intellectual capabilities have not been fully integrated into the culture."

A Catholic biblical scholar, Assistant Professor Bernadette Brooten of Harvard Divinity School brings a startlingly new focus to the study of the New Testament. On occasion she pulls the rug out from beneath the patriarchal canon. Consequently, challenges to traditional thinking abound in her classes: the old artifacts of knowledge shift first, then the larger pieces get shuffled, forcing students to rearrange their mental furniture. By the time her courses draw to a close, some pieces are discarded, no longer needed, and others still may not fit into their original places. Questions about the religious foundation for the exploitation of women surface with surprising clarity in her

173

courses. Questions of anti-Semitism are also sharply focused, forcing students to confront many forms of prejudice in the New Testament.

Born in Coeur d'Alene, northern Idaho, Bernadette is one of four children. Her great personal passions: love of travel and love of "old" things, which dovetail with her dedicated scholarship. Old for Bernadette is not a Tiffany lamp, or discovering one of Shakespeare's lost sonnets. Rather, "old" is ancient, such as fragments of papyri from a 200 BCE (Before the Common Era) Egyptian manuscript. The infinite care and endless enthusiasm with which Bernadette fingers her fragments of the past is combined with a forward-thinking dedication and energy, which she brings to the vision of a new church—a church that challenges some of the sexist attitudes inherent in the Christian biblical tradition.

BACKGROUND INFLUENCES

You are a young biblical scholar whom people often quote and admire. What are some of the forces, the culture, the education that led you to become the person you are?

Brooten: I think that my Catholic education was very important. I had parochial and Catholic education from grade one through the end of college. The religious education in the Catholic schools which I attended from a young age was very critical. I was taught quite early on, for example, that one should not understand the Bible literally, that the creation account in Genesis was not meant to be in contradiction to the theory of evolution. The author of Genesis was speaking at a different level, I was taught. It was a view of reality different from that of a natural scientist.

In the midst of Vatican II, our catechisms were changed so that we had some teaching about world religions as part of our religious education. In comparison with Protestant friends, I felt my education was more critical than. . .they were getting. Theirs was more—I'm not sure one would say fundamentalist necessarily—but a more conservative understanding of the Bible. In college at the University of Portland in Oregon, I took the required theology and philosophy courses. Some students were not happy with these requirements, but for myself I found them very helpful. These courses made it possible for me to think about theology.

At the University of Portland, when I was an undergraduate from 1968-71, a female theologian taught at the school. I never had a course with her, but I knew that she existed. I saw her at faculty meetings from afar, and I knew that it was possible to be a woman and be a theologian. And her presence that one year made a deep impression, just because it was my first year. I then went for a year abroad to Salzburg, Austria, and when I returned, she no longer taught there. Yet she showed me the possibility, in a very concrete way, of becoming a theologian. So I decided to go on and to study theology, and I went to the University of Tübingen [Germany] in 1971 and studied there.

At that time there was a very strong ecumenical spirit at the University of Tübingen. I took courses in both the Protestant and Catholic departments of theology. In 1973, I entered a doctoral program at Harvard. During the time of my doctoral study I continued to go back to Tübingen. I also studied at the Hebrew University [Jerusalem] for a year, [in order] to have broadly-based training.

My training at Harvard was very ecumenical, with its strong tradition of studying the New Testament in its cultural environment. My training at the University of Tübingen was affected by its long tradition of both Catholic and Protestant theology. At the Hebrew University in Jerusalem I studied Hebrew. Those were some of the focal points of my education.

You wanted to be a theologian, but ended up being a biblical scholar. Is there a difference?

Brooten: Well, some people would say there is a difference. The way the term "theologian" as usually understood in this country is in the narrower sense of philosophical theology, or constructive theology, or systematic theology, or dogmatic theology. I think that theology is the study of what is most important to people. A more traditional way of putting it is to say theology is what is of ultimate significance. I don't think that one has to be a theologian to study the New Testament. There are many ways we can study it: as literature, as history, or as a set of historical documents. We can study it from the standpoint of anthropology; one can study it simply to understand the language. And there are many things one can do with it. One can understand it as part of the history of religions. I have an interest in working with it theologically. Working with the New Testament theologically. . .does not mean describing the theology of the New Testament and then making that theology my own. Working theologically with the New Testament for me means trying to understand what is the most important thing that a given author wanted to say, deciding for myself what is most important for me in life, and bringing to discussion what the author thinks is most important and what I think is most important.

PAUL: A PRODUCT OF HIS TIMES
Could you give an example to clarify the distinction?
Brooten: Yes. For the apostle Paul, the hierarchical structures of society were not so important to him that he wished to change them. I think that he believed that slavery was inevitable; I think that he distinguished sharply between women and men; and I think he felt that there were different roles in life for women than for men. In some ways, he felt that slaves and women could be taken into the community and could be equals within the community, were equal before God. However, when a runaway slave by the name of Onesimus had come to him, Paul in the end sent him back to his owner. He didn't grant him sanctuary, he sent him back to his owner, Philemon. He writes a very diplomatic letter to Philemon saying that he should receive him as a brother and that he's more than a brother. Nevertheless, the person Philemon, from whom the runaway slave had escaped, then receives the former slave back and we do not know from the letter [whether or not] Paul was calling upon the slave owner to emancipate the slave. There is no clear indication that he was no longer to serve as a slave.

But there is an indication that later on Paul urged slaves "to be subject to your masters."
Brooten: Well, that is not Paul probably, but a student of Paul's. In the letter to the Colossians, and the letter to the Ephesians, there are statements like that, also in the so-called Pastoral Epistles. These statements about the subordination of slaves, as well as those about the direct subordination of wom-

en, were probably written by a student or students of Paul rather than by Paul himself.

The reasons for thinking this are that the language is quite different from the language of the writings of Paul, the unquestionable writings of Paul. In certain of the letters attributed to Paul, the theology and language are somewhat different, and there are some biographical details that don't fit into what we otherwise know. There are, therefore, a number of reasons for thinking that some of these letters were not written by Paul himself. Nevertheless, even within the writings that clearly were written by Paul, there are statements that move in the direction of subordinationism. The so-called Deutero-Pauline writings, that is, the writings by students of Paul written in his name—[the students] certainly must have felt they were writing it in good faith, that they were accurately representing his views—moved his thought in a slightly different direction. But they didn't necessarily make a radical break with his thinking.

I think, therefore, that Paul felt that there were certain hierarchical structures within society that simply are that way. I think that in this respect also his call for women to veil themselves, and for men to have short hair, and women to have long hair, and his view that love relations between women and women and between men and men are a result of a fundamental alienation from God, show that he accepted certain hierarchical structures within society.

Do you think Paul was challenged on his views?

Brooten: I think that some women questioned him. I think that the Corinthian women who were not wearing veils had a different theology than Paul's. It's not that he did not have an opportunity to see a different theology, but when he saw it, he rejected it. So he writes that God is the head of Christ, and the Christ is the head of man, and man is the head of woman. I think that the women in Corinth who were removing their veils or who were wearing short hair did not have that theology. I [would argue that] it was not important for him theologically to make any change in those structures. He felt that they were in accordance with God's will, and they were significant enough [for him] to try to give a theological underpinning to them. So that he's not just a passive recipient of the world around him, he actually tries to give a theological reason for maintaining certain societal customs and structures. . . .I think that for Paul justification by faith, the significance of the belief in Christ as the crucified and risen one, and a change of life on the basis of this belief, are what are most important to him. Theologically, I'm not in agreement with this focus.

A SETTING FOR VIOLENCE AGAINST WOMEN
How do you handle these two things: your questions about, and your theological disagreement with, Paul?
Brooten: If I assume that God is the head of Christ, Christ is the head of the man, and the man is the head of the woman, I have set up the basis for a structure of violence. I am of the opinion that adult women will not submit [to this kind of reasoning] without some sort of force, which may be psychic violence or physical violence or economic restrictions.

So essentially what you're saying is that in some ways Paul's theology has hurt women?
Brooten: Yes. The view that the man is the head of woman is the view that keeps the leadership abilities, the intellectual contributions and capabilities of women from being recognized, appreciated and integrated into society. It is an enormous waste for our culture that women's leadership and intellectual capabilities have not been integrated fully into the culture.

You devote much intellectual energy to clarifying the fact that psychic or even physical violence is built into the New Testament. How did these writings, so discrimatory toward women, come to be preserved?
Brooten: The New Testament writings were written within a male-dominated, patriarchal culture. To make the writings that have emerged from that culture normative means to make that culture normative. Many scholars and lay people feel that this study of women in the New Testament is the study of a peripheral matter, that it is off of the main theological core.

Will you explain?
Brooten: Well, one looks at Pauline theology and sees justification, the crucifixion, the resurrection, understandings of grace and sin, and sees that women do not fit into these things. Women are not important. One imagines that we can have a gender-neutral understanding of justification by faith, of sin, or of be-

lief in Christ. And yet, when Paul says that God is the head of Christ, Christ is the head of the man, and the man is the head of the woman, then we see that the Christ about whom he is speaking fits in a certain way into the hierarchy which he has constructed to keep women from developing fully. So that, in fact, the way that Paul uses Christ is not gender-neutral.

Now one has to be very careful here. Paul has tension in this respect. He also says there is not male and female in Christ, and there is neither slave nor free, neither Jew nor Gentile. And he also works well with women colleagues. For example, a woman apostle is mentioned by him in his letter to the Romans.

Who was she?

Brooten: Junia, in Romans 16:7. Prisca was also a woman with whom he worked closely, together with her husband. Aquila and Prisca taught in the synagogue, as stated in Acts. And so it's not the case that he clearly says women should not be allowed outside of the home, should not be involved in the leadership of the church. He has a complex understanding, but nevertheless, in the end, he is not interested in seeing a basic change in societal structures. Not with respect to slavery, not with respect to women.

He rejects and condemns same-sex love. He is very condemnatory of all non-Christian religions so that his theology. . .if one accepts, for example, without question his theology of justification which seems to be gender-neutral, one will have to ask from which sins is one justified? In Romans, one of the sins from which one is not justified is for women to love women or for men to love men. And for him, that kind of a love relationship represents a fundamental alienation from God. So that justification is not an abstract concept in Paul; it is a concrete concept. Justification and the condemnation of same-sex love are thus interwoven with each other. Now this does not mean that Paul's understanding of justification might not be useful theologically today. It means that one cannot take Paul's theology and make it the theology of the church without bringing along with that theology a number of the aspects of the patriarchal culture from which he comes and in which he participated.

SAME-SEX LOVE IN THE NEW TESTAMENT
I think it would be useful to talk more about same-sex love since

I'm on that subject. Let me give a short summary. On the basis of my research I have found that Paul's condemnation of same-sex love is closely related to his view that the man is the head of the woman. And if one studies his words in the context of other ancient writers on same-sex love, one finds that those who rejected it in antiquity, in the ancient world, often did so out of the belief that female roles and male roles are very different from one another. Therefore, for a man to express his love for another man sexually is for one of the two men to become like a woman. That is, to sink to the level of a woman. For a woman to express her love for another woman sexually is to try to become like a man. This is an unacceptable crossing of gender boundaries and is seen to some ancient writers as contrary to nature. Paul describes such love relations as contrary to nature also, so that we cannot take his rejection of same-sex love out of the context from which it came: the understanding of what is masculinity and what is femininity. . . .And therefore it would be inconsistent, for example, for a church to call for the equality of women while at the same time rejecting love between women and love between men.

THE BIBLE AND AMERICAN LAW
In your teaching of the New Testament, is a focus on something like same-sex love novel?
Brooten: Well, that's one thing I've done a lot of work on. One way in which the Bible continues to function today is through laws that have a biblical root, even though the Bible may no longer be quoted in them. For example, many of the early sodomy laws in this country quoted the Bible, usually Leviticus, occasionally Romans. The laws today don't quote the Bible, but the root of the recent Supreme Court decision on the Georgia sodomy laws is biblical and religious [see Appendix D for details of the case].

In ancient Rome, in the pre-Christian period, there was not any kind of a general prohibition of same-sex love. Under Christian influence, there came to be more restrictive laws. This continued into the Middle Ages, when the ecclesiastical courts had jurisdiction. Henry VIII and Elizabeth I also took over from the ecclesiastical courts into their own royal courts—the secular courts—jurisdiction for sodomy. Later English common law came to be the basis of American law. In some cases, however, the Bible was actually quoted in the case of colonies which did not take over English common law.

In the state of Georgia, English common law was the law in effect at the time of Georgia's existence as a colony. The recent Supreme Court decision on the sodomy law in Georgia upholding the sodomy law gives as its primary argument the antiquity of the sodomy laws. Justice Burger in his concurring opinion refers to "Judaeo-Christian moral and ethical standards." The legal brief of the state of Georgia explicitly mentions the Bible. They mention Romans; they mention Leviticus; they also mention Thomas Aquinas. So if one knows both the history of these laws and if one looks at the legal discussion that led to the Supreme Court decision and the opinion itself, one can see that religion has been very important in this decision. Religion in general, and the Bible in particular.

In the Supreme Court decision, the majority opinion does not contain an explicit mention of the Bible. It speaks of the antiquity of the laws. But if one knows legal history, one recognizes the reason that these laws go back so far is because of biblical and other religious influences. Ancient Greece did not have laws outlawing same-sex love. Roman pre-Christian society did not, but under Christian influence they did. There were some tendencies in that direction within Roman pre-Christian society and there was a law that apparently was primarily against homosexual rape. But it would be very misleading to suggest, or it was very misleading of Burger to state in his concurring opinion, that according to Roman law sodomy was a capital crime. It was [in] this Christian period that it was introduced.

So that the Bible and history are being used inaccurately in this case. . . ?

Brooten: Yes, that's right. And I think it has important implications for biblical scholars. I think biblical scholars have a contribution to make by pointing out this biblical background and by questioning this use of the Bible.

So you cannot take something acceptable in the first century, or in early Christian times and apply it word for word or law for law to this time without taking that period's history into account.

Brooten: Yes. It's not clear that what Paul wrote was always accepted in the communities which received his letters. We don't know what the women in Corinth did when they received the letter about veiling. We don't know what the communities in Galatia did when they received his letter that dealt with circumcision and dietary laws. So we do not have the whole picture of Christian communities. We have the very powerful letters of Paul, the gospels and so forth. But we don't always have other Christian views.

For example, take the gospels—there are Jewish-Christian gospels that are not included in the New Testament. Now the gospels included in the New Testament may well have been written by Jews. There are, however, gospels [such] as the Gospel of the Ebonites, also a gospel of a Jewish-Christian community, which did not break with Judaism but continued to see itself as Jewish. The early Jewish-Christians in the second or third or fourth centuries apparently called their churches synagogues, rather than adopting the term "church." They maintained the structures of synagogue leadership and stayed in closer contact with Judaism. These are some of the writings that we have not included in the New Testament canon.

WOMEN IN THE NEW TESTAMENT
Do you think that these writings originally may have been more favorable to women? Or is that in dispute?
Brooten: To take the question of the Ebonites, it's difficult to say. I like to encourage people to read as widely as they can in early Christian literature and not restrict themselves to the New Testament canon. I'll give one example that relates to the history of women. The Acts of Paul and Thecla is a writing by a person who seems to be a follower of Paul. The date is not clear. It may be from the first century, it may be from the second century. In this writing a woman becomes a convert to Christianity through Paul and she refuses to marry her fiance who is the leading man of the city. Instead she goes out, she follows Paul, she runs into grave difficulties with the authorities. The story ends, with the words, "Having enlightened many with the word of God, she slept a noble sleep." She is thus depicted as an active missionary: a woman who is active as a leader and who refuses to marry, which causes great consternation in her own family [and] others in the city.

If one compares this writing with some writings within the New Testament, perhaps written about the same time—the Pastoral Epistles, such as First and Second Timothy, or Titus—one reads that a woman should not teach or have authority over a man. In the Pastoral Epistles, men are depicted positively as teaching, but women will be saved through childbearing, and thus as wives and mothers.

Yet Thecla refuses to marry.

Brooten: In fact, she refuses to marry. So we see that there are differing views [among] people who were associated with Paul. And the view that came to be accepted within the canon was that women should be subordinate. This other writing which depicts a woman as not subordinate and an active leader was not included. Now I wouldn't say that the Acts of Paul and Thecla is a feminist writing. I think that it was written within a patriarchal context, but did present an alternative vision for women. The alternative vision was celibacy. That was an important alternative vision within early Christianity for women. Celibacy had the possibility of calling into question the subordination of women within marriage.

Do you mean celibate women need not be subordinate to men?

Brooten: Well, if a woman can be a teacher as a celibate woman, then a married woman may ask why she too cannot be a teacher. The existence of a woman as a thinking, active, traveling person calls into question the subordination of women within marriage. Also, giving women an alternative to marriage might cause the institution of marriage to change in order to keep women in it. What has happened, however, through Christian history, was that celibacy was not ultimately allowed to call marriage into question. And I think that the way that this worked most effectively was to make celibacy like marriage so that a religious woman came to be considered the bride of Christ. In other words, this woman is not without a man over her. There is a man over her.

Namely, Christ.

Brooten: Namely, Christ. So then celibacy is seen to be like marriage, which allows marriage to remain as it is.

What would have happened had there been a different view of celibacy?

Brooten: Take, for example, the institution of spiritual marriage in the early church. Spiritual marriage was marriage in which the couple did not have intercourse with each other, yet lived together, supported each other in their Christian lives, and apparently had a different understanding of the roles of women and men than was traditional. For example, the Church Father, John Chrysostom, writes that the men in such marriages sit down and spin with the women, while the women take up business activities and the men support them in this. He says that the men should remember that they are soldiers of Christ and not behave in this fashion.

In other words, "Straighten up."

Brooten: "Straighten up!" So I think that that kind of celibacy showed that women and men could live together without any particular role division. If they showed it [worked], then others might think they could do this too. The celibacy in a community showed that it was possible to live as a full human being and not be lonely. You don't have to live within marriage; you can live with other members of your own sex. Or celibacy; as the so-called anchorites, that is, people who lived alone in the desert or lived alone in cells elsewhere, showed, it was possible to live alone and be a full human being. You don't need a member of the opposite sex to complement you. If, therefore, a woman is a full human being who does not need a man to complement her, which celibacy shows, then might not one think that within marriage a woman is a full human being and does not need a man, and a man is a full human being and does not need a woman? That could have changed the understanding of marriage. But what happened within Christian history was that [leaders were] essentially able to domesticate celibacy, to make it like marriage so that marriage could remain as it was.

And not upset the structure.

Brooten: And not upset the structure.

Was it an accident that the canon of the New Testament, the four gospels and the epistles, was chosen?

Brooten: It took a number of centuries before the canon as we know it became fixed. The New Testament writers were writing letters to particular congregations, or they were writing accounts of the life of Jesus. The New Testament canon arose over a period of centuries. There were some books of the New Testament that were in dispute for quite a number of centuries: the Revelation of John, the Epistle to the Hebrews, some of the so-called Catholic epistles; Second Peter and Jude are examples. There were other writings that some Christians included in their canon, such as the Acts of Paul, the Jewish-Christian Gospel to the Hebrews, the Epistle of Barnabas, or the so-called Didache. And there was not a uniform New Testament that was used everywhere in early Christianity.

JESUS AND DIVORCE: CHURCH AND ANNULMENT

Divorce in the New Testament is forbidden. From a scholar's viewpoint, will you interpret this prohibition?

Brooten: I think I'll start with the contemporary policy. The Catholic church does not allow divorce. It only allows annulment. In order to obtain an annulment, one must establish that marriage in the fullest sense did not take place, that is, that the marriage was not valid from the beginning. In recent years there's been a so-called liberalization of the Catholic annulment policy, whereas previously very few annulments were granted. The number has increased significantly in recent years and one might think that this is an improvement. I think that it is, but the annulment, the policy of the Catholic hierarchy on divorce, is still very problematic.

Why is that?

Brooten: In the first place, the annulment procedure is a very intrusive one. Detailed questions of sexual relations within the marriage are asked, and the person requesting the annulment and the respondent, the former spouse, are asked in the form of a questionnaire, or through an oral interview, detailed questions of their intimate life. This is the basis upon which an annulment is granted or is not granted. This intrusiveness is seen to be quite normal. The marriage tribunals are to a large extent all male, and women are expected to appear before them or to present in writing to an all-male or nearly all-male tribunal, details of their intimate sexual life for review. Then on the basis of particular legal grounds within canon law, the annulment will or will not be granted. The basic principle, that the marriage had never really taken place, is totally hypocritical.

For the Catholic hierarchy, the origin of this annulment policy is the strict adherence to Jesus' divorce prohibition. Jesus did not allow divorce at all and [many are] unwilling to depart from this divorce prohibition. The divorce prohibition occurs in several forms, in more than one form in the gospels of Matthew, Mark, Luke, and in First Corinthians written by Paul. There is no doubt that this is an original saying of Jesus, that in some form he prohibited divorce. To be sure, this prohibition of divorce has in some cases through history protected women from arbitrary dismissal by their husbands. It has protected women sometimes. However, it has also kept women within violent marriages. It has kept women in marriages to men who incestually abuse their children. It has therefore changed the character of marriage.

An institution from which there is no exit becomes a different kind of institution. Not to allow divorce means that women experience marriage in a different way. If there is never the possibility of the dissolution of the marriage, then violence and other forms of abuse can continue in a much more unhindered way than if there were a way out. The practice within Christianity has in fact not always been as rigid. The Eastern church, for example, has had a different policy toward divorce than the Western church. And now this policy of annulments in the church, in fact, constitutes something like allowing divorce.

However, it also requires that people deny a part of their history—that the marriage ever really took place—by looking back to the period before they married. They must find a reason for the marriage not being valid, which becomes a very strange way of rewriting one's own history. Further, the reason that more annulments are now granted is that one has defined marriage in a much different way than previously, so that the spiritual aspects, the emotional and psychological aspects, are much more strongly emphasized.

You mean in the Catholic church. . . ?

Brooten: Especially in the Catholic church. So that now one must say that in the truest sense of union, the marriage never took place. There is a different understanding of marriage than had been current previously. Under that previous understanding, very few annulments were granted. This newer understanding allows for a new kind of intrusiveness. For example, one may require psychiatric examinations or [have to answer] psychological questions concerning one's personal history.

ANTI-SEMITISM AND THE NEW TESTAMENT
Isn't it possible that Jesus may have been thinking of the protection of women?

Brooten: Well, I think it's difficult to know what Jesus was thinking because he doesn't say it. The argument that he was thinking of the protection of women, I believe, is an anti-Jewish argument. That is, one argues that within Judaism women did not have the right to divorce their husbands, and that therefore Jesus was protecting women from being divorced, women who did not have the right to initiate divorce themselves. The second argument is that women in those times who were divorced by their husbands were destitute and probably had to become prostitutes or vagrants. These two arguments are based upon a one-sided, negative view of the situation of women in Judaism at the time of Jesus.

There were circles within Judaism in which women could not initiate divorce and there were circles in which women could initiate divorce. There were situations in which women who were divorced were destitute, but there is evidence that not all women within Judaism who were divorced would have been destitute. There's more evidence of the economic activity of Jewish women than one had previously thought. This is thus an example of the way scholars of the New Testament may rely upon an inaccurate picture of Judaism in order to defend a saying of Jesus with which they do not essentially agree. You see, it's liberal scholars arguing for liberalization of divorce policy who say that the intention of Jesus was to protect women, so that if that was his intention, we could allow divorce today.

The problem is that that argument is based upon a. . . negative view of women in Judaism. It's inaccurate. And so it's an argument that's built on the backs of Jewish women. If we carefully study the history of Jewish women in this period, we will not see that the situation of women in Judaism was radically different from the situation of women in early Christianity. There were women within Judaism who were leaders in the synagogue, there were women within Christianity who were leaders. There were some Jewish women who were active in the economy, and there were some early Christian women who controlled funds of various sorts to be able to donate to churches.

There were some Jewish women who were educated, there were some Christian women who were educated. An important part of working against Christian anti-Semitism is learning to be more accurate in understanding the history of Judaism: the situation of Jews today and the situation of Jews in the past.

Could you talk further about anti-Semitism. Rosemary Ruether writes that the roots of the New Testament are essentially anti-Semitic. Do you agree? Also, will you explain why the Pharisees received so much cristicism from Jesus?

Brooten: The early Christians were extremèly disappointed that most Jews did not accept Jesus as the messiah. From what we know of Jewish literature in the post-biblical period, Jews were not especially interested in the messiah. They did not write very much about the messiah. Because of the fact that a number of Christians still remained within synagogues and preached within synagogues, there were great conflicts between those Jews who believed in Jesus as the Christ and those Jews who did not. And these conflicts escalated and became more than simple conflicts. Out of this anger on the part of believers in Jesus toward Jews who did not believe in Jesus, we come to a very distorted picture of certain aspects of ancient Judaism in the New Testament.

For example, if one were to read only the New Testament, one would think that the primary characteristic of the Pharisees was hypocrisy. If we look at other ancient texts from the first century and at later texts, we will find that the Pharisees were a group which in some ways democratized Judaism. That is, they strove to make it possible for common people to make their daily lives sacred so that a person could learn how to follow the law, the Torah. Through the educational programs instituted by the Pharisees, a Jew could learn how to follow these complicated laws which before they may not have thought possible. A person who didn't wish to follow these laws would consider that a burden. A person who did wish to follow them would consider helpful an educational program on how to do so.

These programs on Torah were not solely for the elite then.

Brooten: No. I might add that studying the Pharisees shows us once again that there is no objective history. We can't take one account of the Pharisees and say this is the accurate account. We also can't take one account of Jesus and say this is the real Jesus. We can't take one account of Alexander the Great and say this is Alexander the Great. Every author writes from his or her own perspective and understanding of the meaning of history or the significance of a given figure. . . .Christians today must be very careful to work toward a more accurate picture of ancient Judaism because there has been a very distorted picture throughout most of Christian history. And accuracy doesn't mean objectivity. In looking at the Pharisees, I would want to look at all the sources. The New Testament documents are a critique of the Pharisees. Other documents present the Pharisees more positively and it's important to look at all of those to try to understand the group, its significance, the opponents of it.

EXPLOITATION OF WOMEN SLAVES

Could you talk about violence and the exploitation of female slaves in the New Testament?

Brooten: Let's go to the sexual exploitation of female slaves and I'll start with slavery in this country. There was sexual exploitation of female slaves in America. How is it possible that this could go on among men who professed to be Bible-believing Christians? There is strong evidence that in the Roman Empire sexual exploitation of female slaves was not uncommon. The New Testament doesn't address this question. There is no explicit discussion of the sexual use of female slaves. Perhaps an indirect reference would be to prostitutes because a number of slaves were prostitutes. But in the passages of the New Testament dealing with slavery there is no explicit reference to female slaves, or to sexual exploitation of female slaves. In the New Testament passages which command slaves to be subordinate to their masters, [we find that] the term used for slaves is a word that includes both women and men. But to command a female Christian slave to be obedient in every respect to a male, non-Christian slave-owner means to allow the continuation of the possibility of the sexual exploitation of that female Christian slave. Not to address the question of the sexual use of female slaves while commanding that female slaves be subordinate to their masters is to allow such exploitation to exist.

INCEST IN CHRISTIAN HOMES

Do you find that this position has continued in the church?

Brooten: I think that it's something that has been tolerated. This kind of sexual exploitation along with other kinds of sexual exploitation, if they are not explicitly addressed, will continue. Let me take the example of father/daughter incest. According to a study done by the sociologist Diane Russell, of 930 randomly selected women in San Francisco, 152 or sixteen percent had been incestually abused as children. This study cannot take into account repression of memories so that if the women had totally repressed the memories of an incest history, they would not have answered positively to the questions in this study. This abuse goes on in Christian families, in non-Christian families; it goes on in every social class, it cuts across all kinds of ethnic and racial lines. It is not the case that only poor, working-class, black or white families experience incest. Nor is it the case that upper class or middle class white families are in any way exempted from this practice. This goes on. . .

Across all social strata.

Brooten: Yes, across all social strata. And the question now is what does this have to do with Christianity? Well, for one thing, if it goes on in Christian homes and it is not addressed as a church issue, it will continue. The Christian churches have practically ignored such abuse for centuries. If leading men in the church can incestually abuse their daughters with no intervention, it will continue. The New Testament does not address itself to this issue. There's one passage in Paul that may be a reference; it's unclear. But, yes, I should say only recently has there begun to be literature on incestuous abuse.

Do you think that this recent literature may be due to the emergence of women scholars in the field?

Brooten: Yes, it is. The women's movement has addressed the question of violence toward women in a general way and on the basis of women having the possibility to speak about violence in a way that had not been previously possible. Women began to speak more. When women began to speak out more, then scholars, feminist scholars, studied what was going on and wrote about it. Previously there had been denial of the existence of incest in psychological literature, psychiatric literature, medical literature, etc. Sigmund Freud was especially important in this development in that in his early practice he encountered quite a number of women who reported incestuous abuse by their fathers. He first believed them. Later he could not accept that so many women could have been incestually abused, and then he turned to believing that they had fantasized it. And this Freudian view significantly influenced psychiatry and the whole mental health profession.

Until the women's movement.

Brooten: Until the women's movement, which changed this situation. For the first time women could be believed. How this sexual abuse within Christian families relates to the Bible is the question I would like now to pose.

First, it is very problematic to [state], as moral advice to a woman who has been sexually abused, [that she] turn the other cheek as the Bible teaches. This is a saying of Jesus that is most likely an authentic saying of Jesus. It is normally extolled as of high moral validity. Women who have been violently abused have been taught to turn the other cheek. I have come to the conclusion over the years that telling women who are beaten by their husbands or forced to have sexual intercourse against their will by their husbands, or forced by their fathers or brothers or uncles to have sexual intercourse as children—in other words to turn the other cheek—is unconscionable.

How would you rectify this?

Brooten: I support what is presently going on, which is that more and more women are coming forth and describing violent abuse toward themselves. Being able to speak about the abuse is a very important step toward stopping it. Some churches are becoming aware of such abuse occurring within families who are members of those churches. And some feminists in church work are writing about and speaking about violence toward women.

A fundamental difficulty is that the churches do not have a history of taking seriously violence toward women, and if the subordination of women is enshrined within Christian tradition, then it is difficult even to see it. This subordination of women has been coupled with violence toward women, violence which has been quite acceptable. It has often been quite acceptable to discipline one's wife; it has, in fact, been considered quite normal. Having intercourse with one's wife when she doesn't wish it has not been considered problematic. Therefore, women speaking about violence is a revolutionary breakthrough and an important step. One must understand the historical origins of violence, and that's where I think the study of the New Testament and of the other sources of Christian theology is important.

CHRISTOLOGY AND WOMEN

I want to ask you about christology. Nuns, as Sister Augusta Neal's study *Catholic Sisters in Transition* notes, are among the most educated group of women in this country. They and other women have indicated some problems with christology. Would you address this problem from your perspective?

Brooten: Christology is the theological understanding of Christ. The maleness of Christ is a strong important strand within Catholic christology and other Christian christologies. A christology which emphasizes the masculinity of Christ is often a christology which is used in the subordination of women or the exclusion of women from priestly office. The Vatican declaration on the ordination of women to the priesthood makes this its primary point. Because Christ was a male, women cannot be ordained, because women cannot represent Christ physically. This is a christology which emphasizes the masculinity of Christ. There have been other examples of this through Christian history.

The question before feminist theology today is whether there can be a christology in which the masculinity of Christ is not significant or is not used in this way. Within the New Testament we already find the beginnings of a christology of masculinity. For example, in the letter to the Ephesians, a wife is told to be subordinate to her husband as to the Lord. The husband is thus compared to Christ. The church is compared with the woman. This image of Christ as the bridegroom and the church as the bride, which has been used as the model for Christian marriage, is a text often used in marriage ceremonies. The text is based upon an understanding of Christ in which it is not possible to exchange the two images, to say that Christ is the image of the bride and the church is the image of the bridegroom. Another way to view Jesus would be to think of him as a brother.   I think that it may be possible theologically to develop a way of understanding Jesus in which his masculinity is not central.   Within the Catholic tradition, however, that masculinity been central and it has been used to keep women from leadership.

How did you obtain this internal freedom to lay your own theology alongside ancient theology and, as conflicts emerged, to raise questions? How did this happen and where do you see your future?

Brooten: It was a gradual process. I have found that there is great strength in understanding how violence toward oneself works. We are taught that to be the victim of violence is a shameful thing. We are taught as women to be victims and I have found that learning to speak about the ways in which women have been victimized gives me, as a woman, strength. That is, the strength that I find is the strength that is not granted to me. Women are not granted power by men. Rather, we learn to accept the power that we have. . . .

More Catholic women today are learning that we do not need to ask the male hierarchy for power. We are learning to accept the spiritual power within us. Accepting the spiritual power that is available to women is threatening to oneself because of the consequences. It certainly causes, and will cause, conflicts with those who perceive themselves to be the only legitimate controllers of power. That's the reason why the Vatican in general, and Cardinal Ratzinger in particular, is so concerned about the power of American Catholic women and how to contain it. There is this power which is a spiritual power within us. We have not had to ask for it or to take it from someone else.

When I speak of the spiritual power of women, I don't mean that the spiritual power of women will necessarily prevail. I think it's possible that the atom bomb will prevail. To the extent to which women oppose the inhumane use of violence, women will prevail. Within the Catholic church there is an increasing number of women opposing the use of inhumane violence. The power that comes from that opposition comes from within and is very great.

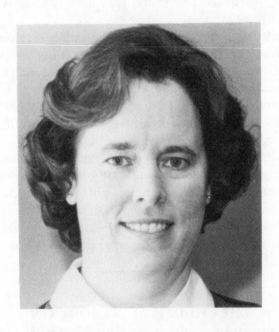

MARJORIE REILEY MAGUIRE

"You can murder the president, you can torture people, you can be a terrorist, blow up a department store, push the button to end the world, and yet you're not excommunicated. You can even kill a newborn baby and not get excommunicated. But if you commit the sin of abortion. . .you are automatically excommunicated."

Marjorie Reiley Maguire is a theologian who attended Catholic schools from kindergarten to Catholic University of America in Washington, D.C., where she earned her doctrorate in 1976. She decided to become a nun while still in high school but her parents talked her into waiting until she finished college. After teaching for a year, she entered a convent and "lasted four months."

Her ambition to study theology began in the mid-1960s. One of her professors was Dr. Daniel Maguire, then a Roman Catholic priest, whom she eventually married, and who presently teaches at Marquette University. They have one surviving son, Tommy, aged eleven.

The resume, writings, speeches, and public services of this educator are impressive, and one asks why is she not employed in a Catholic university. "You'd think," she says, "that Catholic institutions would want to give an example to others by hiring family teams who were competent in the same area. It would demonstrate solidarity of the family and avoid commuter marriages. But this isn't the way they operate."

The difficulty of getting a job in Catholic academe, she believes, is partly the market, and partly the difficulty encountered by women of independent thought. After spending many years of preparing to teach theology, Dr. Maguire now feels she must salvage what is left of her life in some other field. In the following interview she dicusses what that life is and how she envisions her future. _____

THE CHURCH AND ABORTION

Briefly and simply, why is the church's position on abortion not "monolithic?"

Maguire: There are a number of reasons. The first reason is because I am the church, you are the church, all who read this are the church. When the press or others ask what does the church teach on abortion, they are thinking of the hierarchy. When I say the church's position is pluralistic, not monolithic, I'm thinking of the Vatican II notion of the whole church.

The people of God. . . ?

Maguire: Yes, and it is a fact that there are diverse opinions on abortion in the Catholic church. The second reason is because (even when you look at the hierarchy) Catholicism always held that the only things you had to believe without question were infallible teachings. No pope has ever issued an infallible declaration on the subject of abortion. In fact, it surprises people that no pope has ever issued an infallible declaration on any moral issue. We know what some of the hierarchy has had to say on moral issues, including abortion. Everybody knows John Paul II's position on abortion. But he has never proclaimed it an infallible declaration. So, if it's not infallible, it's fallible. Fallible means it could be wrong. Therefore, Catholics who disagree with his statement have an obligation to the church to say where they disagree. They have an obligation to let their pluralism be known. The pope's position on abortion is monolithic, but not the church's. [The third reason is that] as a theologian, I know the history of church teaching on abortion.

Will you review it?

Maguire: The bishops often say it has been "the common and constant teaching of the church that abortion is morally wrong," a heinous crime. But when I review the history, I find a much different picture than they see. First of all, they are right in holding that the church always taught that abortion is wrong. But the reasons why it was wrong are not the reasons these bishops give. Bishops today tend to treat it as murder. The tradition did not treat abortion as murder. The reason abortion was condemned in the tradition, by St. Augustine and others, was because it was seen as anti-contraceptive, anti-procreative. Anything considered anti-procreative was condemned. Very early, Christianity got the idea that the only thing that could make sex acceptable was that it issue in procreation. Reproduction, therefore, made sex acceptable.

Christians were contaminated by the Stoics (early Greek philosophers) who believed that we must always act according to reason. Any time emotions or passions entered in, they clouded reason and made a human being lesser, closer to an animal. This was not a Jewish idea (our birth parents as Christians); this was not an early Christian idea. This was a pagan idea that came into Christianity.

Could you elaborate?

Maguire: This was a pagan notion in the atmosphere at the time, and it's interesting that early Christianity allowed it to seep into Christian thinking, allowed it to distort our thinking on sexuality for two thousand years. Because the Stoics said you could only have sex if it was oriented toward something reasonable, then contraception became evil, homosexuality was evil, abortion was evil, all because they kept the sex act from issuing into reproduction.

St. Augustine did not believe that abortion was wrong because it was murder. In fact, he says in his commentary on the Book of Exodus that the fetus cannot yet have a soul if it is not formed as a human being in the flesh. His words are [On Exodus, 21.80]: "The law does not provide that the act (abortion) pertains to homicide, for there cannot yet be said to be a live soul in a body that lacks sensation, when it is not formed in flesh and so is not endowed with sense."

Thomas Aquinas teaches the same thing: until you have a body formed as a human body, you can't speak of a human soul. Now, the objection is sometimes raised that these people did not know today's biology. However, their teaching was philosophical, not biological. They had a valid philosophical insight that you cannot really speak of a human being before it looks like a human being, before it can function like a human being. I think if they knew our modern biology, and they were basing personhood solely on biology, they would say there is no possibility of a soul until you have the cortex of the brain. That is the basic thing you need [in order] to have a functioning human body. The cortex comes late in the pregnancy, the end of the second trimester. Thus, I don't think they would change their basic philosophical position today, even knowing our biology.

Besides being considered anti-procreative, a second reason why abortion was considered wrong [is that] it was seen as a way somebody could cover up other sexual sins, such as fornication or adultery. But the tradition rarely taught it was wrong because it was murder. Until 1869, for the majority of theologians in the Catholic church, it was a "way out" opinion to think that the embryo, the fetus, was a person from the first moment of conception. There were a few people who thought that, but it was considered a minority opinion.

A DIFFERENT UNDERSTANDING OF PERSONHOOD
What happened in 1869?

Maguire: The pope at the time bought into this theory. Pius IX was a very authoritarian pope who gave us the doctrine of infallibility, also defined the Immaculate Conception of Mary. When you put all these things together, you can see he had a political reason for buying the theory that personhood begins at conception. What I will say in his defense is that biology had newly discovered the existence of the ovum, and hence woman's part in conception was recognized. Before then it was always thought that man contributed the totality of what became a person and that woman only provided the growing place. But when the ovum was discovered, fertilization was discovered. However, in 1854, Pius IX had defined the dogma of the Immaculate Conception, that Mary was free of sin from the first moment of her conception. But if you were the pope defining this dogma, you wouldn't want to have everyone else's personhood beginning later than conception.

An interesting point, though, is that Pius IX never explicitly said that personhood begins at conception. However, in 1869, he issued legislation making excommunication the penalty for abortion at any stage of pregnancy. Thus, he implicitly endorsed the idea that the soul entered at conception. Yet he did not issue an infallible document on abortion then or later. (Infallibility was defined as a dogma in 1870 at Vatican I.) There had been only one other time in the history of the church when excommunication was the penalty for abortion. That was in the three year period from 1588-1591.

Why then?

Maguire: The pope at that time, Sixtus V, made excommunication a penalty for abortion because there was a large number of prostitutes in Rome. He thought that if he made excommunication the penalty for abortion, he could cut down on prostitution. It didn't work. The next pope, Gregory XIV, took away the penalty. It was the only time in history until 1869 that excommunication was the penalty for abortion.

It has stayed that way since?

Maguire: Yes. Now, the real interesting thing about the [recent] changes in the Code of Canon Law is that the number of things for which one can be excommunicated dropped. Perhaps thirty or forty cases came down to six. One of those six is the sin of abortion. I'll come back to why I say the "sin" of abortion. But first it is important to realize that you can murder the president, you can torture people, you can be a terrorist, blow up a department store, push the button to end the world, and you're not excommunicated. You can even kill a newborn baby and not get excommunicated. But if you commit the sin of abortion, they say you are automatically excommunicated.

Excommunication as a penalty has no meaning if it isn't applied to things people really see as sins. Also, people mistakenly think that if a woman walks into an abortion clinic, has an abortion, she is automatically excommunicated. It is not true. Excommunication is only for the sin of abortion. Remember, the Catholic cathechism told us there were three things necessary to commit a mortal sin. It had to be seriously wrong; secondly, one must know it was seriously wrong; thirdly, one had to believe it was seriously wrong and still do it, thus flying in the face of conscience, and in the face of God. But a woman who goes into an abortion clinic, thinking she's doing the right thing, has not fulfilled that second condition. She, therefore, has not committed a sin. Hence, she is not excommunicated. Automatic excommunication only means that your bishop is not going to write and tell you you're excommunicated. If you think it's a sin, excommunication is automatic. If you don't think it's a sin, there is no excommunication.

Why do you think abortion is such a charged issue?

Maguire: I think it's fear of women. It's fear of the power women have over their bodies. The hierarchy is trying to control that power. I think it's basically tied into birth and pregnancy and it's sort of a "uterus envy." Freud spoke about "penis envy" and there are women psychologists who have spoken about uterus, "womb envy." I really think these men have that envy at the subconscious level. We need a psychologist to further probe this anomaly. They think that women have too much power over the life processes, and they don't want them to possess such power. Moreover, if these churchmen have control over someone's sexuality, they then really have control over [that person]. So for the hierarchy of the church to give up control in the sexual arena is to make them feel like they have no authority whatsoever.

Do you think their emphasis and intransitory position on this issue may be due to lack of experience?

Maguire: They have unrealistic, celibate ideas about sexuality. Benedictus Merkelbach, the author of one of the old, influential moral manuals, wrote that couples should not have sex more than three or four times a night. Now, how many married couples do you know who have sex three times a night? The problem is that bishops have been trained in this kind of male, celibate, unrealistic, and romantic view of sex.

Let us take the state of Rhode Island: The population is sixty-four percent Catholic and sixty-eight percent of the

people having abortions at the state's largest maternity hospital are Catholics. Do you believe they think abortion is wrong?

Maguire: I think many Catholic women who have abortions do not believe it's wrong. The problem, however, is that some of them are not quite sure. In their heart they don't believe it's wrong, but they've been taught all their lives that it is, hence, they go on a guilt trip. With our first child, we did not believe in a magical notion of baptism, or that our baby would go to limbo if he weren't baptized. We waited four weeks because we wanted a ceremony with grandparents present and with an uncle who is a priest. But one tiny part of my being was worried: suppose he dies and there is a limbo. I was trained as a theologian and I still had to overcome that emotion. Now pity the poor woman who doesn't have all my training and who's been told all her life that anyone who has an abortion is a sinner. Her whole experience tells her: no, this is not a sin, this is what I should do. But there is a conflict going on in her being because of this guilt trip that's been laid on her.

In addition, many feel guilty about using birth control, which is also considered sinful [by the institutional church].

Maguire: I heard that Catholic women have abortions rather than use birth control, because abortion is only a one-time sin. Using contraception constantly, that would be a sin every time. Or a sin, three times a night, if you follow Merkelbach. This is crazy thinking. Yet, it is the kind of thinking fostered in Catholic women.

HOW CATHOLIC WOMEN CAN BECOME FREE

As a trained theologian, how can you help women confronted by such teachings?

Maguire: Well, the only way is by speaking out and making people know the history. I've gone through this history and I believe as people hear it, they become freed. They will come to realize that the bishops either don't know or are covering up this history. I don't think all the bishops are evil; I think that some are ignorant. Others have only seminary training, which is a little bit more than a bachelor's degree. They are not trained in theology. Or they haven't been trained in theology since Vatican II; and they are not philosophers. . . .Many never stopped to ask, "What is a person?" "When does personhood begin?" and "What does personhood beginning automatically at fertilization say about God?" Yet these questions have to be asked and they have to be asked from the woman's point of view, from the woman's experience. When they are, they will then reflect womens' experience. And the idea of personhood beginning at fertilization does not reverberate with most women's experience.

Nobody thinks abortion is great, nor have I ever met anyone who is pro-abortion. However, I do not call life sacred, because then I would mean inviolable, and I'm not a vegetarian pacifist, so obviously I do believe life is violable. Even human life, I believe, is sometimes violable. I can justify self-defense; I am less comfortable with war and capital punishment. I [do not] say life is inviolable, nor does the church. Consequently, it is dishonest to say life is sacred. I believe persons are sacred, and their life is the most basic gift they possess. Thus, it is extremely valuable. Life can never be taken lightly.

THE NEW YORK TIMES AD

You were involved in the controversial ad on "Pluralism and Abortion" that appeared in *The New York Times*. How did this advertisement originate?

Maguire: People often ask, "What would have happened to the ad if the Vatican didn't come down on the twenty-four nun signers?" Some say we'd only be wrapping dead fish in *The Sunday New York Times* of October 7, 1984. But because the Vatican has kept it alive, it has now become "the famous ad."

It was conceived by my husband Dan and me as a statement to be signed by theologians. We thought it might eventually be used in testimony before Congress. Both of us were at the meeting of the Society of Christian Ethics in January 1983 where I presented a paper called "Personhood, Covenant and Abortion." Putting the final touches on the paper, I talked with Dan and Frances Kissling of Catholics For a Free Choice, who were also at the meeting, and suddenly we got the idea. Wouldn't it be a great time, we mused, to start a statement on abortion and circulate it to a few of the theologians present.

We sat and brainstormed about ideas. We had our little

nine-and-a-half-year old retarded son, Danny, with us, fearing to leave him with babysitters because he had started having seizures. He died nine months later. It's sort of ironic. We sat in the hotel room writing that statement while we tended to our son Danny.

Anyway, we circulated the statement and got about ten signatures. Frances Kissling asked to release it to the press. She did so on January 22, 1983 and there was little reaction.

In the next year and a half, as a Fellow in Theology and Ethics at Catholics for a Free Choice, I worked on gaining additional signatures from theologians. I got the mailing lists from the Catholic Theological Society, the College Theology Society, and the Catholic Biblical Association. Mailings to these groups gathered more signatures for what was called the "Catholic Statement on Pluralism and Abortion." By the summer of 1984, Governor Cuomo and Geraldine Ferraro came under attack for their positions on abortion. Then it occured to us that the press kept talking about the Catholic position on abortion, but we knew that there is no one Catholic position on abortion and we had at least seventy-five theologians who had signed the statement to prove it.

First, though, we wrote to all the signatories to let them know we would release the statement and the list of signers to the press. Not only did we want them to know, but we also wanted new names. We did get another group of signers besides theologians, including quite a few nuns. By the same token some previous signers had second thoughts and took their names off. There were also quite a few theologians who had indicated on a questionnaire that they agreed with the Catholic Statement but could not sign it because their jobs would be in "jeopardy." We also indicated that support when we published the ad. Finally, on October 7, 1984, the ad: "A Diversity of Opinions Regarding Abortion Exists Among Committed Catholics" appeared in *The New York Times* [see Appendix A].

Two signers still withhold compliance with the Vatican: Barbara Ferraro and Patricia Hussey. What are your thoughts on their actions as well as those of the other nuns?

Maguire: Well, I admire Ferraro and Hussey's courage greatly. This kind of resistance is needed to change the Vatican in the long run. It may not come in our lifetime, but each of these little acts added together lead to change. But I don't want to commend them and act like I'm criticizing the nuns who accommodated. Early on I thought all the nuns should just sign something. Why ruin their lives over an ad in *The New York Times*? It's not that important. The issue of abortion is important, woman's right to choice is important, but I questioned, Should they give up their lives over an ad? What I since have realized is that all the nuns took this issue more seriously than I did, realizing that if they [gave] in right away, it would have been a message to women that this issue is not important. Thus, I can understand accommodation with the Vatican and I also appreciate that the nuns held out as long as they did.

AFFECTS ON FAMILY

How did the abortion debate affect your husband and family?

Maguire: Besides the ad, my husband Dan Maguire was involved with the abortion debate in another way. He, on behalf of Catholics for a Free Choice, had briefed congressional leaders in 1982 and 1983 on Catholic theology and abortion. These breakfast meetings were sponsored by Geraldine Ferraro and two congressmen. His talks showed that Catholics can have attitudes on abortion that depart from those of hierarchy. "We are pluralistic, not monolithic," he said. Geraldine Ferraro used this phrase of Dan's to describe his talk to the participants at the briefings she sponsored. During the Presidential campaign in 1984, Archbishop [John] O'Connor [of New York] critized her for saying the Catholic position was not monolithic on abortion. Dan wrote to *The New York Times* saying that these were his words and not Ferraro's, and that the Archbishop should fight with him and other theologians who hold this [position] and not with Gerry Ferraro. With this and the ad and a lot of talks on abortion, he felt great stress and tension during the fall of 1984. He thought he could lose his job, and suddenly, we would be without support. The end result was that he wound up in the hospital in December 1984 needing three blood transfusions, because of a bleeding duodenum [small intestine]. Stress does affect people's health. Recently Sister Marge Tuite died supposedly of cancer, but studies show that cancer [may be] caused by psychological problems. The Vatican beat up on her so much that. . .it ate away at her. Sister Margaret Traxler, another signer, had a stroke, possibly brought on by this tension.

The other stresspoint for the family is that Dan had a series of invitations from academic institutions for 1985. He was scheduled to give workshops and courses in four places: St. Scholastica College, Duluth [Minnesota]; St. Martin's College in Lacey, Washington; Villanova University, Philadelphia; and Boston College. They were all cancelled over Dan's participation in the abortion issue.

Not only that, but invitations from Catholic academe for the future dried up. So there was a great deal of stress and it still continues. [Recently] the Creighton University in Omaha. . . invited him to speak. Later, the president cancelled the invitation saying Dan disagreed with the magisterium. Some faculty [at Creighton] disagreed with their president on the basis of academic freedom. They asked if any speaker who disagrees with the magisterium could be disinvited. For example, a general who bombs hospitals, or people who make nuclear weapons. We were told that the president of Creighton answered that there was no church teaching against bombing hospitals.

VIEWS ON PRESENT STATUS IN CHURCH
How do you perceive your relationship to the church?
Maguire: I'm a cradle Catholic and I'm not about to join some other church. I attended Catholic schools all my life and decided in high school I wanted to be a nun. My parents talked me out of it until I finished college. I taught for a year and then entered the convent. I only lasted four months. I wanted to study theology. I received a Ph.D. in religious studies at Catholic University in Washington, D.C. While there, I met my husband, Dan, a very liberal teacher. Gradually, my ideas changed. I saw his teaching was correct. I'm still the same nice Catholic "girl" that I always was. In that sense, I haven't changed at all.

Yet, how does my Catholicism today differ from when I was a child? It's not the same. I feel the church is my ethnic group, my family, something to identify with, but it's something I like less and less. Morris West puts my feelings well in *The Clowns of God:* "I cannot be quit of the church any more than I can be quit of my mother or father or my furthest ancestors. I cannot dispense with traditions that have shaped me. I cannot adopt another man's history or fabricate a new mythos for myself. I loathe what this family does, often, to its children; but I cannot leave it and will not traduce it. So I wait. . . ."

What are your thoughts on the woman-church movement?

Maguire: I went to woman-church when it met in Chicago in 1983 and was very moved. It's the way of the future. And yet I'm not active in any woman's prayer group in this city. In a sense, maybe I am trying to disengage from the church because I feel very rejected by this church which formed me. It makes me feel alienated.

A MALE-CONTROLLED CATHOLIC PRESS

Could you discuss your experiences with the Catholic press?

Maguire: The Catholic press is mostly unwilling to touch the issue of abortion from the pro-choice point of view. The Catholic press is controlled by men. Even if laymen, they are part of the hierarchy. They are part of the boys' club which doesn't see abortion as an important issue. Their attitude is illustrated by what a theologian said to me, "Why dwell on pro-choice? You take away from all these important issues: hunger, nuclear war, and, in fact, you're getting liberal bishops into trouble." These men who run *Commonweal* or *National Catholic Reporter,* both lay presses, have for years been pushing social justice. You have to give them credit. Finally, they now have in their corner the bishops, who for years couldn't care less about social justice issues. Suddenly, we women enter the picture and ask about women's ordination, and about abortion. These press men are finally so happy to be part of the old boys' club with the bishops turning to them for leadership on these social justice issues that they feel to take women's issues on would lead to a loss of credibility with the bishops.

My experience with the press is this. *National Catholic Reporter* is very anti-choice on abortion, but they have allowed a few pro-choice articles to be published, and will publish letters of a pro-choice nature. However, they were not supportive of the nun signers. They didn't see the issue. *National Catholic Reporter* has a long way to go, but it has shown at least a little willingness to discuss abortion. *Commonweal* is so ideologically closed that they have published only one pro-choice article. It was a marvelous article by Joan Callahan on abortion and public policy. But *Commonweal* couldn't print that alone. They had to print a rejoinder by Sidney Callahan, whom they called a feminist-for-life. She is anti-choice.

America is run by the Jesuits. They had an article by Richard Doeflinger, who heads the pro-life office for the bishops, questioning who really are Catholics for a Free Choice [CFFC]? He wrote a long article in *America*, attacking Catholics for a Free Choice. [He also attacked the Maguires.] He implied suspect funding sources for CFFC and [suggested] that CFFC had trapped the poor nuns into signing the ad. Who, he questioned, are the theologians who hold a different view from the bishops? I answered his questions in an article and sent it to *America*. They refused the article. The editor stated that it "would likely confuse our readers (and perhaps some ethicists I know), no end." My article, laying out the diversity in Catholic thought, would confuse people! In other words, the truth would confuse readers. He said he would allow a long letter up to a thousand words as a response but not the article. I wrote the letter. They didn't publish that either. I then sent the article to *Commonweal*. In a long, contorted letter they first considered it, changed their minds, reconsidered, changed again. People who have read it in *Conscience*, where it was finally published, agree it should have been published by *America*.

Was it frustrating for you not to be able to respond to Doeflinger in *America*?

Maguire: The editors of *America* are very anti-choice on abortion. They weren't concerned about truth. They were only concerned about ideology and about Doeflinger's connection with the bishops. When I came forward with evidence contrary to the assertions in his article, they could neither admit nor publish it.

Their magazine needs to survive; it's published in New York City. Do you think their funding situation and their setting had something to do with their decision not to run your article?

Maguire: Maybe that's it. Perhaps they really thought their readership would not tolerate my article. But it's sad, because the Jesuits had a reputation for excellence. They had a reputation for wanting to follow the truth. If they had printed the article somebody else could have come back and refuted it, or written another article or a letter. No, I don't think it was economics. I think the Jesuit reputation for intellectual excellence is false. That's sad.

Do you think that these men running *America* and *Commonweal* and *National Catholic Reporter* find it difficult to acknowledge, or to even know, that they are sexist?

Maguire: I don't think it's asking too much of them. It would be asking too much. . .to expect that they have to overcome it tomorrow. It would be asking too much to expect these men to fully feel what a woman feels. For instance, I don't think that I could feel what a black feels. . .in a white country. All we can do is hope is to get close to black experience, and to support their civil rights. These men will never completely feel what it feels to be a woman in the church, but they could care enough to try to be concerned. But when an article comes to them, when it is sitting on their desk, for them to turn it down on spurious grounds is sexism.

Do you have any reservations about the use of abortion in this country?

Maguire: In this sense. . .I wish we had a society which would work on social issues so that women would not have to make that choice. That is the only way I'm content to reduce the number of abortions. Even if the number of abortions doubles, I don't want to have a law outlawing abortion. Ultimately, it has to be the woman's choice.

TWO CONVERSIONS

You are a feminist theologian. How did you reach this position?

Maguire: I had two conversions: one is my abortion conversion, one is my feminist conversion. I'm a recent convert to feminism. I used to think feminism was crazy, and wonder what was wrong with these women. What made a feminist out of me were the funerals and inaugurations of two popes in 1978. I remember watching Paul VI's funeral, and it suddenly struck me that there were no women on the TV screens. I knew there were feminist theologians like Rosemary Ruether and Arlene Swidler, even though I hadn't read much they had written. I suddenly thought, why aren't these TV stations asking some of these women about what the pope's election means for the future of the church? Instead they asked men like Fathers [Andrew] Greeley, [Richard] McBrien, and [Vincent] O'Keefe in Rome.

But no woman. . .

Maguire: There was one: CBS had a panel with Sidney Callahan. Even Barbara Walters, who has interviewed shahs, kings, and queens was not sent to Rome by the networks to see what. . .she could get on who would be the new pope. I realized they would never send her, not so much because the networks were sexist. Rather, they knew that in this sexist Catholic organization, she would get no news. She would get no scoops. This church was a closed organization to women. I didn't even have feminist theory at the time this new reality awakened within me. Besides this observation about the networks, I was also changed by observing my son as I watched the papal coverage on TV. I thought, suppose I had a daughter? What would it be like having a daughter in this church?

Well, the first coverage ended. Then in a month, John Paul I died. When I heard the news (it shows how naive I was), I thought, "Oh! the networks should not repeat the mistake they made the last time. I have to enlighten them!"

I put in long distance phone calls to the news directors of NBC, CBS, and ABC. Of course, I didn't get through to them; I reached secretaries. I gave my spiel about how I noticed a month before that they had no women on the news coverage and I hoped they weren't going to do that again. This time, I urged, they really ought to send women correspondents. Well, of course, they did the same thing again. My little boy this time was running around the house and my niece was visiting. They put cereal bowls on top of their heads, as they chanted, "I am the pope." They were so annoyed at me watching all this church stuff while they couldn't see Sesame Street. Finally, they got into the spirit, chanting "I am the pope" and suddenly, it was like a revelation, a transforming moment. I thought: Tommy can see this pageant and he can be a pope someday, but

Jandy, my niece, can never be pope. Somebody has to tell her, "Dear, you cannot dream that dream, because you're a girl." It was like a revelation; it was my moment of conversion. I clearly realized what being a feminist means. Imagine, just four months before, I had negatively answered a feminist questionnaire sent to Catholic women. There was a question in it asking, What do you think about sexist language? Is it important? I answered, How silly; we should not be hung up on this. Four months later I had this conversion, and all of a sudden, sexist language and all the other feminist issues were transformed for me.

My other conversion was in graduate school. In the master's program, Dan Maguire brought up abortion, mercy death, and similiar life issues. I had learned previously that it was acceptable not to take extraordinary means to preserve life, but any direct intervention to end life was absolutely forbidden. I was a good devil's advocate in class, objecting to any direct termination of life. One day, as I was arguing, Dan said to me, "You're a pacifist." I said, "No." (Today I would answer yes.) It struck me suddenly that my principles were not absolute. I had taken the principle "Thou shalt not kill" and I applied it so that I allowed war, capital punishment, and so on. Yet I was unwilling to discuss abortion and mercy death. With that insight, I realized all these others were discussable too. I could then accept abortion on the intellectual level. But when I heard of a young woman who had had an abortion, I thought, How could she do it? So on the affective level I had not changed.

What changed me on the affective level was my first pregnancy. I realized pregnancy wasn't a great romantic thing whereby I felt a partner with God, carrying this new person. It's only meaning was what I brought to it. We saw in the pregnancy our future child because we wanted this fetus. However, there was no great flash of meaning that came saying, "I'm a person" or "I'm a creature of God." I realized then how awful it would be to be pregnant if I didn't want to be. Then I realized how a woman can choose to have an abortion. I changed on the affective level. A couple of years later, when I was three months pregnant with our second child, we learned that this. . . first child had a serious genetic disorder and [that] I'm a carrier of the disorder. I had to then face abortion on a practical, personal level. I had an amniocentesis. Fortunately, the fetus was healthy so that today we have an eleven-year-old son who is the delight of our life. However, I would have aborted if the diagnosis had been different.

As a theologian, a woman, I then had to ask myself: Do I have a moral right to become pregnant in the future? There was a twenty-five percent chance of my pregnancy ending in abortion. I agonized over that, and finally decided I did have that moral right. Unfortunately, I never again became pregnant.

So feminism and gradual insights into the church's stand on abortion changed you.

Maguire: Abortion, combined with my feminism, made me passionate on this issue. If women cannot have a choice in this area, they have no choice about their lives. It isn't just a matter of property rights. People often criticize the expression "rights over your own body" as if your body were your house. Everybody has a right over their house, but you can lose your house and still be yourself. But for persons, our body is the fabric of our personhood. We cannot be a person without our body; we're not angels. If I don't have a right over my own body, I don't have a right over my person. I have no self-determination.

Do you think men have control over their bodies?

Maguire: For men it's not an issue. They have control over their own bodies, and over their lives. It never becomes a question whether they should have control over their bodies. Women never had control, and now are achieving control—that is what frightens the hierarchy. Additionally, men can dream dreams and realize their fruition. They can dream of going to Harvard, Yale, or Brown, and compete with other men. Yes, more and more women are getting into these places, but men still have a better chance of gaining admission. Once men graduate from these prestigious institutions, they will get a job almost anywhere. Women, even graduates of those places, are going to have to prove themselves. In the church men can also decide what they want to be. People are not setting up roadblocks all along the way as they do for women, or blacks, and other minorities or ethnic groups. These roadblocks make the difference.

Are you optimistic about the future?

Maguire: No, I'm not, especially since this pope is young. Things are not going to get any better. He has authoritarian people in office, and they are not going to make it easier for the people of God.

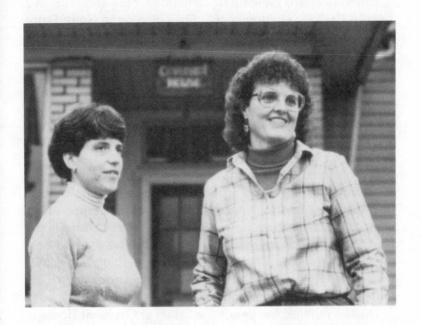

BARBARA FERRARO AND PATRICIA HUSSEY

"The biggest challenge to Rome, to the institutional church and to the hierarchy is that we women feel very Catholic, and very religious, and very much within our rights to challenge the church. That's why many of us will not give up; we will not walk away because it is our church. And our church is a community of believers. It is not merely the hierarchy."

Two sisters of Notre Dame, Barbara Ferraro and Pat Hussey, were among the twenty-four signers of the statement ad, "A Diversity of Opinions Regarding Abortion Exists Among Committed Catholics," which was printed in *The New York Times*, October 7, 1984. They remain the only two who have not signed a required retraction by the Vatican. They are asked to declare that they abide by the church's position on abortion. Because of their persistence in refusing to accept the church's position, they are threatened to be expelled from their order.

Barbara Ferraro grew up in Cambridge, Massachusetts, in a "totally Catholic environment." She entered the Notre Dame sisters in 1962, obtained her degree and taught elementary school for eight years. Realizing that a large Catholic population of youngsters attended public schools, she went to Loyola University in Chicago for a masters in pastoral studies to prepare herself to meet their needs. From 1970-78 she did parish work and found deep fulfillment in relating to women, listening to their "stories," counselling, them and providing a woman's presence for them on a parish level.

She obtained her doctoral degree in pastoral counselling at McCormick Presbyterian Seminary in Chicago. She realized then that she could no longer work in a parish because, in her words: "[I was] hearing the 'no-no' from the clergy with whom I worked. They felt my place was either behind a desk teaching. . .or pushing papers. . .doing the normal things a religious woman should do. Only then, I realized I did not want to continue to fight that system and use my energies there."

She has pursued her pastoral vocation at Covenant House in Charleston, West Virginia, where, with Patricia Hussey, she is co-director, working with homeless and poor people.

Pat Hussey grew up in a Catholic family in Springfield, Massachusetts, and attended Catholic schools throughout her early education. Through contact with the Notre Dame community she saw these nuns dealing with "marginal students, the ones that were 'loose,' the ones engaging in sex at a very young age." She entered the community in 1967 and finished her degree in special education at Southern Connecticut State College.

After teaching fourth to sixth graders Pat realized that teaching "was not my. . .gift." Rather, her gift was working with delinquent youngsters in a Connecticut state institution from 1973-76. These youngsters were status offenders, runaways and a few murderers. She also worked with many women on the staff and, through her encounters with them, awakened to the "incredible commitment" of Jewish, Protestant as well as Catholic women who challenged her conception of who constituted the preserve of religiously committed women.

Pat attended the Jesuit School of Theology in Chicago, receiving a Master of Divinity degree in 1979. "It formed me so well," she notes, "that I chose to work in a jewelry factory in Providence, Rhode Island, for two years. The factory was key in helping me decide what work I wanted to do." She greatly admired working women, many of them single parents dedicating their monotonous lives to "stringing and racking Pierre Cardin jewelry" all day long. She was also horrified by working conditions of the men, one of whom she often would see coughing up blood as he worked over tanks filled with cyanide.

When Advent House for the homeless was founded in Providence, Pat began to volunteer there. It was her experience in this setting that transformed her and launched her career in a new direction.

EARLY RELIGIOUS LIFE

Barbara, you entered the convent in 1962 and Pat in 1967. Do you recall your thoughts at the time?

Hussey: When I entered I was very clearly challenged by our [the Notre Dame] constitutions. They spoke of commitment to the poor in the most neglected places. At the state institution, I worked with an incredible black woman, Ida Billingslea, who challenged all my stereotypes of women. Interestingly enough, when I made final vows, the woman who gave the homily at the ceremony was Ida: a black woman; a Protestant married woman. Yet it was she I chose.

Barbara, you seem moved by this...?

Ferraro: It's really significant that Pat speaks about Ida who is not a nun, yet who challenged Pat while working with delinquent youngsters. Ida is a simply extraordinary woman— extraordinary in her ordinariness. She is one of the women who have spoken to both of us over and over again. It's not the women who are prominent out there, but the women who day by day rub shoulders with us. They speak a whole lot to us. Ida has suffered a great deal, having had open heart surgery. Equally significant, she wanted to speak at Pat's final vows...when in fact, the models in front of us have always been Sisters of Notre Dame. This is the emergence, the breaking out, of the old forms of community.

Hussey: Well, I'm certain we broke the whole religious "ghetto" mentality and. . . .When we began to talk about challenges to the abortion issue, and when I reflected on the experiences of kids who were victims of rape and incest, I healthfully challenged my whole Catholic mentality. I questioned church teaching which says anybody who has an abortion, or considers an abortion, is evil or immoral and is in need of forgiveness. In fact, these girls we're dealing with were the ones who have been violated and victimized, by fathers, pimps, so-called Johns or tricks as they are named. These are twelve- to eighteen-year-old kids.

COVENANT HOUSE FOR THE HOMELESS
As I understand, Barbara, there was a national search for a minister and his family to direct Covenant House. Why did Covenant House in West Virginia hire the two of you?

Ferraro: I think it's probably part of the phenomenon of people today realizing what women religious, educated women who are in touch with reality, have to offer. Since we both studied together, and our time in Chicago overlapped, we realized that we had complementary skills and that it would be very good for us to see if we could work together. My experience had been working alone in parishes, struggling along with my ideas and my philosophy. Wouldn't it be good, we reflected, if we could work as a team and begin to act on social justice issues together? When we heard of this search, we had already put together our philosophy, some of our goals, and what we would like to do. Besides, we were very much interested in looking at long-term changes which we with others could accomplish, not merely "Band-Aiding" desperate situations. When we went for our joint interviews, they were impressed. The search group consisted of lay people and clergy in the Charleston area. We had a three-day interview; the committee took us around the community. We met with some of the "street people" at the local soup kitchen called Manna Meal. They observed us in action and apparently liked what they saw. They offered us the job, creating a time-and-a-half position which meant that Pat, for four months, worked part-time in a supermarket. . .as a cashier. We began our new project, which was not connected with the Catholic church. We felt we could be freer to get involved in social justice issues. Moreover, it was a good entry point into a community. We were excited, particularly about the ecumenical adventure which is now funded by twenty-seven churches and temples.

[Even though] the project was undefined [in its early stages], lay people as well as religious were very much committed to Covenant House. They were very supportive of our idea, our non-Band-Aid long-range view. They were impressed with what we had to offer. One of the founders has stated that he is continually amazed at what we are capable of doing, and what we have accomplished these last five years.

Eventually they employed both of you full time. . . ?

Ferraro: After four months Pat came on full time. What is real important is we operated as equals from the very beginning. We two team together and call ourselves co-directors.

Could you describe the clientele whom you serve?

Ferraro: First of all, we never refer to them as "clients." We say the people we work with, or we talk about "the folks" we are with. Every place they go in the community they're seen as "clients," and placed in that subservient role. We try to work with people who come to Covenant House as equals. They are our equals; we are there together. They are people who are homeless, people who are on low or fixed income, people who have been institutionalized or classified as falling between the cracks and lost in the system. Nowhere in the system can they find the resources needed, nor do they have the ability to find any relief.

Hussey: When we refer to folks on low and fixed income in West Virginia, we're talking about welfare benefits ranging from $201.00 [a month] for a family of two, to a maximum of $477.00 for a family of eight or more, which is way below the poverty level for the United States. People who are mentally ill or mentally handicapped will receive maximum benefits of $336.00 a month, again, well below the poverty level. Therefore, they don't have a chance. Many of them are on the streets, homeless people. Yet, Charleston has nowhere the population of homelessness of cities like New York, or Washington, or Chicago.

Ferraro: [There are] manageable numbers [of homeless people]; we can work well with them. We pretty well know all the people in the community who are homeless and our center is in the downtown area. Folks can take showers, do their laundry, and prepare for job interviews. We have an iron and ironing board, a shoe kit, and access to a free telephone. We do lots of advocacy work, crisis intervention, counselling, referral and resource work. We have an emergency fund for rents and utilities; we have clothing and a food pantry. Everything depends on volunteers; we're the only two staff people, with 150 volunteers who work with us consistently. During our vacation, these wonderful people from all the churches and temples assume responsibility for Covenant House and keep it open. The reasons we do that is to involve the community; it's a community project, it's not ours. And one of our goals is to try to get the religious community involved in assuming leadership for what happens in their community. Working at Covenant House is an effective and moving experience for community members.

CHANGES IN THE 1960s

When you entered the convent (1962 and 1967), the early 1970s were times of flowering in the church. How were nuns affected by Vatican II?

Ferraro: I entered in 1962, on the cusp of change. I wore the long habit, and lived all the old rules. Then, with Pope John XXIII in the 1960s and Vatican II, many new things emerged. Fresh air came through the open windows. It was an exciting and expanding time. . . .It is now twenty-four years since I entered. I've known nothing but change and it has been very challenging. Women religious took seriously the documents of Vatican II, and [we] took seriously the recommendation to look at our roots as a congregation of Notre Dame Sisters. Women also became educated, we are now extremely professional, and we are involved in the realities of the world around us. Nuns allowed liberation theology and feminist theology to seep in, take hold and transform us. Consequently, we changed our lives and our works.

I know that's what happened to me and the last twenty years have been the most exciting in my life. Sixty-two people entered Notre Dame in 1962; now nine of us are left. . . .As Pat has said over and over again these last twenty-two months: we are where we are today. . .because of the challenges of Vatican II. We've taken our constitutions of the Sisters of Notre

Dame very seriously; we've taken the challenges of the Scriptures very seriously, and our education over the past ten to fifteen years—all of it has challenged us to take the stands and brave the risks we've taken.

Hussey: What's interesting to know is that the older sisters in our community. . .were women who fought for education, and fought for people to finish their degrees before they went out teaching. They felt it was very important that nuns be professional, competent, and educated, to provide the best for their students. Today, it is interesting to know all of this search for excellence has come under fire. Because we are professional, and because we are educated, Cardinal Ratzinger, head of the Vatican Congregation for the Doctrine of the Faith, describes this as the *problem* of religious women in America. I find his critique appalling and frightening for women religious. The questions I would ask of him are, "Is ignorance better for the church then? Is it better not to be educated? Is it better not to be professional? Is it better to be unwitting so that blind obedience can be invoked? And ultimately, does he want ignorance so that the so-called daughters of the church will be blindly obedient to the church fathers?

Your Catholic feminist sisters are saying: the church has always tried to keep women barefoot and pregnant. . .

Hussey: I think that's true, especially if we closely examine the different doctrines and teachings of the church. The official church speaks of submission to the husband; deals abysmally with abortion, and any number of sexual issues. I believe the church wants to be in a position of dominance and domination to keep women submissive.

Ferraro: They not only don't deal well with women, but they don't even invite women's experiences. They do not invite women around the table to make the decisions that form the church's teachings on women's issues. That to me is a great farce, since Vatican II called us *all* to take responsibility as a community of believers to challenge and to search for the truth together. The only thing that seems to enter into the church's official teachings today is what the magisterium (bishops, cardinals, and pope) says. Some theologians have challenged teachings where the experiences of people are denied and these theologians have gotten into trouble with the Vatican. This is especially true on sexuality. The biggest challenge to Rome, to the institutional church, and to the hierarchy, is that we women feel very Catholic, and very religious, and very much within our rights to challenge the church. That's why many of us will not give up; we will not walk away, because it is our church. And our church is a community of believers. It is not merely the hierarchy.

Do you think that the current Vatican is having "second thoughts" about the new directions promulgated by Vatican II?

Ferraro: I don't know if the hierarchy ever, ever felt that it [Vatican II] would bring women to where we have come today. I feel there's a complete denial of our experiences within the Vatican, because what we're doing is challenging the status quo, and we're saying to these men that we are going to shake up the system they have kept so tight; we're going to shake up what you have known and we are challenging your understanding, because our understanding of God is very different from your understanding of God. Pat refers to it often as two parallel churches: the church of the people of God and the church of the hierarchy. Both exist side by side, but we are continually on a collision course. Religious women, particularly in the United States, are in a collision course with the Vatican, and history shows it very clearly over the last ten years. What Rome wants us to do is to become quiet little women who do our little thing, go to school every day, teach, go home, and close our doors at night. . .[or] dusting the altar as in Poland, as it was recently reported in the papers. I don't think you'll ever get the women in the United States to turn back. What's that song? "There's no turning back. . . ." We cannot turn back on what has been challenging, nourishing, and life-giving for us.

THE NEW YORK TIMES AD

Your collision course with the Vatican was ignited by your participation in the *The New York Times* ad [see Appendix A]. How did your involvement with the ad come about?

Hussey: We were at a meeting one weekend, September 1984, with Marjorie Tuite, who came to an area church meeting. The group meets once every six weeks, and we had Marjorie in for the weekend. Before boarding the plane she said, "Oh, by the way, Pat and Barbara, I have this statement which speaks of the diversity of opinions on abortion in the Roman Catholic church. Why don't you read it and see if you can sign it?" And both Barbara and I read the ad, read the statement and felt, "Oh, absolutely, yes."

At that point in 1984 it seemed very clear the public and vocal hierarchy members were staffed with Republicans basically. Some of these men were definitely on Reagan's team, buying his death-dealing policies, hook, line and sinker, and yet judging Geraldine Ferraro for her single issue of pro-choice abortion.

In view of that political climate, and because we work day-in and day-out with people who are poor and affected by Reagan's policies, absolutely we would sign the ad. We would say . . .that we who are Catholics, that we who are Catholic nuns, supported the reality that good Catholics could vote for a pro-choice candidate. And we felt it was very important to put our names with the incredible list of other names. Seeing the printed release later we chuckled: "Here we are, two little peons in West Virginia signing an ad with a number of great people." We were very glad to do so.

Ferraro: Marjorie. . .has since died. She was a mentor for both of us in many ways and an incredible strategist in social justice. Before she died she said to us, "And they dared to call us unfaithful. . .the hierarchy dared to call us unfaithful." Marjorie was with us [that September], helping us to do an analysis of what had recently happened. . .when we asked the church a question. We asked why it was putting money into a building which ended up being a 6.2 million dollar boondogle, when West Virginia was the state. . .highest in unemployment. Marjorie was helping us analyze when do you say "no" to the church, and when do you give in?

Pat and I were also key in organizing a concert that was to come into town. We never even realized that the ad appeared in *The New York Times* that same day, October 7, 1984. We were busy organizing a Holly Near and Ronnie Gilbert national concert with the theme being "Vote for a Change, the Whole World is Watching." It was an energizing event to defeat Reagan whose policies terribly affect the people with whom we work.

Besides, Geraldine [Ferraro] was running in 1984, and I saw that finally a woman might take a leadership role in society. I had that same excitement in 1975 when women first voiced the word "ordination" and I said, "My God, maybe in my own lifetime we will see women in leadership positions in the church." I was also elated that Geraldine had the same last name as I did; possibly her family is from the same area of Italy as mine. It was thrilling. . . .I was real excited for her.

VATICAN BACKLASH
What happened after October 7, 1984? What was the sequence of events?

Hussey: Things were pretty quiet for at least two months. Barbara and I never saw the ad in *The New York Times* until weeks later. [Things] began to explode [around] December 17, 1984, when we received a call from one of the members of our general government in Rome saying that she had received a letter from Cardinal Hamer, Vatican head of the Congregation for Religious and Secular Institutes [CRIS]. The letter informed her that we had signed this ad which appeared in *The New York Times*, and that we must retract our names or else be threatened with expulsion from our religious communities. Threatened with dismissal from our religious communities! At the time, it was described as a rather harsh letter. . . .Moreover, it is interesting that when we sisters deal with each other, we always communicate as equals. Yet, Cardinal Hamer in this instance was communicating with the main superior general, and not directly with any of the signers, which is another basic indictment of the hierarchial church.

How so?

Hussey: Because they want to maintain and preserve the hierarchy. I do not sense that many members of the hierarchy and Vatican believe the church is a community of equals. They do not accept that we are all believers in this community called church. They maintain their positions as superiors with twenty-four nun signers of an ad as inferiors. There is a chain of command, and they operate within that chain of command.

Ferraro: Which is very unlike the way we have operated women's communities in the last ten or fifteen years. We worked as collegial groups, with the understanding that authority resides within the membership. The way we were treated in this process, the process the hierarchy chose to use, was a process very foreign to us and to our experiences over these last years.

Hussey: Vatican officials did not engage in dialogue with us. It was very clear that they simply treated our superiors as "messenger girls." I mean that with all the disrespect that goes along with it. I regard my leadership person as a woman, but they regard her as a messenger girl. [One particular sentence from the letter] sticks in my memory: "Tell them that they need to follow this; they need to retract, or you will begin the process of dismissal."

In December, as you can imagine, there was a flurry of activity just before Christmas. We gave Christmas greetings to each other at a meeting in Washington, D.C., on December 22 for the nun signers and other signers and a couple of superiors. Basically the questions were: What's going to happen? What are we going to do? What kind of action should we take? As nun signers we felt that it was important to act in solidarity with one another. Bonding together was very important. What has happened, though, over the past months is surely a breakdown in that solidarity. There was an isolating factor where many communities believed that they should work as an individual community instead of bonding across fifteen different commmunities. We were twenty-four different signers from fifteen different communities.

Ferraro: In January 1985, we met again in Chicago: nun-signers, lay-signers, and a group of superiors. There were three distinct meetings going on, with a strong movement from some of us to really bond together across lay and religious life. But for some time now there has been a real contention about mingling lay and religious women. We let Rome separate us; we allowed Rome to individualize us; we were afraid and separated the lay signers from the nun signers. Still, this was a wonderful opportunity to model what we had been verbalizing over the decades. We never carried it out. We did a real disservice to our lay women who signed that ad, when we did not bond with them.

Anyhow, in Chicago we started to do some strategizing as to where to go from there, what to do next. The second ad on

"Freedom to Dissent Within the Catholic Church" [see Appendix B], started in January 1985 with the lay signers and the nun signers. Leadership people were not involved when we planned to publish a second ad of solidarity with people who were experiencing reprisals. Simultaneously, stories were surfacing as to what was happening to some signers.

We planned hearings on women's lives, and these sessions were held in Washington, D.C. and Chicago in March and April 1985. Incidentally, these meetings were life-giving because we attempted to look at some of the positive ways we could respond to what was happening in our lives.

Hussey: You might want to say, Barbara, what was very clear to us in Chicago [was that] we heard the expression of fear. Leadership felt that now is not the time to fight; abortion is not the issue. What we described repeatedly was that it was not *we* who made an issue of abortion, not *we* who went to the media, not *we* who made it the public thing that it is. Rather, it was the Vatican which is interfering and intimidating us and we have to name that. If the time is not now, we asked, *when*? We began to describe the whole picture and to make connections. "What happened to Agnes Mansour? Nobody came to her side, We did not stand firm and strong then. It did not happen when Liz Morancy and Arlene Violet were in their political ministry. You say again, now is not the time for religious communities to stand firm and strong. . . . "We kept voicing these sentiments. And we said if *now* is not the time, and abortion is not the issue, when are we going to stand firm? Is homosexuality going to be the issue that will get us to stand firm? Is ordination of women the issue that will make all of us stand firm?

Ferraro: What they were looking for was a safe issue. What they said was [that] abortion was not the issue; it's too volatile; it's too emotional. But once again, as Pat pointed out, the fact that each time an issue comes to the forefront, it is not the right issue. Our question is when will it be the right issue? When will the right time be?

REJECTION OF APPEASEMENT
Both of you are against appeasement then?

Ferraro: Obviously we're against compromising our values. The models we had in front of us, and from whom both of us learned a lot, are women who have gone before us, women who are walking with us. Cases like Agnes Mansour, Liz Morancy, and Arlene Violet—all three left voluntarily. They did not capitulate; they continued to do what they were doing, but they left voluntarily. And we felt we had limited choices . . . .As Mary Jo Weaver said very well at that meeting in January, "Either capitulate to something that's dying or allow something to die in order to create new life." I believe the latter. We did the latter—we allowed something to die in order to create the new, and I think it's time that as religious women we say "no more" to Rome; we say "no more interference in our lives." We are grown, educated, well-respected professional women and we have a right to determine what happens in our lives. We have a right to question, we have a right to dissent, and we have a right to speak from our experiences, and both Pat and I realize that we will not capitulate, we will not compromise what we believe, and we will not voluntarily leave. So the only thing we have left is basically to stand by what we believe and see where that course brings us.

So now you are at the point where all the other nuns involved in the ad have signed some sort of retraction. . .?
Hussey: Twenty-two of the twenty-four have in some way been cleared, or their cases have been closed. Some of the women did sign statements. They signed statements that in their eyes did not say that they publicly adhered to the Roman Catholic teaching on abortion. Yet it was clearly interpreted or misinterpreted that way by Vatican officials. They deliberately miscommunicated their statements to the general public, insisting that they publicly adhered to the Roman Catholic teaching on abortion. Barbara and I kept saying during the course of the year that we are not going to play word games; we are not going to put in writing what *they* want; we are not going to retract our names from the ad. Because how can you retract a call for dialogue? It doesn't make sense. Some signers are unaware of what their leadership people put in writing.

You mean they didn't read the document themselves. . .
Hussey: They did not have access to read the document that their superiors submitted to the Vatican and for which they were cleared. You see, the so-called dialogue was actually a dictate from Rome to our superiors, and our superiors were the

ones communicating with Rome, with the CRIS [Congregation of Religious and Secular Institutes] office. The communication was between both of them; it did not happen through us. What leadership was supposed to do was to get statements from us, and communicate our positions back to Rome. So, yes, some people did not see the communication nor do they realize what was written.

What do you think of that?

Ferraro: What I feel is tragic in all of this is women working against women; Rome is accomplishing, or trying to accomplish, ways to divide women against women, and it's sad that leadership people were put into a position where they felt they had to do something less than what they believed in. . . .

Hussey: Just to go along with that, Barbara, I think what happened was leadership people were interested in the institutional survival of their communities. Therefore, in order to protect the majority of nuns they bent over backwards to accommodate Rome and Vatican officials. Personally, I don't understand it. I think there is an incredible amount of fear there. When we are very afraid, we do different things to accommodate the person who has power over us. I think that that has been very clear during the past two years, that the Vatican has the power to obliterate women's communities according to provisions in canon law.

What can the Vatican do?

Hussey: I think there is a whole lot of economic power, sanctions that can be brought to bear. If, for example, in an archdiocese a bishop can dismiss the Sisters of Notre Dame from teaching in schools, or dismiss religious educators, that would affect us economically. I think if we are a canonical order then they could seize the property of Sisters of Notre Dame, the little property we have. Talk about justice. . . . Another angle is many sisters consider it important to be part of a canonical community and have the pope's blessing. Were we non-canonical, and not have that relationship with the pope, it would not be good for some women in our community. I don't consider that official relationship a great thing, especially in light of what's happened in recent history.

Were you non-canonical, would your property belong to the local bishop rather than to Rome?

Ferraro: What's the difference between that and the analogy right now that we, as religious women, are the property of Rome? Symbolically, we're their property, because they can dictate to us what we can do, what we can't do. I think the analogy has been repeated again and again this past year as one looks at our situation, and that of other battered women. (One thing I exclude is the fact that we at least have the luxury of walking out.) The women we work with day in, day out, don't have the options we have. Yet, as religious women, we do have options to walk out of this battering. As we listen to the studies that have come out, *The Wall Street Journal's* showing that although nuns have given their lifeblood to the church for minimal money, the bishops do not feel any obligation to these women in their retirement. Economically, we are trapped and need to re-examine our relationship with dioceses and the church. Should that not raise some questions among us? Why are we being tied to the institutional church?

What are you gaining from this?

Ferraro: What are we gaining? Nothing from my perspective, other than to be property, and to be told what we can or what we cannot do. And not to be treated as adult women.

Hussey: One of the frightening things for me has been—I think actually it's written in canon law—that nuns, as public witnesses, are to uphold the official teachings of the church. Whether that's in canon law or certain Vatican rhetoric. . .it is a quote that has been used against the two of us. As public witnesses, we nuns are to uphold the official teachings of the church. My question is, If we are to be serious about what is truthful, how can we blindly accept official teachings of the church? Be it the issues of abortion, ordination, birth control, homosexuality, or any issue that is controversial at this time I, as public witness, am not going to blindly and obediently be submissive to "church fathers" whose teachings are wrong and evil. And I refuse to be a partner in that. I think that is what we are healthily calling ourselves to examine.

THE REAL PROBLEM OF HIERARCHY

While we are on the hierarchy, I have one question. Why do you think the hierarchy is so emphatic in it's response to this issue?

Ferraro: We have been talking about fear a lot in this interview; and I believe they are frightened we are going to upset their apple cart. They have lived very safe and very comfortable lives; many of them claim they have the absolute say on what happens or does not happen to the institutional church. They have had the control and the power. As women, we have become educated and we understand the history of the Roman Catholic church. We have listened to the Spirit in our lives, and have become professional and *really* know the experience of people out there in the pew. We come with all of that and we challenge the hierarchy of the church, and it has upset them because they can no longer stay comfortable. . . .If they can quiet us, if they can perpetuate the myths they have perpetuated for themselves, then they will survive. If, however, we continue to be what the church should be all about, if we remain and challenge the church—the church is our church, it's not the men's church—if we continue to do that, it will upset them. I'm happy for the challenge, and that's where we women need strength to work together.

CONFRONTING VATICAN REPRESENTATIVES
You have been in the same room with some very powerful ecclesiastics who tried to change your position. Who were they and will you describe the experience?
Hussey: On March 22, 1986, Barbara and I met with two representatives from the Vatican, Sister Mary Linscott who is a member of our religious community, and Archbishop Vincenzo Fagiola of CRIS. We also met with Archbishop Pio Laghi who is the Vatican ambassador to the U.S. In March, there were eleven of us nun signers whose cases were not resolved. These meetings, therefore, were set up with Vatican officials. You can imagine there was some trepidation associated with meeting these officials until the time we met with them face to face. We were there under the guise of dialogue. Revealingly, Archbishop Pio Laghi stated, "We are here for dialogue, discussion; however, I must insist that after our time together you must put in writing. . . ." Barbara and I then knew what we were dealing with.
Ferraro: The strength we had going into that meeting was certainly the people who stayed with us, the women who stood with us, the faces of women we had known who have been op-

pressed by the church, who have had to face the question of abortion in their own lives. Our one goal in going into that meeting was to try to speak clearly from our experience, to speak truthfully, and not play word games. I characterized that meeting as extremely manipulative, paternalistic, and seductive. I felt that the men of the church present, Archbishop Pio Laghi and Archbishop Vicenzo Fagiola, tried to break us intellectually, but we could match them. We knew exactly what we were speaking about when. . .

Hussey: They said the church was always consistent . . .

Ferraro: I insisted it was not always consistent. They tried to break us on the whole emotional level by asking what would our "mommies and daddies" think if we were no longer religious. Then they tried to break us psychologically. Emotionally they tried to break us, particularly in their actions. . . .Fagiola came over and started to stroke Pat's arm, and held her hand. This sort of seductive thing was uncalled for. I'm sure he wanted us to be unclear in our thoughts. He told us he would pray for us, blessing us when he was leaving, and putting us in "little girl" positions. He handed out coins to the three leadership people only. Our clear goal was to present ourselves as intellectual, professional women who knew what we were talking about. I think we accomplished this goal very clearly. I think we undid them. They did not realize that we could be as strong and vocal as we were at that meeting. Basically, what it accomplished for us was [that] we did not submit to their wills. We did speak clearly of the experiences we have had, the experiences of women who have had to choose abortion, and what our position on abortion was. . . .They were not successful in extracting loyalty oaths from us, pledging our belief in the church's teaching on abortion.

Did they leave you with any ultimatum?

Ferraro: They put a time line on us to prepare a statement showing our adherence to the Roman Catholic church's teaching. We clearly said to them we did not believe in the Roman Catholic position. Clearly, they were not hearing our experiences at all; all they wanted was to have something in writing, that we believe in the church's position on abortion. Pat and I put together a statement clearly expressing our position; and clearly expressing what we felt was the interference of the Roman Catholic church around this point in women's lives, and how this interference continues.

Hussey: Let me cite how that meeting cleared my thoughts: we said constantly to the members of our religious community and to our leadership that the repression will not stop here. The Vatican will continue to intervene and interfere in our lives. One of the nun signers has been very committed to working with the gay community. She received a letter also from Cardinal Hamer of the CRIS office saying he was aware of her commitment to the gay community, and of some of her positions on homosexuality. Therefore, she would have to write a statement that she supported and adhered to the Roman Catholic teaching on homosexuality.

We have Pio Laghi's interference with the orders who support women's ordination. Further, we continue to hear about cardinals, archbishops, and bishops who have a fixation on the whole abortion issue. Most recently, I became aware of a situation where a woman who had worked with a mentally handicapped, heavily-medicated schizophrenic youngster who became pregnant, and decided to have an abortion. Now there is a great amount of confidentiality existing between hospital chaplains and patients. This young woman went to a confessor, confessed she had had an abortion—a young mentally handicapped, let me reiterate—and the woman chaplain who had counselled her received a call from the bishop saying that he wanted to see her the next day in his office. She consulted a canon lawyer and appeared the next day before the bishop. He stated his concern about her position on this youngster who had an abortion. She said, "Bishop, my relationships with patients is a matter of confidentiality. Therefore, I am not going to discuss this situation with you. However, if I were you, the bishop, I would be much more concerned that the seal of confession has been broken. And you should have that priest before you and talk to him." Again, we see that there's this fixation on the abortion issue, and this is a confidentiality in which bishops have no right to interfere.

He tried to remove this person as a chaplain, appealed to her boss in a secular hospital, trying to take away her job, over which he had no control.

Did the boss let her go?

Ferraro: No. The boss said she was an excellent chaplain and he, not the bishop, would decide whom he fires.

This incident can be multiplied by the hundreds. They are not going to stop here. Today it's the ad on pro-choice; yesterday it was Agnes Mary Mansour; we thought it was going to end with Liz [Morancy] and Arlene [Violet]; we thought it was going to end with Father Fernando Cardenal in Nicaragua when he decided to stay in his ministry of education. It's not going to end here. The church is clearly reversing itself. . . .

Does this sadden you, barely twenty years after the advances made through Vatican II?

Ferraro: I think the hierarchy is afraid of the life in the church.

Hussey: I think the hierarchy is afraid of challenge. What will be sad is if people give up in despair.

Ferraro: It saddens me because the church has become very life-giving, particularly to men and women who for the first time in their lives are beginning to realize there is a God who cares; there is a God who accepts them as they are, and their understanding of God in the church has taken a new, a revolutionary outlook. They believe they are free people; that's what the women in the church believe and have done for one another. The hierarchy resents all that.

TEAM COLLABORATION

You have talked about working together. It looks like the solidarity you two have and continue to share as a team has helped you through your trials and tribulations. Could you talk about this team relationship, as well as why you are able to hold out in these trying times?

Hussey: There can be no doubt during the past two years, it has been due to the support of the people we work with, as well as our work together which has given us strength during these trying times. Because of the work we do together, and our attempt on a daily basis to analyze what's happening within city government, state government, national government. . .it's not unusual for us also to analyze the structure of the Catholic church. We realize that politics is as alive within the church as in city, state, and national government. Therefore, it has been good to analyze together what is occuring in the church.

At times, if either of us had less than an energizing day, we have been able to support each other. We have been able to laugh together, and our laughter has been critical for maintaining our sanity. Because of the work we do which is daily "hands on," it helps us stand strong and firm in our position. The people I work with have challenged me to stand firm, constant, and faithful during these trying months. It makes me strong in some way to name the reality which oppresses women, or religious communities, or anything that challenges the status quo. It is important for our community of Charleston that we challenged the status quo.

Ferraro: I think if we had not had praxis previous to this. . .

INFLUENCE OF LIBERATION THEOLOGY
Would you define praxis?

Ferraro: Praxis is basically living so that our lives are not all theory. We try to live out what we have read, in practical everyday life. Had we not the *experience* and *practice* in previous years of working through the Women's Ordination Conference, or of working in the local situation in which we challenged the diocese as it built a multi-million dollar complex, we would not have been able to stand firm and strong. We watched two priests in the diocese who challenged local people to confront oppressive systems and yet, when oppression from their own church hit them in the face they were not willing to say "no" to the powers. These two ended up walking away from the community. Then the issue of the right to dissent struck us two years later. We had already walked through the other experiences; we had already done an analysis, and we realized that there is no way we can turn our back and walk away from the oppression in our own church. We walked with people for the last four years and urged them to say "no" to the systems that oppressed them.

In theory, we talk about the fact that we should not have security. We should be equal people among the people. [This means we have] to look at a lack of security if we are to lose our "status" in the Roman Catholic church as nuns, and be reduced to "lay status" as a penalty! What does that say about lay people in the church? Does it not, then, give us the opportunity to say we truly are equal among equals? Does it not put us in a position to really live out what we had been saying? We now understand we are equals in this church of ours. And so to lose my status as a nun is not frightening. . . .But as I asked earlier: What security do we have as religious women in the church? Certainly not an economic security!

When you signed this ad, this "Statement on Pluralism and Abortion," what were you signing essentially? What are your beliefs about abortion?

Hussey: There are two distinct questions there which have become more clear over the years. I signed an ad which simply described the diversity of opinion on abortion in the Roman Catholic church. And we needed to talk about that diversity. . . period. What has happened over the course of the twenty-two months. . . .I was going to say twenty-two years! [Laughter]

It's been a long time. . . .

Hussey: . . .It's been a long time. . .has been clarifying my position. That is the one spoken of as pro-choice and which I happily claim as my own position. Because of my meetings with different members of the hierarchy, my pro-choice position has been clarified.

Ferraro: That's right.

Hussey: Marjorie Maguire wrote in *Conscience* about the difference between pro-choice and pro-abortion. I don't believe anyone is pro-abortion. I don't believe that people recommend abortion as a procedure for every woman. I believe women are adult moral decision makers; women are very responsible. When a woman comes to struggle with abortion within the Roman Catholic church, all of a sudden, according to the hierarchy, she loses her adulthood; she loses her sensibilities; she loses the sense that she is a moral person. I believe, and I claim for women, even at that most difficult time that they are, in fact, adult moral decision makers. And I will stand with the woman who has to make the choice if she has to have an abortion. It is this insight which has become very much clarified for me over the past two years. I thank people like Cardinal Hamer for forcing that kind of clarity on me. I now feel that I have begun to speak very much in the open as a Roman Catholic woman, a Roman Catholic nun for the pro-choice position. Nor do I think it's something we can walk away from.

Ferraro: I want to say that the Vatican has done Roman Catholic women a favor by forcing this issue, because it has helped many of us sharpen our position on the issue of abortion. When we had to meet with Vatican officials in March of this past year, and they had been pushing us to make a statement that we adhered to the Roman Catholic church's teaching on abortion, it forced us to sharpen our position. We clearly support womens' right to choose; women are good moral decision makers, and clearly, we will stand with women in that choice.

We realize that any moral issue out there certainly can be abused. Abortion can be abused, and has been abused; we are not so naive to say there are no abuses. We confront the Roman Catholic church to accept women as people who have certain rights, and they have control over their bodies. What we ought to be working on are other options for women: birth control, adequate day care centers, adequate jobs and benefits, and health benefits for all people. Then women with more choices may not find themselves forced to choose abortion. The Roman Catholic church has done a great service for Roman Catholic women in forcing some of us as Roman Catholic nuns to sharpen our position. It has been a great sign of hope to people in the Catholic church.

We have had Roman Catholic women from all over this country write to us. They said, "Thank you for what you are doing: I support you in your decision." One woman wrote to us early on and said, "I believe I may even find God again." And I believe that is extremely important; it has touched me very deeply. For whatever reason, both of us are in the situation we are in--sometimes it's hard to deal with it—why we are the only two and why there are not others standing with us. It is a humbling situation; it's one that I would not have chosen. But here we are: why, we do not know. . .why are we the ones speaking out at this point.

You two stand alone in your decision. . .?

Ferraro: It would be much better if we worked together as a collective team of twenty-four. Individual action is good; collective action is much more powerful. If we work together—twenty-four, forty-four, or one hundred—we could change the church. But at least there are two, and we are not standing alone in that sense.

Why is the hierarchy so obsessed with sexual matters, both with the women you describe and with some men, like Charlie Curran?

Hussey: Dan Maguire has a great line where he says he believes the Catholic church is stuck in the pelvic zone. I believe this is true. With regard to sexuality and female concerns, I think the hierarchy is interested in the control of and power over women. That's the bottom line: I don't know how else to say it.

PRESENT STATUS IN COMMUNITY

Where do you stand within your order? Are they going to back you and resist pressure from Rome to dismiss you?

Hussey: On June 17, 1986, the Sisters of Notre Dame General Government Group issued a statement saying they would not begin the process of our dismissal based on our signing either the first or the second ad. They did not believe that signing the ads was sufficient reason for our dismissal. At the same time, their statement to the press indicated a second part requesting that "We enter into dialogue together about our public pro-choice position." Our superiors were women of courage in that they stood up to the Vatican. We are the only congregation standing up to CRIS officials, saying publicly they would not dismiss us based on our signing two ads.

At the same time, they have difficulty with our *public* pro-choice position. I don't know exactly where that will lead us. I hope, in fact, they are serious about having a dialogue. We are to meet with three of our general government people later on and I don't know what will happen. There is as much diversity and split about abortion within the Sisters of Notre Dame as there is in the U.S. population, or possibly in the world community. There is a great amount of fear within the Sisters of Notre Dame surrounding the abortion issue, because abortion is the red flag with the Roman Catholic church. There are some Sisters of Notre Dame who want us to leave, and feel we would be doing the community a favor; others say the Vatican should not interfere in our lives. Only we can determine who are and who are not members. All of this ambivalence is jumbled up in the Sisters of Notre Dame, in the United States and internationally.

Ferraro: We demanded our group to make all correspondence between us and our general government public for our provinces in Boston and Connecticut. We held open meetings in both provinces to talk about the issue, and to hear both sides. We tried to use it as an educational moment. . . .We always did it together. We invited both provinces together, because Boston and Connecticut are very close. We had an open meeting in Worcester and another in Springfield during the course of the first year.

How did these meetings go?

Ferraro: They went well in the sense that many people who wanted to, came. Interestingly, people did not come who felt that their presence meant they were in support of us. We know [that] not everyone agrees with us. So there was fear on all levels. But for the people there it was a good education.

Hussey: There were probably 150 at each meeting, which out of five hundred nuns showed sizeable interest.

FAMILY REACTIONS

Could we discuss your families? Pat, what is your family background and how has your family responded to your situation?

Hussey: I have two brothers, one sister, all younger, and my mother and father are living. For my parents it has been a roller coaster of emotions during the past two years. There has been some sentiment of "Why can't you sign a statement that is expressive of your view points, and still respectful of the church?" At the same time there is an incredible amount of anger toward John Paul II and his intervention in our lives. The reprisals they feel that have befallen me and a number of nun and lay-signers shows there is an incredible amount of repression within the Roman Catholic church. That is not healthy for the church. They felt so strongly about it that they signed the second ad which was a Declaration for Solidarity. A brother and sister signed the statement as well. A second brother was surprised his name was not there, and then he realized he is a procrastinator. Siblings have been very supportive. My parents, though—as I said, it has been a roller coaster kind of effect, though they are very supportive.

Barbara, you come from a large family. How have your parents responded?

Ferraro: I am one of eleven; the second oldest of eleven children. Similar to Pat, it has also been a roller coaster for my parents. They are very staunch Catholics; we were brought up strictly within the Catholic faith. My parents taught us all to be independent, and to say what we believe. My dad had experienced that in his own work as a public figure in Cambridge. I learned from my parents—even though it's very difficult for them to deal with the public nature of this episode. The publicity has been extremely hard for my mother. My dad has been very supportive. Both parents support me as a person, love me as a person, though it's very hard for a parent when a child's life (no matter how old) takes on a different public position because of the situation one finds in life. I say to them, "This is history; I am part of it." But to say that, and not to come across as someone trying to promote oneself, requires a solid knowledge of oneself. In fact, we have not promoted our own publicity. My siblings are extremely supportive; some of them disagree, but most of them agree with me—and feel I have a right to speak. They certainly have followed my education for the last ten to fifteen years, and my own experience of women being oppressed in the church, and they speak out loud and strong about that.

Hussey: When the press comes and refers to us as the "pro-abortion nuns"—which obviously it has—oh! a gasp in my parents' lungs, "Are they saying that about my daughter? What is her real position?" At the same time we say to our parents, "Look, you are the ones who nourished our faith; you are the ones who taught us our faith within the church; you are the ones who have taught us to speak the truth, to rub shoulders with people. *Your* lives have, in fact, nourished ours, and this is where we are, in great part because of *you.*" I think it's that silent pride and, at the same time the feeling, "Oh! we didn't mean for you to go this far."

Ferraro: It has particularly forced my mother to look at abortion and what it means. Certainly a mother of eleven kids never believed in birth control: she was always taught that was a "no-no!" I have brothers and sisters who support her. My mother had to learn, both parents had to learn, that their children had grown and emerged to a different reality. I know my mother has searched out and joined some groups in church to try to understand. . .

Hussey: She went to the bishops' hearings and. . .

Ferraro: . . . .And then she went to one of the meetings and asked her group what they felt. Did they feel that Rome had issued a hard statement to those women who signed the ad? And everyone agreed, and they started a discussion. Though she did not want to be identified as a mother. . .

Hussey: . . .And at that point someone said, "Oh, are you Barbara Ferraro's mother?" She said, "I don't want to be identified;" yet, she was willing to explore and hear what others had to say. But the publicity, the public nature of it, has been difficult.

STATUS IN THE CHURCH

Is it becoming irrelevant to you whether or not you belong to the church? To the people of God?

Hussey: I hope I'm at least among the people of God. What was interesting for me this year in terms of my identity as nun—I know that I've been nourished and challenged by the Sisters of Notre Dame, but at the same time my identity is not as a nun. Therefore, if I am not to be a nun, it is okay. In terms of church, whatever church means, I believe I am a person of faith. I believe it was the Scriptures that challenged me, and my Christian faith which constrained me to stand with the poor, the marginalized, and to be concerned about setting people free. Working toward people's self-determination whether they be the poor or homeless, or in Central America: these I consider my commitments for the future. And, I hope, they will become stronger as a result of these last two years.

Essentially, then, you view yourself as part of the people of God?

Hussey: That's correct.

What about you, Barbara?

Ferraro: I would say likewise. Certainly the church is my church. I'm proud of that. The institutional church, no. I made the decision five or six years ago not to work for the institutional church because I felt it very confining. The church, to me, is certainly the people of God, and I am where I am today because of—I have had the privileges of my education and my experiences as a Sister of Notre Dame. I certainly am in a different position from any of my siblings. Because of my education and my experience as a sister, I have the strong commitment to work with oppressed people, and to confront the institutional church which oppresses women particularly. I continue to be aware of issues in Central America. Both of us visited Nicaragua in 1984 and made a connection with the work we do.

So, my identity is not wrapped up in being a nun; I feel that I am very much a woman, very much a religious, and I can continue with my commitment. One thing I feel very secure about in all of this, and one thing I can say is that my commitment will continue to be what it is and will not change. I feel I can continue to live out that commitment whether I am a nun or not a nun.

In his interview with Robert Coles, Dan Berrigan claimed his activity against the war in Vietnam was a "no." He also argued that in a more profound way it was a "yes" to Christian love and concern for the human race. How in light of the ad do you view your life as a "yes"?

Hussey: It's interesting to view ourselves at this point of history, not because of choice, but because of the ad. We were thrown into it. Since December 1984, Christmas. . . .I think every day has been a "yes" to pursuing the truth, to pursuing the church as a community of believers, to pursuing and clarifying and making it necessary for the church to listen to women's experiences which have been ignored and denied with regard to abortion. This has been important in a daily "yes" for me since December 1984.

Ferraro: I would say our "yes" is one which is creating a new model: saying "yes" to the fact we are women who can make decisions, who can think, and who can remain within a community of believers. I wish we had the models out there for us; models of women who have said the kind of "yes" we are attempting to say, because then we would have someone as a model. . . .It is to take each day and to remain "clean and clear" about what this "yes" means and not to compromise our values. To say "yes" to the challenges day in, day out. . . .

Hussey: I think, Barbara, the model is there for us. I think if we were to look at the number of people who supported us during the past two years. . . .I would not discount a Fran Kissling; I would not discount a Mary Hunt, who were also lay signers of the original ad; I would not discount Maureen Fiedler who has certainly stood with us in her signing the statement which she has since seen used against her.

What I'm saying about a new model, Pat, is that the folks who have gone before us like Agnes Mary Mansour, Liz Morancy, and Arlene Violet, all voluntarily left. The others who ["recanted"], in a sense capitulated one way or another. To consistently say "no" to a compromise and "yes" to the reality [of women's experience]--that model is really not there for religious women who are caught in the institutional church (except maybe in a Fran Kissling or a Charlie Curran). It is not yet [apparent] in the women who are in the same lifestyle as ourselves. How do you. . .stay within that lifestyle, [but say] "no" to the institution and "yes" to the reality. Somehow or other, you and I are caught up in that reality, wishing there were more people with us to make it a lot easier.

THE FUTURE

How do you see the future?

Ferraro: I think the future is open to a new creative church, already emerging in the United States: a church of women and men, but particularly women. A whole new women-church movement has emerged. For me, that is the church of the future, which I want to be part of, am part of, and will continue to be part of.

Hussey: The church which is life-giving for me is the church which does not rest on the status quo; a church which aligns itself with the poor of our earth; a church which honors people's experiences; a church which is open to dialogue and expression; it is a church which is viewed as a community of believers. All of that will continue in spite of the repressions, because it is that which challenges all of us, who view the church as a community of believers, to be strong, to unite with each other, to stand up against the repressions, to claim what we know is the truth and to go on.

Ferraro: I think the new church has already emerged in Latin and Central America: a church of liberation which people have taken into their lives and these people have begun to determine what happens to them. It is certainly in contradiction with the hierarchy in the Third World: that's clear in Nicaragua. It is for me a wonderful model; it gives me hope. In fact, it is my only hope—when people who have enough courage to determine their own lives. . .hope for new life and struggle for this new life. This gives me hope. In our own country we will see that kind of revolution. It will happen here.

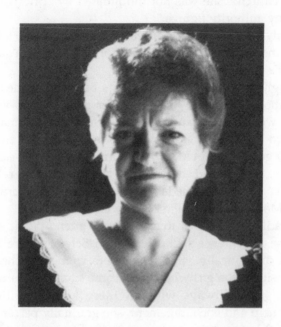

MARY ANN SORRENTINO

"They can throw out a Curran, throw out a Mary Ann Sorrentino, and a Marge Tuite can die, God rest her soul. But for every one of us, there are ten in the wings, if not 150 in the wings, just dying to come out. . .We are part of a chain, a catalyst for the next link, the next person to speak up. More and more people will not take it any more."

Mary Ann Sorrentino, formerly Executive Director of Planned Parenthood of Rhode Island for many years, was born in Providence, Rhode Island, of an Italian immigrant father, and a mother who was "a very strong woman." Her father, a successful businessman, was much more religious than was her mother. Her memories of him—he died when she was nine—are fragmentary, yet she knows that he was a "softer person than the spirited strong whirlwind" vision she has of her mother.

"Pooh-poohing" formal structures of religion, Mary Ann's mother had a "careful attitude" toward people who were always in church. She was not intimidated by "priests, hierarchy or any authority figures."

An only brother, seventeen years older than she, tells her, "You're more like Mama, and I'm more like Papa. You know what? It's better to be like Mama."

For eight years she, at her father's behest, attended a private Catholic elementary school. Her relationships with the teachers were stormy, and weekly sessions of her small class conducted by the mistress general seemed always to end with, "All very good—except Mary Ann Sorrentino." At an early age, therefore, she found herself deprived of such religious "rewards" as sodality medals and opportunities to crown the Blessed Mother or be the First Friday Guard of Honor.

Persuading her mother to allow her to attend public schools, she chose Providence's Classical High School where her life changed dramatically. She remembers women teachers who were sensitive to a girl who had become silent and terrified of walking "the hallways with all these kids." With these teachers help and encouragement, she gradually perceived her worth and her abilities and went on to Elmira College [New York] and the University of Florence [Italy]. Married in 1965 to an attorney, she has one daughter. The event which cast this Catholic woman onto the national scene was the summoning of her daughter to the parish rectory for an examination of the child's views on abortion. During that session, she also learned that she was excommunicated.

You are in the heart of a conflict that has had national and ecclesiastical repercussions. What do you perceive as the real problem in all the public furor over Mary Ann Sorrentino and her position as Executive Director of Planned Parenthood of Rhode Island?

Sorrentino: The real problem, as I perceive it, has less to do with the church's teaching on abortion than with the frustration of the hierarchy. What's happening to other Catholics like Father [Charles] Curran, is that the hierarchy gets frustrated because they cannot (if they ever could) whip people into shape and force them to toe the party line. On the other hand, lay people and even some clergy are saying, "If I think this is wrong, I have to say so." Beyond that they add, "Let the chips fall where they may."

I don't care how many threatening letters are sent to me from Rome, or if I am excommunicated, or if I cannot marry in the church, or my daughter cannot make her confirmation. I do not care, and this is the truth as I see it. My posture must be aggravating to the powers. I was talking to a priest recently and I raised the question of what priests are doing in their lives that is not right. He said, "That's not an issue. The church learned centuries ago to close its eyes to scandal, especially within its own ranks. We always had priests who were getting married, priests who were having children without the benefit of marriage, or whatever they were doing that was 'wrong,' and the church learned to live with it. What they never will learn to live with is anyone threatening their power and their authority."

Were I just another sinner in the moral sense, somebody would be able to deal with me at the hierarchical level. To stand defiantly and say: "I will not accept your authority in this area" is the worst crime in the church, and that is what they're angry about. They're angry with me, they're angry with [Rev. James] Provost, they're angry with [Rev. Charles] Curran, they were angry with Liz Morancy and Arlene Violet. They're going to be angry especially if one is a woman. Bad enough a man should question, but women are supposed to be ironing priests' vestments and cooking their dinner. They don't see us in any role beyond that. A couple of weeks ago a priest said that it was a privilege to iron their vestments. I said, "Well if it's such a privilege, why don't you do it and let us do some of the less privileged stuff like giving out communion?"

You mentioned the frustration of the hierarchy? What do you think they are afraid of?
Sorrentino: Loss of power and control. It's all about power and control, and then beyond that, I suppose if you wanted to say, power, control, money, and workload. But it's about power and control.

But the traditional, stereotypical view of women is that they are weak. How can weak women threaten these very self-confident and high level clergy?
Sorrentino: They know in their hearts that we're not weak and

they've always known it; they know "La Popessa," the nun close to Pope Pius XII in the Vatican, was not weak. They know from their own history that certain women, without the benefit of public recognition, ran the Vatican. Now women at various levels are actually saying, "I want to run the Vatican. I don't want to be some lackey in a low position, but the one who in fact makes all the tough decisions." Men know, history knows, that women are strong. Now women are coming out and saying, "I'm tired of being the ghostwriter, the backseat person; I want to be right up front."

THE CAUSE OF THE CONFLICT
Mary Ann, will you briefly describe what happened and how your conflict came to a head?
Sorrentino: On May 24, 1985, I received a phone call in my office at Planned Parenthood from my pastor's assistant. A prior call from my daughter's religious education teacher demanded that I bring Luisa to the rectory that afternoon. Luisa, my daughter was then fifteen years old. It was the Friday before her scheduled Sunday confirmation, so I asked what was wrong. She said, "I can't discuss that with you, but it's urgent that you come here as her confirmation is hanging in the balance." I called my husband and he was incensed that this was going on. He said, "Forget about it. I'm not going to let them interrogate our child. I don't care if she never makes her confirmation." I then called a priest friend of ours and the three of us held a conference call. We decided to go and find out what was going on, because we didn't want Luisa to be robbed of the opportunity to have this sacrament. She had worked for it for eight years; she deserved it.

Coincidentally, Andrew Greeley had just written an editorial in *U.S. Catholic* the previous week saying [I paraphrase], "Don't let these folks at the CCD classes intimidate you as parents. Demand the sacraments for your children. They have no right to impose these conditions, like attending eighteen meetings. It is baloney and don't take it." He went on to say, by the way, that he believed a lot of such behavior has to do with people's need to reinforce their own sense of power and masculinity.

With Greeley cheering us on, Luisa, my husband, and I approached the rectory. Luisa was quite intimidated and shy, naturally, a fifteen year old brought up in a fairly traditional Italian-American Catholic home. We have those values. The image of this priest all in black, especially an older, respected priest sitting behind his desk in this darkened office telling you you can't make your confirmation if you don't denounce abortion—and that really meant renouncing your mother—was horrifying to her, and to us as adults. On my way out the door of my office to the rectory, I thought, "Something important is about to happen here. I don't really know what, but something . . .so let me put this tape recorder in my purse. I ought to document this conversation." And I did. It was very fortuitous, as it turned out. Luisa was interrogated, and she satisfied the priest that she was not an abortionist—or whatever he wanted to know from her.

What did he want to know?

Sorrentino: He wanted to know if she thought abortion was wrong, and whether or not she specifically would have an abortion. My husband, an attorney, was arguing that he wanted every child to be asked that question, if things are to be this way. "Only Luisa," the priest responded, "will be questioned. She has been brought up by your wife in that same atmosphere." As if I sent out poisonous gases!

What did your daughter say to those questions?

Sorrentino: Luisa was very good. The most important thing about this interview from a mother's point of view was that I, like every mother of an adolescent child, had experienced the feeling they give you that you don't know anything. They know everything. You wonder if anything you believe is really ingrained into them at all. In that moment my daughter let me understand that what I am and believe was part of her, and she wonderfully resisted this big power figure. She said repeatedly, "Father, I don't know what I believe. I've never been pregnant. I don't know." Finally she said, "I wouldn't have an abortion if I were pregnant, no, but I don't know what someone else should do or whether I think it's wrong, I don't know." And he finally accepted that.

You didn't feel betrayed?

Sorrentino: Never. She was wonderful. She gave the best choice of responses; she just kept saying, "I don't think any woman who doesn't want to have an abortion should be forced to have one, I don't think *that*. . . ." It's right on the tape. And he said, "Well, forget about other people; I'm just talking about you." And she said, "Father, there are women who have had abortions who go here to this church." She was terrific.

[At this point Luisa enters the room] Luisa, could you describe how you felt during the interview?

Luisa: Well, I was upset because my mother had been hurt by the church. I didn't want a lot of attention drawn because of me. Now when I think back, I think that was selfish of me. Of course, I want everything to be done for my mother, for her to be able to go back to church. You know people think it was more traumatic than it actually was for me, because it wasn't that bad. I got a lot of attention, but not too much. My parents supported me. I try to support them as much as I can.

So where are you now, in light of the church?

Luisa: Nowhere. I don't go any more. I don't want to go. You know, I just feel the only time I'll ever go back is when I'm married. I'll teach my kids to be Catholics, but. . . .

Do you feel sad about this, Luisa?

Luisa: Not really, because I don't think church ever really helped me believe in God any more than anything else. I think my parents taught me more. I have a pretty good knowledge of what God wants me to do, and what's right, what's good. I don't think church ever taught me that. I know how to be a good person. I don't think that a priest can tell me because they're not that great, either.

Mary Ann, could you return to the interview and explain what happened. . .?

Sorrentino: It was all very anger-provoking. . . .After Luisa left the room, my husband and I had an opportunity to thrash around a bit with the priest. It was a very ambiguous situation for me, because several times in the course of the discussion I said, "Father, I don't want to argue with you because I know you are a good man." And he is. He's an eighty-year-old priest who can barely see and who hasn't been well, and I knew clearly that this was not his doing. It was an example of the terrorism of the hierarchy who had sent a phone call from the chancery. He was asked to do this dirty work and I knew his heart, somehow, was not in it. I'm sure he does not believe in abortion. But he's too good a man to hurt a child; I was very torn about him. But I was also angry at having this happen to my child. It certainly put a pall on the whole confirmation. We went through it because Luisa deserved to have the sacrament, and we wanted her to have the best day possible. But as you just heard, it really was the death knell of her faith. Now she says, "I will probably only return to church to marry." That is really her Italian culture speaking more than any religious obligation.

It's the thing one does. . .

Sorrentino: We celebrate, in our ethnic background, each important step in our life, every passage, with a religious ceremony. It is usually a Catholic ceremony. It is inconceivable to my daughter that she might get married outside of the Catholic church. Maybe when she gets married. . .she might be just as happy to get married in the chapel of a local university, or in some non-denominational ceremony. It will be her decision. My husband and I have no further demands to make on her, or no further wish to subject her, at this early point in her life, to what we see as a long road of fighting in the Catholic church. We brought her through fifteen years of Catholic upbringing. I think she now resents, in some ways, my trying to stay in the church. In some ways she would be relieved if I would abandon it.

Feeling that you might be hurt further?

Sorrentino: She thinks I continue to be hurt. And she's right. She cannot at this young age understand that my commitment to staying in the church has to do not only with religion and faith, but also with commitment to issues of justice and of women. It's easy to leave. But you're never as effective a fighter from the outside. And we know that from history. Someone wrote to me early on and said you must never leave. You must stay on the inside and bother them. And I'm going to do that.

LIVING WITH EXCOMMUNICATION

Where are you in light of the excommunication? How does it make you feel?

Sorrentino: Well, it still makes me feel very angry. . . .The priest had indicated to me on the phone that day that he also wanted, beyond speaking to me about Luisa's confirmation, to speak about my own position. I said, "Father, you had something else you wanted to tell me." He said, "Yes. Don't come to communion Sunday at her confirmation because you won't be given communion." And I said, "Why?" "Because," he said, "you're excommunicated." And I said, "I haven't been notified of that by the bishop." He said, "You don't have to be. It's automatic." And of course I didn't know anything about canon law at that point. I was shocked. I didn't know we had this self-destruct mechanism called *latae sententiae*. I said to him, "I will not further embarrass my child by challenging your authority because she's been through enough. But I will pursue this through every ecclesiastical avenue open to me."

Right after the confirmation, I wrote letters to the bishop; to Pio Laghi, the Pro Nuncio in Washington; to anyone who would listen to me. I tried to get answers first to what had been done to my child, which was clearly indefensible. Secondly, I wanted to know about this [my] excommunication. We know that there are Catholics around the world involved actively in abortion, as indirectly and more directly than I am. They have never been singled out this way. I wanted an answer to that, which of course I never got. Now, we continue this correspondence, you know, my husband and I and Father [James] Coriden [canon lawyer at Washington Theological Union Seminary], who became [my] canonical advisor. In the midst of all this correspondence, Father Randall of the Providence Charismatics went on cable television on January 21, 1986—nine months later—and publicly announced my excommunication on television. That's how it became the national and international issue that you described earlier.

This public trauma was very disappointing, seeing that we had done everything to keep Luisa out of the public meat grinder. . . .The rest is history. Beyond that, the good thing that came out of it was that their foolishness soon became apparent to Catholics and non-Catholics alike. I have never met a person, or read anyone's opinion from anywhere, who thinks that what happened to my daughter is justifiable. Forget about me. The abuse of a child because of her mother's or her father's behavior is unheard of in the church. That was then—now we have eleven-year-olds being thrown out of parochial schools because they express an opinion on abortion. . . .I mean, it's getting crazier instead of more rational, so I don't know where it's all going to end. James Coriden continues to be my major link to the church; he has written another opinion, a legal opinion.

I'm aware that he wrote an article stating that you have not been "automatically" excommunicated.

Sorrentino: Canon 1398 does not apply in my case. Therefore, no self-excommunication occurred, according to his best reading of the law, attested to by seven of the top canonical lawyers in the country. So I accept, obviously, Father Coriden's opinion. I know that the bishop is under no obligation to read that opinion, let alone abide by it. Unfortunately, we still have a feudal system where the emperor may wear no clothes and even if someone points out that he's wearing no clothes, [but] we all pretend he is, then life goes on.

Have you, or has Father Coriden, shared with the bishop the findings of these scholars, these clerics?

Sorrentino: Oh, yes. And the bishop's response, in *The Providence Journal*, is that he's under no obligation to Father Coriden. He claims that Father Coriden does not know the "local" situation, and only the bishop is in charge here. Just like [former U.S. Secretary of State] Alexander Haig said the day the president [Ronald Reagan] was shot, "I'm in charge," so, in fact, in our church, it's true that he's in charge here just as Cardinal Cody was in charge in Chicago. Only after they die is the church able to say maybe this priest or bishop or cardinal did a bad thing. While they're alive, they never have to say they're sorry.

Have you received other clerical support?

Sorrentino: Yes. It often comes in the form of intimidated, yet supportive priests who are afraid that it will be known that they are pulling for me. But there have been some brave priests in Rhode Island, who have said fairly publicly, in the context of their own pulpits, what an embarrassment this whole thing was for them and for our church. Certainly I have received support from nuns, and Catholic lay people have responded in huge numbers.

All seven hundred-odd letters came mainly from Catholic lay people who are just beside themselves. There is also the downside, which is that people can support privately, but. . . .I was invited to come to Genesis's community at the outset by some people there. And I started to attend.

Genesis is a parish without walls?

Sorrentino: It's a chaplaincy of the bishop and it operates at the pleasure of the bishop. The people in the Genesis community like to think that they are there because many of them are in some ways disillusioned with the routine kind of hierarchical bureaucracy of other kinds of normal parishes. But what I've found is that the bishop has threatened the current chaplain if I participate. He meant to shut Genesis down if I were to receive the eucharist in any form from anyone. Some people in Genesis have been so terrorized by my presence that they have behaved in less than Christian ways. After my last conversation with the Genesis parish council I decided not to return because it was creating a painful, divisive spirit.

Have you been asked to leave this new parish?

Sorrentino: Well, I wasn't asked to leave. If you ask anyone from Genesis, they'll say, "Oh no, we didn't ask her to leave because Genesis is a welcoming community." When people say to you, "Your presence is the most divisive thing that ever happened to this community," it is not very welcoming.

I understand that some of these same parishioners at one point were bringing communion to you.

Sorrentino: Yes, they were. I've never talked about it publicly because I was trying to protect Genesis. . .[but] I think at this point I don't feel the same loyalty as I did. . . .I knew the first time it became public knowledge the bishop would get hysterical and do something rude. But yes, people brought communion to my seat which was a very moving experience. People started sitting in solidarity with me at mass and not going to communion themselves. I think some of them are still doing it, even though I'm not there any more—mostly women trying to make a statement.

You must understand that in Genesis, for example, there's an officer from a health accrediting agency who licenses my clinic, and there are some non-Catholics. I asked the priest at Genesis what I asked the other priest on the day of Luisa's interrogation, "Please tell me about justice. How can you give communion to this person and deny it to me?" I don't want anyone to be denied, but I don't want to be selectively denied. The question is very difficult for the priest at Genesis. I've been told ridiculous things such as: the person who licenses your clinic spends a smaller amount of his time working on abortion-related activities. My answer to that is that I didn't know God worked on percentages. I don't believe the difference between good and evil had to do with whether or not you had been on the [Phil] Donahue show. Does God think more of a sinner who is on the front page of *The New York Times* than the private sinner no one ever knows? I think the sin is in the act and not in how many people read about it. I have lost faith in this system.

Is it possible for you to walk into any church where you are not known and receive communion?

Sorrentino: I don't know if it is possible in this state any more. In Rhode Island, I've been public, and I have been in the papers and on television for a long time. From the reaction of people on the street, I doubt I can walk into any church without being recognized by someone. Even if the priest didn't recognize me, some parishioner would, and call the bishop. "She was here today and she received communion" and then the boom would lower on the parish.

It is certainly possible in the country and in the world. I travel a great deal. Excommunication is totally unenforceable, because even if I don't receive the eucharist at mass, I'm entitled to go to church anyway. If someone takes part of his or her host home and gives it to me an hour after communion, I don't feel any different than I do in church. Excommunication is an empty gesture; an empty name. I have no concern about [how it affects] my relationship with God.

WHY REMAIN?
Why do you stay in this church?

Sorrentino: I stay for a set of different reasons. I stayed all these years because it was my church, my family's church, the church I had known, the church I had always believed in. I had some differences with it and I basically felt that no religion was perfect. I want to be in this church; there is something exciting about it, and especially now with all this questioning going on. Beyond those reasons I remain because I have an opportunity to make a difference. I will *not* give them the satisfaction of leaving. I will stay in there and bother them; as long as I am there, [this] "bother" will never go away. The issue is of women fighting back; this fuss is not about abortion, it is about women fighting back. I thought of going to the rail every Sunday at Genesis parish, and being refused communion, just to stand there for the whole hour. It would be an important gesture for myself, for the priest, and for the community to experience what it feels like.

Do you think any of the women of Genesis would walk with you?

Sorrentino: Some would; when I left the Genesis parish council one night, I said, "I just have one thing to say to you, Mr. F. (he was the most brutal person there, the one who said my presence in Genesis was the most divisive thing that had ever happened), "If you think my presence in Genesis has been divisive, then my absence will certainly not be healing." I will not go away because I am not in the room. What happened to me will not go away from the community just because I am not in the room. He will soon learn this.

How would he learn that?

Sorrentino: I think by the courage that other women and men will gain to speak out because of my absence. If he is in that community, he will hear about it. People will be troubled that I am not there. I know that the public has a short attention span, and that after a certain amount of time I may be forgotten. I am not so egotistical that I can't recognize reality. But there are a few strong people who feel I was abandoned by the community, and who will remember me every Sunday. And in some way, during the Offertory intentions, they will speak, they will pray for me, for Luisa, and for other women like us. The issue is in the air; it won't go away. It is naive to think that by casting me out, or throwing out enough folks who don't toe the line, the issues will go away. It has not worked; and it will not work.

FAMILY SOLIDARITY
How has your family responded to your excommunication?

Sorrentino: My wonderful brother is my biggest fan and we are as close as ever. The sad experience has bonded my husband and Luisa and me in a way that might never have happened otherwise. You heard my child; she certainly has a strong sense of loyalty and even a sense of protectiveness, as it were, about her mother and her father. Nothing can ever destroy that outcome. It has not been a completely negative experience. Parts of it were certainly positive, even very enjoyable, but other parts are a burden for me. I'm not free to live my life, and I resent the intrusion. But it is a small price to pay, given what I have I accomplished. When I speak at a campus young women say adulating things to me such as, "I want to be like you when I grow up." I cannot tell them how painful that is. It is so much responsibility. You want to say, as Barbra Streisand once said, "Don't envy me; I have my own pain."

MODELING FEMINISM FOR OTHERS
Do you think that imitation is the highest form of praise?
Sorrentino: That's exactly what is so frightening and so wrenching because they know only a small part of me. They don't know that I failed as a feminist when I was not a feminist, when I was not an independent thinker. They don't know what the road has been like to get to where I am. If they could just emerge, spring full-blown feminists from the forehead of Gloria Steinem, it would be one thing. But, part of what enables one to be where I am, or where Liz Morancy is, or where Marge Tuite was, is all the painful experiences of life up to the point where we have the courage to speak out. It comes from years of pain, many incidents so painful that you finally explode and say, "I'm mad, and I'm not going to take this any more."

Where do you see the future for yourself, for women generally, and for women in the church particularly?
Sorrentino: Women in general are on a good road to equality. We've made progress and we are going to make a lot more inside the Catholic church and outside of it also. We have learned all the things we have to do, and now we must take time to do them. I, for example, just bought some stock in a water supply company in Maine.

This company has a very good public relations department.

They immediately started to bombard me with what appeared to be very personalized letters which probably came out of a computer somewhere. Nevertheless, it is very flattering to receive letters that welcome one as a new shareholder, [as well as] the glossy annual report, and every week something else. Yesterday, I got a letter from the president of the company, asking again if "there is anything we can do for you. . . ." I sat down and wrote, "Since you keep asking me, I am going to answer you. I notice in your Annual Report that there is only one woman on your Board of Directors: she is a token and that's not enough in 1987. I'm sure there are plenty of women in Maine and around the country who can help this company, and if you don't know who they are, call me. I also notice in your Annual Report that the female staff of the actual company is mainly clerical. I do not see any female faces in the executive level and I want to know why. As a shareholder, you asked for input and I'm giving it to you and I want an answer." That's the kind of thing that five or ten years ago we did not do. We did not buy stock, and we did not take time to answer. Now we do.

Men [may] rue the day they ever asked us to say anything, because now we in fact speak it. We do not just smile and say, whatever my husband says is fine.

Further, in the church, I see this flood. . . .They can throw out a Curran, throw out a Mary Ann Sorrentino, and a Marge Tuite can die, God rest her soul. But for every one of us, there are ten in the wings, if not 150 in the wings, just dying to come out. Every time they think they're putting a nail in the coffin, they in fact are giving a shot in the arm to those hundred people in the wings. Catholics who never spoke out about abortion rights have come to the forefront because of what happened to me. For them it was the last straw. Hence, the sad experiences happening to us Catholic oppressed women—women like Liz Morancy and me—are the very things that enable others to take a stand. We are part of a chain, a catalyst for the next link, the next person to speak up. More and more people will not take it any more.

Look, for instance, at birth control as a perfect example. More than ninety percent of the church is saying, "Forget it. I don't care what you clergy say." Struggling to stop the flood is just an exercise in absurdity, never mind futility. On television recently with a wonderful young Franciscan, I said, "Look at all this terrible stuff that's happening with Curran and Provost and others. Where will it end?" He said, "I still believe that the ultimate destiny of our church is the dream of Vatican II. I have to believe that." And I believe it too.

There is a reason why this is happening to me, and I may never know it in my lifetime. Some of it is told to me through my daughter. My crisis may be for personal reasons, as well as for universal reasons. This is the kind of traditional Catholic I am: I believe that God gives crosses to those whom he believes can bear them. So, it is a privilege for those of us who are tested; we are tested because he knows we have the strength to withstand the test and not cave in. That is how God speaks.

GOD OR GODDESS
I notice you keep calling God "he."
Sorrentino: Among many of my sisters in the church, there is a movement to refer to God as "she." Even theologians and cardinals have referred to God as "she." I have no trouble with that. I don't know what gender God is, or if God, in fact, has a gender. In any case, I have this very traditional model in my head. I need that model. I need to think about Jesus Christ as a man, and of God as the father; that is what makes me comfortable. I don't have any discomfort with other people's definitions, but I resent as much a feminist Catholic telling me that I must refer to God as a "she" as in telling me how to live in other parts of my life.

A young feminist said to me, "If you are a feminist you must call so-and-so by her first name." Well, that woman was the mother of a childhood friend of mine. I had always grown up calling her Mrs. X. I could not call her by her first name, but I went to her and said, "Do you mind if I call you Mrs. X instead of using your first name? This other woman says I'm not a feminist if I don't call you by your first name." She said, "That's baloney. Being a feminist means being free to do whatever makes you most comfortable." I, therefore, do not consider myself less of a feminist if I attach a male pronoun when I speak to God. I don't know what God is, but I like that image.

THE STRUGGLE TO FIND A PLACE IN THE CHURCH
How will women come into their own place in the church?

Sorrentino: Not easily. By fighting, by. . .it will be even worse than that: by dying.

By dying?

Sorrentino: Yes. I mean that Marge Tuite's death has as much if not more power around it than her life. That is saying a lot. In her death is the need to fill the void. The void she leaves is so great it will take four hundred of us to fill it, if not a thousand. Hence, her death is as important as her life.

I think Marge Tuite was a martyr of this movement of women speaking out in the church. She was older when she signed the ad [see Appendix A], yet the exercises in punishment and the vitriolic torment that this woman underwent because of that singular action is inconceivable. It, of course, addressed their anger about the way she lived her life in general. It was another way to nail her. It did not help her health. We feel she is a martyr to the movement of women's liberation in the church. Marge Tuite was not old enough to die, and if she had been left in peace, she might not have [died].

We have no medical evidence, but there's no question that they create stress for us that we need not face otherwise. Damn it, then we need to create stress right back because maybe we have a better shot. There's a hell of a lot more old dotty hierarchy men than there are women. We are younger, stronger, and, I hope, we can withstand the stress. If it is going to be a battle of wits, then let it be. We are really at the point I said earlier, "Let the games begin, and let the chips fall where they may." We're ready and we're not going to go away. For some of us our greatest statement will come in our death, because we will die for this in one way or another. Not in the same way that Saint Maria Goretti died, not in that kind of classic martyrdom. But it's a different martyrdom; even the banishments are a form of martyrdom. I mean Liz Morancy is a martyr because as a woman she was forced into exile from a community that she chose and loved, while her community is helpless to do anything. That is a form of death. The Mercy Order was a part of her, a childhood dream that she had to sacrifice. Her dream was killed by these men.

Mary Ann, are you optimistic?

Sorrentino: Well, if optimistic means that I think eventually we will win, yes. If optimism can be defined as ultimate victory in a few thousand years, yes. I don't think that I will live to see these changes. I doubt that Luisa will. Maybe Luisa's daughter will start to see change. It will take a long time. We could get a good head start if this particular pope were not around much longer, but he appears to be in excellent health. This man is certainly never going to give us any respite; he will try, God forbid, to put us back a hundred years before he is through. He is just making the road longer. I don't know if God will ever give us another John XXIII in my lifetime.

I have talked with women who speak of woman-church. What do you think of women-church?

Sorrentino: I don't belong to sexist organizations, whether they're male exclusive or female exclusive. I have no interest in exclusive societies. I'm looking for equality.

I'm interested in changing the Catholic church. I am not interested in setting up offshoot churches which are not legitimately recognized as having an impact on the Catholic church. The answer is not in leaving the church. I have less respect for the people who went to Canada and Sweden during the Vietnam War than for those who stayed in the streets and fought to bring it to an end. Escape is not bringing pressure from outside. If I go to the Unitarian church tomorrow, or some other offshoot of the Catholic church, not recognized as a legitimate part of the Roman Catholic church, then it may solve a lot of my spiritual or psychological pains, but it will be dismissed by the very hierarchy that I am trying to bother.

THE ABORTION ISSUE

Early on in your work it seems you were able to shed guilt about abortion. You are now able to hold hands of women who are having an abortion How did that happen?

Sorrentino: I'm not sure I ever had much guilt about it. I was told that abortion was the terrible thing; no one ever talked about. That's how I grew up and that's what I thought. Then, in 1963 while I was a student in Florence, I had a friend who became pregnant. Like me, she was twenty, but quite worldly. She yelled at me constantly, saying I was living in another century. One day she told me, "I think I'm pregnant." "What are you going to do if you are?" I asked. "You'll have to marry him." She said, "Oh no, no. Marriages that start off that way are never good." I said, "Well, then you have the baby and put it up for adoption." And she said, "No, no, no."

I realized then that she was thinking about having an abortion and I was horrified and frightened. She did. She was very self-sufficient; she found a place to have it, and someone to get her there. I had been asked to accompany her and I would not because I thought it was the man's responsibility. I told him, "Listen: I'm not going to go and hold her hand through this. You should." I worried lest she hemorrhage or die. Besides, we had an honor system in my college: if she got thrown out, I was going to get thrown out too. And if she died, would I have to tell her mother?

She came back to school, and years later she married this man and they had a beautiful daughter. He is a wonderful, honorable man. In the context of her life, her values, and her experience at that moment, abortion was a "do-able" thing. I resisted making judgments about it, and I accepted it.

When I came to Planned Parenthood, abortion was still kind of an esoteric concept. At first, as director, I thought it was important for me to know about abortion. I recall telling the medical director that I wanted to come into the room. I stood behind her, right at the foot of the table where the woman's legs were in the stirrups, and I was facing the wall. Watching this, as I think back, was the worst possible introduction—my knees, weak beneath me from the whole physical experience of blood even though I was no stranger to gore, bones, and people dying when I worked in the Peter Bent Brigham Hospital.

But as a woman, there was something different about this experience. I understood it was not only physically discomforting, but emotionally I understood what it meant to the woman, to me, and to the physician who was also a woman. Further, I trained myself to go there, hold the hands of patients, and experience this moment with them. I got to know these women as women; that is what made me overcome everything. What became primary was not the speculum, the specimens, or even the patient's anguish and physical pain. What was primary was that these women experienced comfort because the option of abortion was available to them. I got to know them as mothers, daughters, people alone, and sometimes poor battered women with no options. That is what brought me to where I am, what I refer to as this "chain of experience." Few people have been privileged to have my experience in Planned Parenthood.

EFFECTIVE BIRTH CONTROL

We have a church which forbids not just abortion but all birth control, except rhythm. . . How do you feel about this?

Sorrentino: There is no question that it's an entirely punitive and ridiculous situation to say you can't use any effective means of not having babies, and on the other hand, if you don't want to be pregnant, yet find yourself pregnant, you must have the baby anyway. It is an unworkable situation. You have to take it one step further. You can't talk about sex either: the church often resists talking about sex education [which would offer] our young people ways of avoiding pregnancy. Catholics are never really supposed to enjoy their sexuality unless they are going to have a baby. The pope keeps telling us that sex is not supposed to be fun. It is not supposed to feel good unless you're going to get pregnant. That's the backdrop against which we're all supposed to be operating and. . .ridiculous. Clearly, few, if any, Catholics pay attention.

Do you have reservations about the perceived mass use of abortion as a contraceptive?

Sorrentino: I don't think that it's being used massively. The overwhelming majority of women who have abortions used another method that failed. We don't have an effective method of birth control. If the world wants to help, it can invent an effective method of birth control for men and women. . . .Very, very few women, in all the years I've been here—I recall only two women who had had more than one abortion—who didn't want to hear about contraception. This, of course, is an unhealthy and irresponsible position. But we can't tell people what to do with their lives. I smoke and I shouldn't: it is not good for my health. But I defy anyone to take the cigarettes out of my purse.

I wanted to say that the church's position on contraception and abortion is a perfect example of the power struggle that I talked about earlier. [It relates to] the first question you asked me, "What's the real issue here?" The only reason that the ception is as Margaret Sanger said, "No woman can truly be free until she can control her own fertility." That's true and basic. These men understand if we can now control our fertility—and we've gotten to be bad enough with no control, in their view— the floodgate will really open. They are petrified of that. That is why they don't approve; it's another sexist issue. Birth control is not a male issue in the church as women prove by paying no attention to the hierarchy. Besides, men don't get pregnant if they have no birth control; women do. The hierarchy will drop dead before they officially allow birth control. They'll know, then, they won't have those last three or four women still ironing the vestments. . . .These men will know it; hence, I believe that power is the bottom line.

APPENDICES

A DIVERSITY OF OPINIONS REGARDING ABORTION EXISTS AMONG COMMITTED CATHOLICS.

CATHOLIC STATEMENT ON PLURALISM AND ABORTION.

[c]ontinued confusion and polarization within the Cath[o]lic community on the subject of abortion prompt us to [is]sue this statement.

[St]atements of recent Popes and of the Catholic hier[archy h]ave condemned the direct termination of pre-natal [life as m]orally wrong in all instances. There is the mistaken [belief in] American society that this is the only legitimate [Catholi]c position. In fact, a diversity of opinions regarding [abortio]n exists among committed Catholics:

• A large number of Catholic theologians hold that [even di]rect abortion, though tragic, can sometimes [be a] moral choice.

• According to data compiled by the National Opinion [Research] Center, only 11% of Catholics surveyed [disapprove] of abortion in all circumstances.

[These o]pinions have been formed by:

• Familiarity with the actual experiences that lead [women] to make a decision for abortion;

• A recognition that there is no common and constant [teaching] on ensoulment in Church doctrine, nor has [abortion] always been treated as murder in canonical [history];

• An adherence to principles of moral theology, such [as] probabilism, religious liberty, and the centrality [of] informed conscience; and

• An awareness of the acceptance of abortion as a [moral] choice by official statements and respected [theologians] of other faith groups.

[Th]erefore, it is necessary that the Catholic community [enga]ge candid and respectful discussion on this diver-

sity of opinion within the Church, and that Catholic youth and families be educated on the complexity of the issues of responsible sexuality and human reproduction.

Further, Catholics — especially priests, religious, theologians, and legislators — who publicly dissent from hierarchical statements and explore areas of moral and legal freedom on the abortion question should not be penalized by their religious superiors, church employers, or bishops.

Finally, while recognizing and supporting the legitimate role of the hierarchy in providing Catholics with moral guidance on political and social issues and in seeking legislative remedies to social injustices, we believe that Catholics should not seek the kind of legislation that curtails the legitimate exercise of the freedom of religion and conscience or discriminates against poor women.

In the belief that responsible moral decisions can only be made in an atmosphere of freedom from fear or coercion, we, the undersigned,* call upon all Catholics to affirm this statement.

SIGNERS

[B]attaglia, Ph.D., Associate Professor, California [Univ]ersity • Roddy O'Neil Cleary, D. Min., Campus [Ministry,] University of Vermont • Joseph Fahey, Ph.D., [Manhattan] College • Elizabeth Schüssler [Fiorenza,] Ph.D., Professor, University of Notre Dame • Mary [C. Segers], author of Final Payments and Company of [Women •]Patricia Hennessy, J.D., New York City • Mary [D.], Women's Alliance for Theology, Ethics and [Ritual • Fr]ances Kissling, Executive Director, Catholics for a [Free Choi]ce • Justus George Lawler, Executive Editor, [Crossroad/]Bookline, Winston-Seabury Press • Daniel C. [Maguire,] Ph.D., Fellow in Ethics and Theology, [Catholics f]or a Free Choice • J. Giles Milhaven, Ph.D., [Professor,] Brown University • Rosemary Radford Ruether, [Ph.D., Pro]fessor, Garrett Evangelical Theological [Seminary •]Thomas Shannon, Ph.D., Professor, [Worcester] Polytechnic Institute, MA • James F. Smurl, [Ph.D., Pro]fessor, Indiana University

College, WI • Maurice C. Duchaine, S.T.D., San Francisco, CA • Emmaus Community of Christian Hope, NJ • Margaret A. Farley, Yale Divinity School, CT • Darrell J. Fasching, Ph.D., University of South Florida, FL • Barbara Ferraro, Sisters of Notre Dame, WV • Maureen Fiedler, Ph.D., S.L., Catholics for the Common Good, MD • Silvio E. Fittipaldi, Ph.D., Pastoral Institute of Lehigh Valley, PA • George H. Frein, Ph.D., University of North Dakota, ND • Lorine M. Getz, Ph.D., Somerville, MA • Kevin Gordon, Director, Consultation on Homosexuality, Social Justice and Roman Catholic Theology, CA • Jeannine Gramick, School Sisters of Notre Dame, NY • Christine E. Gudorf, Ph.D., Xavier University, OH • Terry Hamilton, Woodstock/St. Paul Roman Catholic Community, NY • Jack Hanford, Th.D., Ferris State College, MI • Kathleen Hebbeler, Dominican Sister of the Sick Poor, OH • Patricia Hussey, Sisters of Notre Dame, WV • Caridad Inda, Council of Women Religious, MD • Dorothy Irvin, S.T.D., Dunbar, NC • Fr. Jerry Kaelin, O.F.M., Cincinnati, OH • Janet Kalven, Loveland, OH • Elizabeth Nelson Keating, Yale University, CT • Pat Kenoyer, S.L., Loretto Women's Network, MO • Joseph E. Kerns, S.T.D., Center for Christian Living, VA • Paul F. Knitter, Th.D., Xavier University, OH • Joseph A. LaBarge, Ph.D., Bucknell University, PA • Eleanor V. Lewis, Ph.D., Baltimore, MD • Wayne Lobue, Ph.D., Gilmour Academy, OH • Agnes Mary Mansour, Ph.D., Lansing, MI • Roseann Mazzeo, S.C., NJ • Bro. Ray McManaman, F.S.C., Lewis University, IL • Kathleen E. McVey, Ph.D., Princeton Theological Seminary, NJ • John A. Melloh, S.T.L., Milwaukee, WI • Joe Mellon, M.A., University of Notre Dame, IN • Diane Neu, M.Div., S.T.M., Co-director Women's Alliance for Theology, Ethics and Ritual, Washington, DC • Jeanne Noble, National Assembly of Religious Women, MD • Sr. Margaret Nulty, Sisters of Charity of New Jersey • Kathleen O'Connor, Ph.D., Maryknoll School of Theology, NY • Margaret A. O'Neill,

Ed.D., Sisters of Charity of New Jersey, NJ • Ronald D. Pasquariello, Ph.D., Marist Brothers, Washington, DC • Richard Penaskovic, Ph.D., Auburn University, AL • Gerald A. Pire, M.A., Seton Hall University, NJ • Stanley M. Polan, S.T.L., Franklin Pierce College, NH • Dolly Pomerleau, Catholics for the Common Good, MD • John E. Price, S.T.L., Evanston, IL • Donna Quinn, National Coalition of American Nuns, IL • Jill Raitt, Ph.D., University of Missouri, MO • Maureen Reiff, Chicago Catholic Women, IL • John G. Rusnak, Ph.D., Phoenix, AZ • Mary Savage, Ph.D., Albertus Magnus College, CT • Jane Schaberg, Ph.D., University of Detroit, MI • Mary Jane Schutzius, Federation of Christian Ministries, Association of the Rights of Catholics in the Church, MO • Ellen Shanahan, Ph.D., Rosary College, IL • Emily Ann Staples, University of Minnesota, MN • Marilyn Thie, Sisters of Charity of New Jersey, Colgate University, NY • Sr. Rose Dominic Trapasso, Lima, Peru • Sr. Margaret Ellen Traxler, National Coalition of American Nuns, IL • Marjorie Tuite, Church Women United, NY • Alan F. Turner, Association for the Rights of Catholics in the Church, Valley Forge, PA • Judith Vaughan, National Assembly of Religious Women, CA • E. Jane Via, Ph.D., J.D., University of San Diego and Superior Court of San Diego, CA • Gerald S. Vigna, Ph.D., Pennsauken, NJ • Ann Patrick Ware, M.A., National Coalition of American Nuns, NY • Sallie Ann Watkins, National Coalition of American Nuns, CO • Mary Jo Weaver, Ph.D., Indiana University, IN • Virginia Williams, S.L., MO • Arthur E. Zannoni, Ph.D., University of Notre Dame Extension Program, IN

*Organizational affiliations are listed for purposes of identification only. Partial listing. This statement has been signed by many other Catholics. In addition 75 priests, religious and theologians have written that they agree with the Statement but cannot sign because they fear losing their jobs.

Reprinted from the NEW YORK TIMES October 7, 1984

We affirm our solidarity with all Catholics whose right to free speech is under attack.

On October 7, 1984 at the height of the 1984 presidential campaign, the "Catholic Statement on Pluralism and Abortion"[1] appeared in *The New York Times*.

Ninety-seven leading Catholic scholars, religious and social activists signed the Statement. Since that time, many of the 97 signers and their families have been penalized by segments of the institutional Roman Catholic Church.[2]

Members of religious communities have been threatened with possible dismissal from their orders if they do not retract.

Academics have been denied the right to teach or lecture at Catholic colleges and institutes.

Social activists have been disinvited from participation in programs on issues of peace and justice.

Signers and their families have been harassed in their workplaces.

Declaration of Solidarity

Such reprisals consciously or unconsciously have a chilling effect on the right to responsible dissent within the church; on academic freedom in Catholic colleges and universities; and on the right to free speech and participation in the U.S. political process.

Such reprisals cannot be condoned or tolerated in church or society.

We believe that Catholics who, in good conscience, take positions on the difficult questions of legal abortion and other controversial issues that differ from the official hierarchical positions act within their rights and responsibilities as Catholics and citizens.

We, as Roman Catholics, affirm our solidarity with those who signed the Statement and agree to stand with all who face reprisals. "The ties which unite the faithful are stronger than those which separate them. Let there be unity in what is necessary, freedom in what is doubtful and charity in everything." (Church in the Modern World: 92)

☐ I affirm the **Declaration of Solidarity** and give my permission for the publication of my name in public advertisement.
 (PLEASE PRINT)

name/affiliation*	signature	address

* For purposes of identification only.

We are requesting that each signer contribute $35.00 towards the cost of the ad.

☐ Enclosed is my check in support of this effort. Make checks payable to COMMITTEE OF CONCERNED CATHOLICS. Return to Box 21404, Washington, D.C. 20009-0904.

☐ $35   ☐ $50   ☐ $100   ☐ Other _____

1 In order to facilitate your judgment of the reprisals taken, we print here the full text of the "Catholic Statement on Pluralism and Abortion."

"Continued confusion and polarization within the Catholic community on the subject of abortion prompt us to issue this statement. Statements of recent Popes and the Catholic hierarchy have condemned the direct termination of pre-natal life as morally wrong in all instances. There is the mistaken belief in American society that this is the only legitimate Catholic position. In fact, a diversity of opinions regarding abortion exists among committed Catholics:

 • A large number of Catholic theologians hold that even direct abortion, though tragic, can sometimes be a moral choice.
 • According to data compiled by the National Opinion Research Center, only 11% of Catholics surveyed disapprove of abortion in all circumstances.

These opinions have been formed by:
 • Familiarity with the actual experiences that lead women to make a decision for abortion;
 • A recognition that there is no common and constant teaching on ensoulment in Church doctrine, nor has abortion always been treated as murder in canonical history;
 • An adherence to principles of moral theology, such as probabilism, religious liberty, and the centrality of informed conscience; and
 • An awareness of the acceptance of abortion as a moral choice by official statements and respected theologians of other faith groups.
 Therefore, it is necessary that the Catholic community encourage candid and respectful discussion on this diversity of opinion within the Church, and that Catholic youth and families be educated on the complexity of the issues of responsible sexuality and human reproduction.
 Further, Catholics—especially priests, religious, theologians, and legislators—who publicly dissent from hierarchical statements and explore areas of moral and legal freedom on the abortion question should not be penalized by their religious superiors, church employers, or bishops.
 Finally, while recognizing and supporting the legitimate role of the hierarchy in providing Catholics with moral guidance on political and social issues and in seeking legislative remedies to social injustices, we believe that Catholics should not seek the kind of legislation that curtails the legitimate exercise of the freedom of religion and conscience or discriminates against poor women.
 In the belief that responsible moral decisions can only be made in atmosphere of freedom from fear or coercion, we, the undersigned, call upon all Catholics to affirm this statement."

2 Details regarding these reprisals are available from the Committee of Concerned Catholics.

THERESA KANE'S WELCOME
TO POPE JOHN PAUL II
(October 7, 1979)

In the name of the women religious gathered in this shrine dedicated to Mary, I greet you, Your Holiness Pope John Paul II. It is an honor, a privilege and an awesome responsibility to express in a few moments the sentiments of women present at this shrine dedicated to Mary, the Patroness of the United States and the Mother of all humankind. It is appropriate that a woman's voice be heard in this shrine and I call upon Mary to direct what is in my heart and on my lips during these moments of greeting.

I welcome you sincerely; I extend greetings of profound respect, esteem and affection from women religious throughout this country. With the sentiments experienced by Elizabeth when visited by Mary, our hearts too leap with joy as we welcome you—you who have been called the pope of the people. As I welcome you today, I am mindful of the countless number of women religious who have dedicated their lives to the church in this country in the past. The lives of many valiant women who were the catalysts of growth for the United States church continue to serve as heroines of inspiration to us as we too struggle to be women of courage and hope during these times.

Women religious in the United States entered into the renewal efforts in an obedient response to the call of Vatican II. We have experienced both joy and suffering in our efforts. As a result of such renewal, women religious approach the next decade with a renewed identity and a deep sense of our responsibilities to, with and in the church.

Your Holiness, the women of this country have been inspired by your spirit of courage. We thank you for exemplifying such courage in speaking to us so directly about our responsibilities to the poor and oppressed throughout the world. We who live in the United States, one of the wealthiest nations of the earth, need to become ever more conscious of the suffering that is present among so many of our brothers and sisters, recognizing that systemic injustices are serious moral and social issues that need to be confronted courageously. We pledge ourselves in solidarity with you in your efforts to respond to the cry of the poor.

As I share this privileged moment with you, Your Holiness, I urge you to be mindful of the intense suffering and pain which is part of the life of many women in these United States. I call upon you to listen with compassion and to hear the call of women who comprise half of humankind. As women we have heard the powerful messages of our church addressing the dignity and reverence for all persons. As women, we have pondered these words. Our contemplation leads us to state that the church in its struggle to be faithful to its call for reverence and dignity for all persons must respond by providing the possibility of women as persons being included in all ministries of our church. I urge you, Your Holiness, to be open to and to respond to the voices coming from the women of this country who are desirous of serving in and through the church as fully participating members.

Finally, I assure you, Pope John Paul, of the prayers, support and fidelity of the women religious in this country as you continue to challenge us to be women of holiness for the sake of the kingdom. With these few words from the joyous, hope-filled prayer, the Magnificat, we call upon Mary to be your continued source of inspiration, courage and hope: "May your whole being proclaim and magnify the Lord; may your spirit always rejoice in God your Saviour; the Lord who is mighty has done great things for you; Holy is God's Name."

SYNOPSIS OF THE GEORGIA
SODOMY CASE

The New York Times on July 1, 1986 (1,18,19) reported the decision of the Supreme Court on the Georgia Sodomy case. The court ruled on the right to outlaw private homosexual acts. In a bitterly divided decision (5 to 4), the Court announced that the Constitution does not protect homosexual relations between consenting adults, even in the privacy of their own homes.

Further, the court upheld a Georgia law forbidding all people to engage in oral or anal sex. This law, it said could be used to prosecute such conduct between homosexuals. The court did not rule on whether the Constitution protects married or other heterosexual persons in these practices.

Justice Byron R. White wrote the majority decision by reflecting on the "ancient roots" which affected his decision. At issue was an 1816 Georgia law which, in concert with all thirteen states, outlawed homosexual acts. All fifty states eventually legislated likewise. But since 1961, when court decisions made private homosexual acts between consenting adults no longer criminal, the laws on homosexuality changed in twenty states.

Chief Justice Burger said, "To hold that the act of homosexual sodomy is somehow protected as a fundamental right would be to cast aside millennia of moral teaching."

Forces of morality he listed through the millennia were Judeo-Christian moral and ethical standards, Roman criminal law, Western Christian tradition, and English common law.

The case was a civil suit initiated by Michael Hardwick, a homosexual arrested in his Atlanta home while having sexual relations with another man.

high blood pressure, wounds, heart attacks, headaches, and anxiety.

They may have thought that they removed prayer from the schools but as long as they have exams they will have student prayers in the classrooms.

A minister decided to do something a little different one Sunday morning to hold the interest of his parishioners and for some, to keep them awake. He said, "Today I am going to shout out a single word and you are going to help me to preach. When I say the word, I want you all to sing whatever hymn that comes to mind."

Then the preacher shouted out "CROSS". Immediately the congregation started singing in unison: "THE OLD RUGGRD CROSS."

The preacher hollered out "GRACE". The congregation began to sing "AMAZING GRACE, how sweet the sound."

The preacher said "POWER". The congregation sang "THERE IS POWER IN THE BLOOD."

The preacher said "SEX". The congregation fell into complete silence. Everyone was in shock. They all nervously started to look around at each other afraid to say anything.

Then all of a sudden from way back of the church a little old grandmother stood up and began to sing PRECIOUS MEMORIES.

A priest was performing last rights on a dying man. "Renounce the devil" he said. "Let him know how little you think of his evil." The dying man said nothing. The priest repeated his order but still the dying man said nothing. "Why do you refuse to renounce the devil?" the priest asked. With a gasp and feeble voice the man said, "Until I know for sure where I'm heading I don't think I ought to aggravate anybody."

People were in their pews talking at church. Suddenly Satan appeared at the altar. Everyone started to scream and headed for the exit, trampling each other in a frantic effort to get away from this evil incarnate.

That is everyone except for one elderly man who seemed to appear completely relaxed about the fact that God's ultimate enemy was staring at him.

The Devil walked over to him and asked "Aren't you afraid of me?"

"Nope" was his reply.

"Do you realize that I am Satan and have the power to either kill you with a word or cause you profound horrifying agony for eternity?"

"Yep" was his calm reply.

Very much surprised and perturbed, Satan asked "Why are you not afraid of me?"

The man calmly responded: "Been married to your sister for 45 years."

Sister Mary, who worked for a home health agency, was out making her rounds, visiting home bound patients, when she ran out of gas. As luck would have it, a gas station was just a block away.

She walked to the station to borrow a gas can and to buy some gas.

The attendant said she would have to wait, for someone had just borrowed the only can that he had.

Since the nun was on the way to visit a patient, she decided not to wait, and returned to the car to see if she could find something to fill it with gas.

She spotted the bed pan that she was taking to the patient. Always resourceful, she carried the bed pan to the station and filled it with gas.

As she was pouring the gas into the tank, two men watched her from across the street. One of them turned to the other and said, "If that thing starts, I'm turning Catholic."

Biofeedback

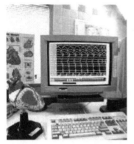

Biofeedback is **a technique that teaches you to control your blood pressure** or other involuntary responses so that you can alter them. In the case of reducing blood pressure you are attached to an electrical instrument that signals high blood pressure by beeping or flashing. You can see on a screen how your thoughts and feelings affect these involuntary processes. This feedback information then allows you to gain control over your blood pressure. This technique is widely used to reduce stress and eliminate its consequences.